Cyriax's Illustrated Manual of
ORTHOPAEDIC MEDICINE

Also by James Cyriax

Textbook of Orthopaedic Medicine, Volume I
Diagnosis of Soft Tissue Lesions (8th edition 1983, Baillière Tindall)

Textbook of Orthopaedic Medicine, Volume II
Treatment by Manipulation, Massage and Injection (10th edition 1980, Baillière Tindall)

Osteopathy and Manipulation (1949, Crosby Lockwood)
The Slipped Disc (1975, Gower Press)
Cervical Spondylosis (1971, Butterworths)
Manipulation, Past and Present (1975, Heinemann)

Cyriax's Illustrated Manual of
ORTHOPAEDIC
MEDICINE

Second Edition

J H Cyriax MD, MRCP

Late Honorary Consultant in Orthopaedic Medicine
St Thomas's Hospital, London

and

P J Cyriax MCSP

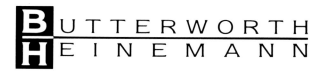

Butterworth-Heinemann
Linacre House, Jordan Hill, Oxford OX2 8DP
A division of Reed Educational & Professional Publishing Ltd

℞ A member of the Reed Elsevier plc group

OXFORD BOSTON JOHANNESBURG
MELBOURNE NEW DELHI SINGAPORE

First published 1983
Reprinted 1984, 1985, 1989
Second edition 1993
Reprinted 1994
Paperback edition 1996

British Library Cataloguing in Publication Data
A catalogue record for this book is
available from the British Library

Library of Congress Cataloging in Publication Data
A catalogue record for this book is
available from the Library of Congress

ISBN 0 7506 3274 7

Printed in Great Britain by Cambus Litho Ltd, Scotland

For Jane Foreman and Holly Nuttall

CONTENTS

PREFACE
TO THE FIRST EDITION

Few conditions are as common as soft-tissue lesions; not many ailments respond so readily to treatment. Yet all too often their care is regarded as a matter of indifference or, little better, as the province of a narrow and complex specialty beyond ordinary reach.

Both views are misconceived; orthopaedic medicine is a straightforward and practical discipline for the profession at large. With the publication of this book, the work has been distilled into terms suitable for ready adoption by the ordinary practitioner, whether a family doctor, physiotherapist or specialist in sports medicine.

This represents an important step forward; orthopaedic medicine may have been born in 1929, but only now is it coming of age. Since the early years tremendous strides have been realized in diagnostic theory but, perhaps for want of a working textbook, the subject has not made its deserved headway towards widespread implementation. To take just two examples, since the mid-1940s it has been possible to abort arthritis of the shoulder, saving the patient anything up to a year's pain; and likewise by a simple injection to deal with many cases of otherwise intractable backache. But in only a tiny proportion of cases do patients needing such treatment actually receive it, and this kind of neglect means that over the years orthopaedic medicine has retained its anomalous status as a discipline that has been overlooked but not superseded. Only its resolute insistence on the virtues of clinical examination, accurate diagnosis and accurate treatment might be termed old-fashioned, but no substitutes can replace these skills.

It is true that all sorts of sophisticated new technologies have developed over the last 50 years – arthrograms, myelograms, ultrasound, blood tests, computerized diagnostic aids and so on. Naturally these are indispensable in the appropriate circumstances, but it so happens that they have no bearing on the ordinary soft-tissue lesion. Thus a patient with, say, a sprained ligament has nothing wrong with his blood or his bones, and an arthrogram may show up an osteoarthrosis that is in reality painless. Procedures boasting the latest equipment, whether diagnostic or therapeutic, are no advance when meted out indiscriminately. The most modern exercise machines or heat delivery systems cannot be regarded as up to date if the patient does not need these treatments; what matters is to establish what is wrong with the patient and then to treat him for that condition.

This was the challenge facing me in 1929. I then found, starting as an orthopaedic house surgeon, that patients were divisible into two categories – those whose defect showed up on X-ray and those whose X-rays were normal. At that time it was the custom to pass the latter on for physiotherapy, consisting of various kinds of heat therapy, general diffuse massage, and exercises. It was a question of divided responsibility. No diagnosis was made or attempted in either the Orthopaedic or Physiotherapy Departments, and the treatments were not given because they were indicated or even specified but simply because they were available. Fifty years later one still hears of patients diagnosed as 'painful shoulder' and batched up for heat therapy or exercise classes.

To be effective, treatment must be an appropriate countermeasure for the condition diagnosed, and this is as much the concern of the doctor as the physiotherapist. The doctor cannot wash his hands of the patient merely by referral elsewhere with some vague label; for he can rest assured that no one else will make good any shortcomings in his initial diagnosis. Whenever a patient is sent for physiotherapy, it must be with the diagnostic certainty not only that physiotherapy is the appropriate recourse but also that the physiotherapist knows the work: that is, how to treat the right tissue in the right way. In such an informed context, the relationship between physician and physiotherapist becomes complementary; he can inject where she cannot; she can take much time-consuming work off his hands by transverse friction or manipulation. Between the two of them, nearly all patients can be dealt with on the spot; generally the last thing needed is to call in a specialist, least of all a specialist outside the field of soft-tissue lesions.

To summarize the basic principles of orthopaedic medicine is now the matter of a few minutes, but from 1929 it took nearly two decades to establish the theoretical groundwork; the findings first saw publication in 1947 in book form as *Rheumatism and Soft-Tissue Lesions*. Over the years this work grew until it now stands as the *Textbook of Orthopaedic Medicine* Volumes I and II, together spanning some 900 pages. These titles are the repository of the sum total of my investigations into soft-tissue lesions and are, I believe, the standard reference work.

But as interest in orthopaedic medicine grew, so a need arose for a renewed publishing programme. One fundamental requirement was an introductory textbook with a broader appeal for the working practitioner, uniting the entire discipline in a single volume. This was the genesis of the *Illustrated Manual of Orthopaedic Medicine*. Nearly all the processes – whether examination, injection, massage or manipulation – lend themselves readily to step-by-step photography; hence the major role in this new book accorded to illustrations, which constitute virtually a complete pictorial presentation of orthopaedic medicine. Indeed, it seemed only logical to press on to make a 'film of the book' and accordingly a companion series of 10 half-hour videotapes has now been completed.

The *Illustrated Manual* sets out to equip the reader to face the great bulk of his patients with confidence. Although it is true that exclusive reliance on this work alone will mean the rare and difficult cases remain obscure, as a rule the material has been not so much simplified as clarified. Everyone sees these cases; with a little effort nearly everyone can diagnose and treat them with gratifying success.

James Cyriax
London 1982

PREFACE

TO THE SECOND EDITION

A decade has passed since first publication of the *Illustrated Manual*. This volume, the second edition, was prepared with the dual objectives of providing a more accessible and better informed successor; design and content have both been updated.

Thus the illustrations have been revised throughout. The most obvious change is the replacement of the old and perhaps rather indecipherable 'live action' examination photographs with new line drawings. This has removed the clutter of extraneous photographic detail, allowing for inclusion of clear directional indicators showing (at a glance) each successive movement. This should make the examination sequences a great deal easier to follow. Similarly, some of the more conceptual illustrations have evolved into diagrams; others have been clarified by the superimposition of overlays. Many close-shot photographs are now presented enlarged, and the new layout brings the captions into closer proximity to their subjects on a page of a slightly more manageable size. All in all, the cumulative tendency of these alterations is towards a more user-friendly book.

As for the text, in some areas – those dealing with equipment and diagnostic aids – the need for modernization was clear. Likewise the occasional error has been corrected, a few sources of confusion eliminated, and a number of procedures (omitted first time round) included. But by and large the basic structure of Dr Cyriax's original text stands intact – in the same way that his diagnostic premises remain unchanged. Nothing has altered the applied anatomy on which diagnosis by selective tension depends. Nor has new research made a more compelling case for concessions in the vexed areas of the facet joint syndrome or the prevalence of sacroiliac strain, and on these particular topics Dr Cyriax's views have been amplified.

At the same time, this new volume refines and extends the original edition. In part this is reflected by a more tolerant attitude towards companion techniques, represented *inter alia* by the first favourable (if qualified) references to Maitland, neck collars, industrial medicine and acupuncture. But more importantly, the text has been comprehensively reappraised, its previous characteristic baldness of assertion modified by a subtler and more informative approach which acknowledges alternative diagnoses, suggests alternative techniques and places increased emphasis on sports injuries. Whether in the form of 'tips', minor complications or additional detail, these refinements reflect the day-to-day experience of working practitioners; and in my endeavours I have been particularly assisted by the expert contributions of:

Malcolm Read MA, BChir, MRCGP
Henry Sanford MA, BChir, DPhysMed
Nigel Hanchard MCSP

whose views have been selectively incorporated. In addition I gratefully acknowledge the assistance of Paul O'Connell MBBS, Dennis Stoker MBBS, FRCP, FRCR, FFR, Andrew Watson MBBS, MRCGP, and further the role of Adrian Pearce MCSP for his most conscientious scrutiny and input throughout. Any improvements in this edition are to their credit; any shortcomings, mine alone.

Patricia Cyriax MCSP

PART ONE

GENERAL PRINCIPLES

CHAPTER ONE

PRINCIPLES OF DIAGNOSIS

Orthopaedic medicine is concerned with the diagnosis and treatment of soft-tissue lesions. These disorders affect a substantial proportion of all patients in general and family medicine; cases are additionally found in departments of orthopaedic surgery, rheumatology, neurology, casualty and, in particular, physiotherapy and sports clinics. Sooner or later nearly everyone suffers some such complaint.

In broad terms these disorders embrace conditions commonly called arthritis, rheumatism, fibrositis, neckache, backache, lumbago, sprained back muscles, sacroiliac strain, sciatica, trapped nerves, pulled muscles,

frozen shoulder, tennis elbow, strained wrist, repetitive strain injuries (RSI), sprained knee and ankle, aches, sprains, inflammation and sports injuries generally.

However, this broad nomenclature encompasses what is in reality a multitude of distinct and readily distinguishable conditions. Once accurately diagnosed they permit the formation of rapid and effective treatment, without which the pain and disability may persist unnecessarily for weeks, months or years.

Soft-tissue lesions are thus a common cause of avoidable pain.

Diagnostic problems

The X-ray

A characteristic shared by the moving soft tissues is their radiotranslucency.

The tissues in question are the joint capsule, ligaments, fasciae, muscles, tendons, bursae and discs; at the spine the dura mater and dural sheaths to the emergent nerve roots are included. Any of these structures can cause pain. None of them, inflamed or otherwise, is visible on the radiograph.

If the pain does arise from a soft tissue, it follows that the X-ray can show only one of two things.

First, it may reveal the bones are normal, thereby playing a negative role except that it lays the patient open to a misplaced diagnosis of neurosis.

In the alternative, the X-ray may disclose some symptomless abnormality which is then incorrectly regarded as the source of pain. In this case the radiograph is positively misleading, a problem not necessarily avoided by recourse to more modern imaging techniques (see page 18).

For example, many patients with a stiff neck display cervical osteoarthrosis or cervical spondylosis. But enquiry reveals that the patient's pain started only last month, whereas the osteophytes have been in existence for a

decade or more. Likewise the osteophytes remain unchanged after the pain vanishes a couple of months later. In fact cervical osteoarthrosis is all but universal to those over 40 and of itself is frequently symptomless. The cause of pain probably lies elsewhere.

To the clinician confronted by a soft-tissue lesion the radiograph is at best of doubtful assistance. This poses a serious diagnostic problem. The patient complains, say, of a painful arm but presents with no objective signs. In fact, the lesion might lie at any one of a number of sites in the joint capsule, supraspinatus, infraspinatus, subscapularis, biceps, subdeltoid bursa, or neck. Correspondingly, the disorder may be anything from tendinitis to arthritis.

The difficulty is compounded because a lesion of any of these tissues can, generally speaking, make the whole shoulder and arm ache, giving rise to apparently indistinguishable symptoms.

Before effective treatment can be administered, the defective tissue must be singled out. If not, any therapy will be directed not at the disordered structure but an adjacent or even relatively distant healthy structure. All pain has a source; the diagnostician's job is to find it.

Palpation

Palpation is often assumed to provide the answer. But nearly all pain from deep-lying structures with the exception of bone is felt at other than its point of origin. Symptoms may be referred by as little as a centimetre or as much as a metre, but in either case the margin of error is too great. Effective treatment must be delivered not just to the right tissue, but the right part of the right tissue: the lesion itself. It is no good working on the infraspinatus if the supraspinatus is at fault, nor are matters much improved if the supraspinatus is treated at the distal site when the lesion lies proximally.

Palpation used by itself regularly deceives. The soft tissues – with one exception – refer pain on a segmental basis. Thus the great majority of shoulder structures refer pain in identical fashion to the dermatome corresponding to their embryological derivation: C5 and C6. These dermatomes do not include the point of the shoulder or scapular area. They extend down the arm. So the painful area outlined by the patient may not even contain the lesion. Any tenderness may itself be referred. Many spots are normally sensitive, the lesion may be buried beyond reach of the examiner's fingers and, in any case, the patient's symptoms may be psychogenic.

The least reliable way to diagnose soft-tissue lesions is to palpate or prod immediately in the area delineated by the patient. Neither the discovery of trigger or myalgic spots nor any description of the nature of the pain – throbbing, burning, stabbing or otherwise – do much if anything to indicate its origin and cause. Like the X-ray, palpation can do a great deal to mislead.

The diagnostic approach: introduction

Like other medical disciplines, orthopaedic medicine relies for its diagnosis on assessment of function. With soft tissues this is relatively easy: a joint moves within certain known limits, certain muscles are responsible for certain movements. It is merely necessary to devise a system based on applied anatomy to detect abnormalities and relate any defect to a specific tissue.

Clinical examination is the key. A healthy structure functions painlessly; a faulty structure does not. Thus each tissue from which the pain could arise is assessed in turn, and as each structure has a known and separate function this presents few obstacles. The tissue that cannot function without bringing on the pain is at fault.

The mechanism of diagnosis is manually applied tension. Each tissue around the suspected joint is subjected to tension in turn. The process is known as 'selective tension'.

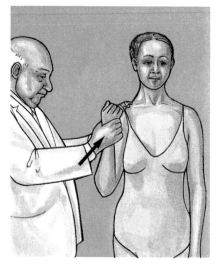

1.1 *A passive movement. Passive flexion stretches one aspect of the elbow capsule. Since the patient is relaxed, the contractile structures are not subjected to strain.*

Inert and contractile structures

A basic distinction exists between contractile structures – the muscle and its attachments – and those which are inert. These latter lack the capacity to contract and relax.

Inert structures are the joint capsule, ligaments, fasciae, bursae, dura mater and dural sheaths to the nerve roots. These can only be put under tension by stretching.

From this distinction the possibility of the clinically pure movement is derived. Tension can be applied manually to assess the contractile and inert structures separately.

Passive movements

If the patient relaxes her limb and the clinician moves it for her (*Figure 1.1*) the inert structures are stretched. But no material strain is borne by the contractile tissues which simply pay out their slack. So when a passive movement hurts, an inert structure is at fault. Inert structures are stretched at the joint's extreme of range; it is then that any pain is apparent.

Resisted movements

If the joint is held still at mid-range while the patient exerts her muscles to their utmost against the examiner's resistance, no material strain falls on the inert structures. Instead it devolves upon the particular muscle or muscle group responsible for the attempted movement. For example, if the patient tries to flex her elbow against strong

4

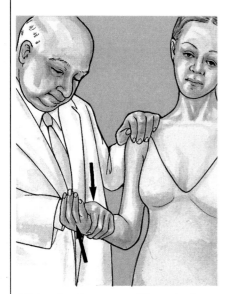

1.2 *A resisted movement. The patient's elbow flexion is forcibly opposed. Resisted movements provide clear information on the state of each muscle group.*

resistance (*Figure 1.2*), tension falls on the biceps and brachialis. If this brings on the pain, one of these two muscles must be at fault and a simple accessory movement will decide which.

The joint must be held at mid-range during resistance to avoid stretching the inert structures.

A suspect joint can thus be assessed by subjecting the tissues about it to a routine of passive and resisted movements. A distinctive pattern of pain and limitation emerges, based on applied anatomy, which allows for identification of the tissue (and often the part of the tissue) at fault.

The state of the structures under examination is thus determined not by palpation but in the conventionally accepted way: by assessment of function. Palpation may or may not follow but will, in any case, be confined to the tissue at fault and even then is conducted only if the structure lies within reach of the fingers.

Finally, many lesions have a distinctive history. Taking

a thorough chronological history together with the clinical examination seldom fails to identify the condition. History is an integral part of the examination.

Examination: an example
When confronted by a patient complaining, say, of shoulder pain the first step, after clarifying the history, is to check whether any neck movements bring on the symptoms. If not, nothing is wrong with the neck or the structures responsible for neck movement. Next, it must be ascertained whether movement at the shoulder girdle or glenohumeral joint elicits the pain. So the shoulder is subjected to a routine of 12 passive and resisted movements which, typically, throw up one of a number of fairly clear-cut findings. For example, a common finding would be painful resisted abduction pointing to a defect of the supraspinatus. A painful arc, if present, reveals the exact site of the lesion in the supraspinatus. Alternatively, painful resisted lateral rotation incriminates the infraspinatus. Individual glenohumeral ligaments do not malfunction, but inflammation of the joint capsule will limit – in different degrees – passive abduction as well as passive medial and passive lateral rotation.

Although history at the shoulder is generally unilluminating, a specific pointer would be if immobility of spontaneous origin came on over three days rather than a more protracted period. This suggests acute subdeltoid bursitis.

Only finally does the examiner palpate. First the patient is positioned so the suspect structure is rendered accessible to his fingers. If assessment of function has revealed only that the lesion is situated in an extensive structure (e.g. the biceps) but not the exact part, it is palpated along its length to pinpoint the lesion's precise site. Otherwise (i.e. if the lesion is known to lie in a small tissue) palpation simply locates the tissue itself prior to treatment.

Sensitivity of neighbouring structures is ignored. For example, even when the supraspinatus is inflamed the tuberosity lying anteriorly is still more tender.

Throughout this book any recommendation to palpate refers to the search for tenderness in a tissue already singled out by assessment of function.

CLINICAL EXAMINATION: SUMMARY I

The moving soft tissues are radiotranslucent. Palpate only after examination along structure already identified as at fault			
A. History/Referred Pain	**B. Assessment by Function**		
1. Take a history	2. Examine incriminated joint by selective tension employing:		
		PASSIVE MOVEMENTS for inert structures: *joint capsule, ligaments, bursae, fascia, displacements, dura mater, nerve roots*	RESISTED MOVEMENTS for contractile structures: *muscles, tendons and attachments to bone*

Structure of this chapter

The theoretical discussion in the following pages deals with basic principles first, commencing with the straightforward resisted movements and ending with the complexities of history and referred pain which refine and complicate the picture. In the consulting room this order is reversed: the clinical examination starts with a history and ends by testing the movements against resistance. In the accompanying charts it is this sequence, corresponding to the actual routine of clinical work, that is adopted. The tables are built up in successive variants and new theoretical findings derived from the text are incorporated, highlighted in white.

Clinical examination

Resisted movements

If one resisted movement proves painful, the likelihood is the other resisted movements will be painless (except sometimes with bursal lesions where the tender structure can be variously squeezed between contracting muscles). Furthermore, the fact that a resisted movement reproduces the pain means a particular contractile structure is the source of pain. The passive movements should therefore be painless and of full range.

The search is thus for a pattern of congruous positive and negative findings; in the absence of a double lesion or a patient with a low pain threshold the symptoms should be referrable to a single source.

There is nothing complicated about testing movements against resistance:

(1) The joint must be held at mid-range (*Figure 1.3*) to keep inert structures off the stretch.

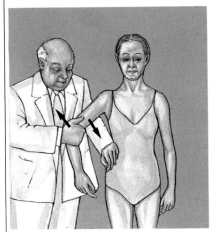

1.3 *Resisted adduction of the shoulder. The joint is at mid-range; the operator's counter-pressure prohibits shoulder movement while his free hand stabilizes the patient's trunk.*

(2) No movement should take place at the joint.
(3) Muscles other than those being tested must not be included. For instance, the examiner must ensure the trunk muscles are not activated when testing resisted shoulder movements.
(4) The patient must exert herself to the utmost.
(5) The examiner pays considerable attention to his positioning in relation to the patient, not least since he is looking not only for increased pain but also for weakness indicating interference with the nervous supply.

Weakness

When strong muscles are tested, minor weakness cannot be detected unless the hands are well placed for resistance and counter-pressure. The examiner's body must be positioned properly. Thus if he stands facing the patient's side when testing the power of resisted shoulder abduction, he will be toppled over backwards. But a true picture can be obtained by standing in front of or behind the patient, one hand at her elbow and the other on the far flank at her waist.

For accurate assessment of muscle weakness a comparison must be conducted bilaterally.

Findings on resisted movements

(1) *Strong and painless:* nothing is wrong with the contractile structure.
(2) *Strong and painful:* This common finding designates a minor lesion of some part of a muscle, tendon or its attachment, in either case almost invariably susceptible to treatment.
(3) *Weak and painless:* this could be attributable to complete rupture of the relevant muscle or tendon but much more often to a malfunction of the nervous system. Impaired conduction along a nerve leads to muscle weakness. Thus if a lesion at the cervical spine compresses the C5 nerve root, then abduction will be weak.

CLINICAL EXAMINATION: SUMMARY II

The moving soft tissues are radiotranslucent. Palpate only after examination along structure already identified as at fault		
A. History/Referred Pain	**B. Assessment by Function**	
1. Take a history	2. Examine incriminated joint by selective tension employing:	
	PASSIVE MOVEMENTS for inert structures: *joint capsule, ligaments, bursae, fascia, displacements, dura mater, nerve roots*	RESISTED MOVEMENTS for contractile structures: *muscles, tendons and attachments to bone* Examine for: (a) pain (b) weakness *Principal findings* (a) pain: lesion of appropriate contractile structure (b) painless weakness: interference with conduction of appropriate nerve (c) strong and painless: normal

(4) *Weak and painful:* serious trouble is present, for example a fracture or secondary deposits. But a patient's understandable reluctance to replicate severe pain may be responsible for apparent weakness.

(5) *Painful on repetition:* intermittent claudication is the probability if a movement is strong and painless at first but hurts after a number of repetitions.

(6) *All the resisted movements hurt:* this could be a gross lesion lying proximally, usually capsular and produced when joint movement is not fully restrained as with the so-called 'muddle pattern' at the acromioclavicular joint. But it is more likely to stem from neurosis.

In practice the resisted movements are tested after the passive movements which take precedence as joint signs.

Passive movements

A lesion of a contractile structure does not produce limitation on passive movement (with the exception of a partial rupture in a muscle or scar tissue and adhesions). Thus if there is limitation of passive movement an inert structure must be at fault and 5° limitation of passive range carries a quite different significance from full range. The exact situation must be determined. In cases of doubt the examiner may have to push fairly hard to arrive at the true picture, and it may take persuasion (or a slight change in angulation) to get beyond a painful arc to establish that pain does in fact cease at full range.

If the movements show the lesion lies in an inert structure, the primary issue is whether the whole capsule or some other inert structure is involved – that is, whether the lesion is capsular or non-capsular. If the latter, the commonest possibilities are internal derangement, ligamentous sprain and bursitis, although occasionally the cause of non-capsular passive limitation may lie extra-articularly.

These classifications are considered below.

Findings on passive movements
Capsular lesions

If an entire joint capsule is inflamed, all or most passive movements of that joint will strain a different part of the capsule. So all or most of the passive movements prove painful and limited.

This constitutes one of the most important concepts in orthopaedic medicine, namely that a lesion of the entire capsule gives rise to limitation in the capsular pattern. In other words, arthritis is designated by the capsular pattern which:

(1) varies from joint to joint;
(2) is denoted by limitation not of a fixed degree but in a fixed proportion.

Thus at the wrist the pattern is equal limitation of flexion and extension with little limitation of the deviations. At the shoulder the pattern is so much limitation of medial rotation, greater limitation of abduction with lateral rotation the most limited.

In a severe case at the shoulder, the limitations would amount

1.4

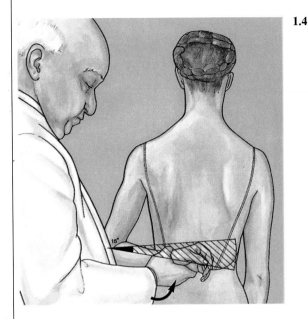

1.5

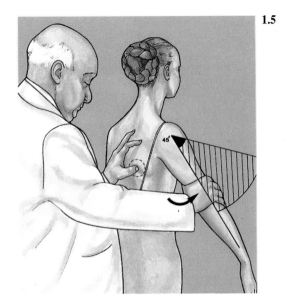

1.6

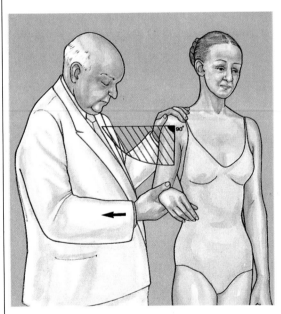

1.4, 1.5, 1.6 *The capsular pattern is the hallmark of arthritis. The approximate degree of restriction for each movement is shown by the hatched area, which depicts a severe case of shoulder capsulitis. Internal rotation is almost full (Figure 1.4), abduction is more limited (Figure 1.5) and external rotation even more so (Figure 1.6).*

of movement in every direction should be substituted the concept of limitation conforming to the capsular pattern for that particular joint. It is a highly sensitive indicator, since arthritis can continue for many months without giving rise to radiological evidence of disease.

The capsular pattern for each joint is listed in Appendix III.

Internal derangement

Arthritis cannot be the cause of limitation of passive movement that does not conform to the capsular pattern. Lesions capable of restricting range, but not involving the entire joint, have to be considered. The principal possibilities are ligamentous strain (discussed below) and internal derangement. Thus a carpal capitate subluxation at the wrist gives rise to painful but full passive flexion, painful limited extension and painless full deviations , easily distinguishable from a capsular lesion marked by equal limitation of flexion and extension (*Figure 1.7*).

Similarly at the neck, in the capsular pattern five of the six possible movements are limited, whereas with an intra-articular cervical displacement the limitation is generally present only on two, three or four movements.

to about 15°, 45° and 90° respectively, and in a less pronounced case perhaps 5°, 30° and 60° (*Figures 1.4–1.6*).

Whatever the cause of arthritis, the pattern is the same. Even in the early cases, where muscle spasm springing into play to prevent capsular stretching beyond a certain joint protects the joint, the restriction of mobility is still in the capsular pattern. The spasm is secondary to the capsular lesion and is itself painless. The reason for the capsular pattern's existence appears to be merely that some aspects of the capsule resent stretching more than others in reflection of the capsule's anatomical construction.

For the traditional notion of arthritis marked by limitation

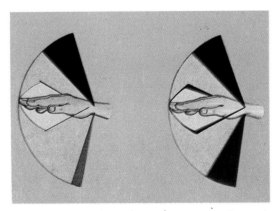

1.7 *The non-capsular and capsular patterns. A carpal capitate subluxation (left) limits extension and hurts (shown red) on flexion , whereas arthritis (right) painfully limits both extension and flexion equally.*

Ligamentous sprains

A sprained ligament will generally cause pain on one passive movement. Thus at the wrist if passive radial deviation is painful, a lesion of the ulnar collateral ligament is suggested, in which case the other three passive movements – flexion, extension and ulnar deviation – prove painless (*Figure 1.8*). The finding is thus of pain at extreme of range in the contralateral direction.

End-feel

The extreme of each passive movement of the joint transmits a specific sensation to the examiner's hands. For example, on extension of the elbow the normal end-feel of the joint is hard: bone is felt to engage bone. Were the end-feel of elbow extension not hard, the joint would not be normal.

The significance of the end-feel is thus the degree to which it corresponds to the end-feel of the normal joint. Different types of end-feel imply different disorders and, with experience, the clinician can frequently sense with his hands what is going on inside the joint. Categories include:

(1) Bone to bone: the standard end-feel for elbow extension but not, for example, elbow flexion (see (4) next page).
(2) A springy block points to internal derangement.
(3) The abrupt check imposed by muscle spasm coming actively into play may indicate severe arthritis, a displacement, for example at the knee, or a destructive

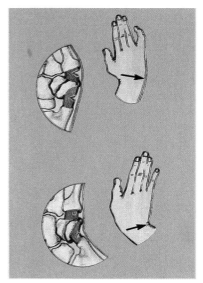

1.8 *A strained ligament causes pain on one passive movement only: passive radial deviation (top right) will hurt with a damaged ulnar collateral ligament (top left). By contrast, passive ulnar deviation (lower right) does not stretch the ligament and is not painful (lower left).*

CLINICAL EXAMINATION: SUMMARY III

The moving soft tissues are radiotranslucent. Palpate only after examination along structure already identified as at fault		
A. History/Referred Pain	**B. Assessment by Function**	
1. Take a history	2. Examine incriminated joint by selective tension employing:	
	PASSIVE MOVEMENTS for inert structures: *joint capsule, ligaments, bursae, fascia, displacements, dura mater, nerve roots*	RESISTED MOVEMENTS for contractile structures: *muscles, tendons and attachments to bone*
	Examine for: (a) pain (b) limitation (c) end-feel	Examine for: (a) pain (b) weakness
	Principal findings (a) capsular pattern: capsular lesion. Pain and limitation in a fixed proportion on some/all movements of a joint	*Principal findings* (a) pain: lesion of appropriate contractile structure
	(b) non-capsular pattern of: (i) ligamentous sprain *or* (ii) internal derangement One/some movements of a joint painful/limited, but not in the capsular pattern	(b) painless weakness: interference with conduction of appropriate nerve
	(c) extra-articular limitation	(c) strong and painless: normal

lesion. Working knowledge of the joint in question refines the possibilities.

(4) Soft-tissue approximation: a normal end-feel when the joint cannot be pushed further because of engagement against another part of the body, for example, on elbow flexion.

(5) Empty feel: this is when movement causes considerable pain before the extreme of range is reached. The sensation imparted to the examiner's hand is 'empty', lacking in organic resistance with further range clearly possible were it not for the patient's pain. Acute bursitis, extra-articular abscess or neoplasm should be strongly considered.

End-feel is an important diagnostic indicator.

Passive movement pain from contractile lesions
This phenomenon should not mislead. Occasionally a damaged contractile structure can produce pain on full stretch where, for example, a tendon is put under strain at the extreme of range. Thus, full passive medial rotation

may hurt in infraspinatus tendinitis, and similarly the extensor and flexor tendons at the wrist may hurt on full passive movements.

Extra-articular limitation
If the amount of limitation at one joint is dictated by the position in which another joint is held, then the restricting tissue must lie extra-articularly. The relationship shows the lesion lies in a structure spanning at least two joints, thus excluding articular disorders. A prime example is straight-leg raising. Limitation of hip flexion is found when the knee is extended but not when flexed.

Occasionally, disproportionate limitation is encountered with gross restriction in one direction combined with full painless range in all other directions. Again this suggests that the joint itself is normal but that movement is prevented by an extra-articular factor. Examples are found at the gastrocnemius muscle (where a partial rupture grossly limits dorsiflexion of the ankle joint), with a haematoma in the popliteal space (limiting knee flexion) and in acute subdeltoid bursitis.

History

After assessing the patient's demeanour and gait as she walks in, the clinician begins the examination by taking a history, which itself must be viewed in the context of the workings of referred pain.

A clear and chronological history is a prerequisite. The patient is asked about the events leading up to the onset of symptoms, what they were then, what brought them on and is then told to recount, week by week or year by year, what has happened since. All the time the patient's account is compared with the clinician's knowledge of the likelihoods of the various conditions and, in particular, with his mental map of the dermatomes. By the time the physical examination is under way he should have some idea of the possible cause(s) of the trouble. Any subsequent diagnosis must be compatible with the known chronological facts. It will be seen that:

(1) Many, if not most, soft-tissue lesions have a distinctive history.

(2) The treatment for many disorders varies according to the stage the condition has reached.

Examples

(1) Traumatic arthritis at the shoulder is confined to those over 45 and causes little or no pain in the first days following trauma. During the first few weeks the entire condition may be aborted by capsular stretching, which in the subsequent stage would aggravate the disorder, by then susceptible to injection.

(2) A cervical disc lesion giving pain on movement down the

arm recovers spontaneously in four months and no treatment avails.

(3) Pain from a tennis elbow generally does not emerge until about two weeks after the causative trauma.

(4) A patient who wakes continually in the early hours with acute pins and needles in the arms, and numbness which persists to the following morning, is probably suffering from a thoracic outlet syndrome.

(5) The patient falls and her knee locks: a meniscus is probable. But if she falls as a result of momentary locking, a small loose body is more probable.

(6) A sharp pain in the heel on the first few steps after sitting is suggestive of plantar fasciitis.

(7) A patient presenting for the first time with a lumbar disc lesion of rapid onset may benefit from manipulation. But regular recurrence following manipulative reduction may indicate sclerosants. If she is over 60, no benefit will accrue from traction. Nor will manipulation succeed where pain from a lumbar disc lesion has been down the leg for six months or more.

Diagnosis and treatment depend on history. Questions include the patient's age and occupation followed by detailed enquiries to cover the condition's onset and subsequent evolution. The examiner should spare no pains to establish what by way of trauma, if any, provoked the symptoms, where they were first felt, where they have spread to since and the general progression of the disorder. Throughout, he will bear in mind the workings of referred pain.

Referred pain

Pain perceived elsewhere than at its true site is termed 'referred'. Nearly all pain (excepting from bone) is referred; the diagnostician's task is to ascertain from where.

The place where the pain is felt is determined by the sensory cortex. This attributes the sensory impulses received to appropriate areas of the body (*Figure 1.9*).

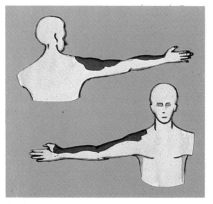

1.10 *The C5 dermatome. Nearly all shoulder pain is felt within this area.*

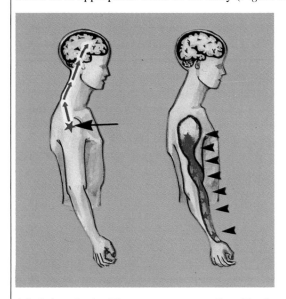

1.9 *Referred pain. The symptoms are attributed by the sensory cortex to the corresponding dermatome. C5 shown.*

With stimuli to the skin, the sensory cortex achieves a high degree of accuracy. Over the years a stimulus reaching certain cells in the sensorium comes to bear the meaning that damage is being inflicted on a certain area of skin.

When a painful stimulus arising from a deep-seated structure (e.g. a soft tissue) is received by the same cells, the sensory cortex interprets this new impulse on the basis of past experience. Pain is referred to the area of skin connected with those particular cortical cells.

This area of skin is the dermatome, and the dermatome to which any given pain is allocated corresponds to the segment from which the structure was embryologically derived. Thus a pain in a tissue of C5 segmental origin is referred by the sensory cortex to the C5 dermatome, and from a C6 structure to the C6 dermatome. So when dealing with a lesion suspected to arise from, for example, a C5 structure, it is vital to know the boundaries of the C5 dermatome (*Figure 1.10*). Pain felt outside that area cannot emanate from a C5 structure, and knowledge of the C5 dermatome shows, for instance, that pain at the back of the elbow cannot originate from a structure of C5 derivation (e.g. the shoulder), whereas pain at the anterior aspect might. It could, of course, also come from any other segment(s) whose dermatomes overlie that area – e.g. C6.

It is with symptoms in the upper and lower limbs that referred pain is particularly important. The dermatomes do no more than represent the original relationship of the limb buds to the trunk at the earliest stage of development of the embryo. The 40 segments in a month-old fetus are distributed horizontally (*Figure 1.11*). At this stage the dermatomes are superimposed directly over their originating segments. But the growth of the four limbs draws the dermatomes out down the arms and legs. At the trunk, however, the original arrangement of circular dermatomic bands remains relatively intact.

1.11 *Embryological derivation. During growth from small to large fetus, the limb projections deform the original shape of the segments as they spread down the limbs.*

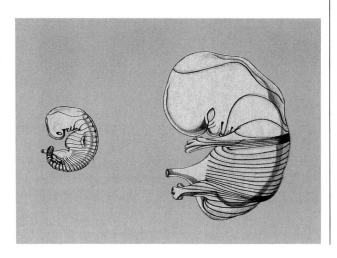

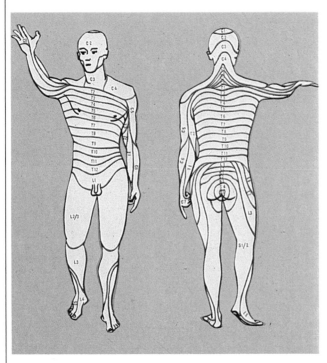

1.12 *The dermatomes. The diagrams give an adequate overall impression of the segmentation of the skin; they do not allow for the areas of overlap.*

This means that the upper limb is covered by the C5, C6, C7, C8, T1 and T2 dermatomes. Pain within the appropriate area of the arm could arise from structures of matching embryological derivation. The L2, L3, L4, L5, S1, S2 and S3 dermatomes all extend into the leg. Thus, when examining for the cause of pain in the limbs, symptoms may originate not just locally but proximally (*Figure 1.12*).

In practice this is simpler than it sounds. For example, the front of the knee falls within (*inter alia*) the L3 dermatome.

Thus in addition to pain of local origin, symptoms there may come from any L3 structure. Primary possibilities are osteoarthrosis of the hip and a disc lesion pressing on the L3 dural nerve root sleeve.

So with anterior knee pain, the first step is to take a history. It should emerge whether the pain is connected with:

(1) Trauma to the knee.
(2) An inflammatory-type disorder occurring spontaneously at the knee.
(3) Pain extending perhaps from the groin to the front of the knee, but arising at the hip.
(4) A history typical of backache coupled with pain down the leg.

CLINICAL EXAMINATION: SUMMARY IV

The moving soft tissues are radiotranslucent. Palpate only after examination along structure already identified as at fault			
A. History/Referred Pain	**B. Assessment by Function**		
1. Take a history. Consider:	2. Examine incriminated joint by selective tension employing:		
(a) the probable lesion and the stage it has reached; treatment is governed by both factors	PRELIMINARY EXAMINATION Where necessary begin by rough outline examination consisting of active movements to establish which joint is at fault. Then proceed to examination in detail of the incriminated joint by a routine of passive and resisted movements	PASSIVE MOVEMENTS for inert structures: *joint capsule, ligaments, bursae, fascia, displacements, dura mater, nerve roots*	RESISTED MOVEMENTS for contractile structures: *muscles, tendons and attachments to bone*
(b) referred pain		Examine for: (a) pain (b) limitation (c) end-feel	Examine for: (a) pain (b) weakness
		Principal findings (a) capsular pattern: capsular lesion. Pain and limitation in a fixed proportion on some/all movements of a joint	*Principal findings* (a) pain: lesion of appropriate contractile structure
		(b) non-capsular pattern of: (i) ligamentous sprain *or* (ii) internal derangement One/some movements of a joint painful/limited, but not in the capsular pattern	(b) painless weakness: interference with conduction of appropriate nerve (c) strong and painless: normal
		(c) extra-articular limitation	

Turning to the physical examination, the various possibilities may be swiftly confirmed or eliminated. If spinal movements are painless, the pain does not come from the spine. If hip movements are painless, the pain does not originate in the hip. But if knee movements bring on the pain, the pain does come from the knee – which is then examined in detail by the appropriate routine of passive and resisted movements.

These principles are duplicated at the upper limb. Most shoulder structures are primarily of C5 derivation. The biceps also has an element of C6. Additionally the arm is served by the nerve roots emerging from the cervical spine. A cervical disc lesion may compress a nerve root at C3 (rare), C4, C5, C6, C7 (common), C8, T1 (rare) or T2

(rare). Pain is then felt in the corresponding dermatome, each of which occupies a fairly well-defined but frequently overlapping section of the arm, elbow, wrist or hand.

As with the lower limb, so with the upper. After a careful history, examination may have to start at the neck, proceed to the shoulder and only ultimately will the structures about, say, the elbow be identified as containing the causative lesion. This is a simple enough procedure and, in fact, knowledge of referred pain simplifies diagnosis.

Pain is referred in compliance with certain rules, understanding of which enables the clinician to define:

(1) from which tissues the pain could arise;
(2) from which tissues the pain could not arise.

Rules governing the reference of pain

(1) Pain is referred segmentally
A C5 tissue refers pain to the C5 dermatome. Subject to (2) below, the pain can occupy all or any part of the dermatome. For example, with acute traumatic arthritis at the shoulder the pain may run all the way down the arm to the wrist. But initially the pain is local and only spreads by degrees to the elbow and finally the wrist. As the disorder wears off, the symptoms retreat proximally. Throughout, the pain is confined to the C5 dermatome.

It follows that the examiner will be particularly on the alert if the patient describes symptoms straddling more than one dermatome at once, or those that migrate from one dermatome to another. Four possibilities arise:

(a) The patient is describing a pain devoid of organic basis.
(b) The lesion itself is shifting – often the case with displacements at the spine.
(c) The lesion is spreading. Consider, for example, metastases.
(d) The pain stems from a tissue that does not refer pain on a segmental basis (see below).

Exception to the rule of segmental reference
The dura mater refers pain extrasegmentally – an exception of the greatest importance covered in detail on page 15.

(2) Pain is referred distally
The source of symptoms must thus be sought locally or proximally. The structures about the knee and elbow stand almost alone in being capable of radiating pain equally in

both directions, but in both cases the patient usually realizes from where his symptoms originate.

(3) Referred pain never crosses the mid-line
Thus a T5 left rib will not cause discomfort on the right of the body. A pain felt centrally must originate from a central structure and cannot be accounted for by a unilateral structure. Similarly, the source of bilateral pain must be sought centrally. A pain alternating from one side of the body to the other must have a central source that can shift from one side to another (e.g. a displacement at the spine).

(4) The extent of reference is controlled by:
(a) The size of the dermatome and the position in that dermatome of the tissue at fault. Clearly, a large dermatome permits greater reference than a small one. Furthermore, a lesion in the proximal part of the dermatome can refer pain further than a lesion in the distal part. At the extremities of each limb the capacity for accurate localization increases. At the wrist, hand, ankle and foot useful results may be obtained from palpation after assessment by function.
(b) The strength of the stimulus. The more intense the pain, the greater the number of cortical cells excited. The spread to adjacent cells in the sensory cortex is regarded by the patient as an enlargement of the painful area.
(c) The depth of the tissue at fault. The deeper a soft tissue lies, the larger the reference to be expected. However, bone sets up a pain that hardly radiates at all.

Symptoms referred from the nervous system

There are four aspects: the spinal cord, the dural sleeve of a nerve root, the nerve trunks and small nerves. Symptoms from each vary in important respects and thus may be differentiated.

(1) Compression of the spinal cord

There is no pain. Pins and needles are apt to be bilateral and to disregard segmentation of the body.

(2) Compression of the dural sleeve and parenchyma of a nerve root

At the point of emergence from the dura, the nerve roots are invested with a dural sleeve. Pressure on this produces pain in all or any part of the relevant dermatome. Thus pressure on the C7 root will give pain down the arm (*Figure 1.13*) while pressure on the L4 root engenders pain down the leg extending to the big toe.

Compression sufficient to affect the parenchyma will produce all or any of the following:

(a) Pins and needles – a compression phenomenon – generally felt at the distal end of the dermatome and often conspicuously occupying an area not supplied by any one nerve trunk (*Figure 1.14*). The paraesthesia has neither edge nor aspect, being felt, for example, within the fingers.

(b) Numbness which, as it comes on, tends to displace the pins and needles. Major pressure on a nerve root causes analgesia. Minor pressure evokes pins and needles.

(c) Weakness, resulting from compression of the dural sleeve sufficiently intense to also impinge on the parenchyma within. This weakness will be discernible on resisted movements.

(3) Compression of a nerve trunk

The results are:

(a) No pain (although pressure on the surrounding dural cladding at the transverse process will hurt).

(b) Weakness. Impaired conduction along a nerve leads to muscle weakness, again discernible on resisted movements.

(c) Pins and needles (*Figure 1.15*) rather than numbness, generally brought on as a release phenomenon. Thus pressure on, for example, the sciatic nerve while sitting causes no symptoms; the pins and needles come when the subject relieves the pressure by standing up. The paraesthesia is concentrated in the distal part of the cutaneous area supplied by that peripheral nerve; the lesion always lies proximal to the upper edge of the paraesthetic area.

(4) Compression of a small nerve

The results are:

(a) No pain.

(b) Normally no weakness because the efferent fibres have left the body of the nerve proximally.

(c) Numbness, rather than pins and needles, occupying the cutaneous area supplied by that nerve (see *Figure 1.15*). The edge is well defined, and towards the centre of the area full anaesthesia is often demonstrable.

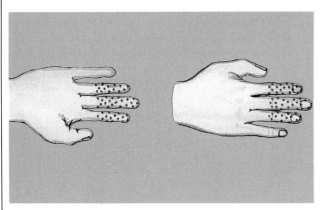

1.13, 1.14 *Pressure on the dural sheath at the cervical spine. Compression of the C7 root (left) can produce both pain down the arm in the C7 dermatome, and pins and needles in both aspects of the appropriate fingers (Figure 1.14).*

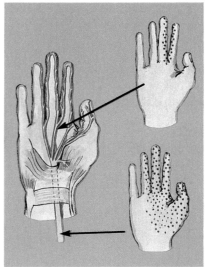

1.15 *Pins and needles. Contrasting symptoms are caused by pressure on the median nerve above and below its point of division.*

Examination of the nervous system

Pins and needles from any source are findings that emerge in the course of the history. Pain from compression of the dural sleeve to a nerve root may be aggravated by spinal movements. In addition, because the nerve roots at the lumbar spine are mobile, any impingement restricting a nerve root's mobility can be tested by indirect traction to the nerve. Thus pain may be elicited by straight-leg raising or prone-lying knee flexion.

Interference with motor conduction will display as weakness on resisted movements. Interference with sensory conduction will show itself as cutaneous analgesia.

An example

Apparently similar symptoms may readily be traced back to source. Thus a trigger finger compresses the two digital nerves at their point of division, engendering numbness of the two adjacent sides of the two relevant fingers. This could not come from the median nerve because the pins and needles would then be felt in the thumb, index, long and the radial side of the ring finger.

If, however, a cervical nerve root is pinched, the pins and needles occupy fingers served by no single arm nerve. The thumb and index finger, for example, are served only by the C6 root.

Exception to the rule of segmental reference

Perhaps because of its plurisegmental derivation, the dura mater does not obey the rules of segmental reference. The dura runs from the foramen magnum of the skull to the caudal edge of the first or second sacral vertebra (*Figure 1.16*) and keeps the spinal cord buffered in cerebrospinal fluid. From it protrude 30 pairs of nerve roots covered by the dural root sleeves.

Whereas pressure on the nerve roots engenders segmentally referred pain, compression or stretching of the dura itself refers pain extrasegmentally. The dura mater is, throughout its extent, adjacent to the intervertebral discs and is thus vulnerable to posterior pressure exerted via the posterior longitudinal ligament.

Pain from pressure on the dura mater at cervical levels (left, *Figure 1.17*) may be felt anywhere from head to midthorax, often pervading many dermatomes simultaneously. It is a frequent cause of scapular pain (but not of brachial

symptoms which may, however, be accounted for by pressure on a nerve root). Symptoms are usually central or unilateral.

Pressure on the dura at thoracic levels (centre, *Figure 1.17*) may radiate pain up to the base of the neck or to the posterior or anterior aspect of the trunk. It often spreads over many dermatomes simultaneously. Symptoms are usually central or unilateral.

Pressure at lumbar levels (right, *Figure 1.17*) may cause pain reaching the lower thorax posteriorly, the lower abdomen, upper buttocks, sacrum and coccyx. Symptoms may extend bilaterally or unilaterally down the legs as far as the ankle but not beyond to the foot. Once again, many dermatomes may be occupied simultaneously.

The mere fact that the patient describes a reference of pain seemingly impossible should focus attention on the dura mater. It is a mobile, inert structure and consequently specifically examined by passive movements.

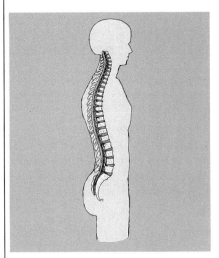

1.16 *The dura mater. Pressure on this structure is responsible for much backache. The pain is referred extrasegmentally.*

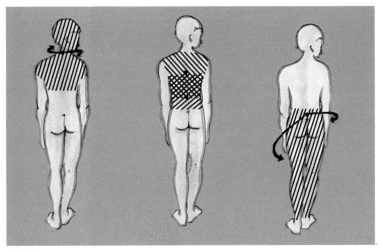

1.17 *Extrasegmental reference. The areas in which pain may be felt as a result of interference with the dura at cervical (left), thoracic (centre) and lumbar levels (right).*

CLINICAL EXAMINATION: SUMMARY V

The moving soft tissues are radiotranslucent. Palpate only after examination along structure already identified as at fault			
A. History/Referred Pain	**B. Assessment by Function**		
1. Take a history. Consider:	2. Examine incriminated joint by selective tension employing:		

(a) the probable lesion and the stage it has reached; treatment is governed by both factors
 	
(b) referred pain. Consider:
 	
(i) dermatome occupied/ segmental derivation, particularly with pain in upper or lower limb
 	
(ii) rules of reference, i.e. referred pain
  – is referred segmentally
  – is referred distally
  – never crosses the mid-line
 	
(iii) site of interference (if any) with nervous system
  – spinal cord: no pain, pins and needles
  – nerve root sheath: pain, pins and needles, numbness
  – nerve trunk: no pain; weakness, pins and needles
  – small nerve: no pain, no weakness; numbness
 	
(iv) extrasegmentally referred pain from dura mater if spinal lesion
	PRELIMINARY EXAMINATION Where necessary begin by rough outline examination consisting of active movements to establish which joint is at fault. Then proceed to examination in detail of the incriminated joint by a routine of passive and resisted movements	PASSIVE MOVEMENTS for inert structures: *joint capsule, ligaments, bursae, fascia, displacements, dura mater, nerve roots*
		
		Examine for:
		(a) pain
		(b) limitation
		(c) end-feel
		
		Principal findings
		(a) capsular pattern: capsular lesion. Pain and limitation in a fixed proportion on some/all movements of a joint
		
		(b) non-capsular pattern of:
		  (i) ligamentous sprain *or*
		  (ii) internal derangement
		One/some movements of a joint painful/limited, but not in the capsular pattern
			RESISTED MOVEMENTS for contractile structures: *muscles, tendons and attachments to bone*
			
			Examine for:
			(a) pain
			(b) weakness
			
			Principal findings
			(a) pain: lesion of appropriate contractile structure
			
			(b) painless weakness: interference with conduction of appropriate nerve
			
			(c) strong and painless: normal

		(c) extra-articular limitation	

Diagnosis at the spine

Diagnosis at the spinal joints follows standard principles but is governed by the sensitivity of the dura mater.

Examination of the spine for backache frequently produces the following findings:

(1) Painless resisted movements, exculpating the contractile structures (e.g. the muscles).
(2) Painful passive movements incriminating the inert structures (e.g. the dura mater).
(3) Painful passive movements in the non-capsular pattern compatible with internal derangement.
(4) Frequently signs of:
(a) interference with dural mobility;
(b) interference with mobility of the dural sleeve to a nerve root, sometimes with signs of impaired nerve root conduction.

(5) A history consistent with an intra-articular displacement.

Clinical evidence thus points firmly to the conclusion that these cases have a single, unified cause: minor and remediable displacements of disc material compressing the dura mater or nerve roots (*Figures 1.18* and *1.19*). This deduction is supported by abolition of the symptoms following:

(1) Manipulative reduction of the displacement (see page 153) or
(2) Reduction of the displacement by traction or
(3) An injection of epidural local anaesthetic, rendering insensitive the superficial aspect of the dura mater and nerve roots.

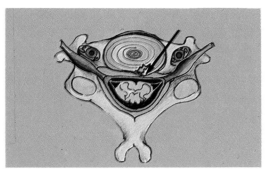

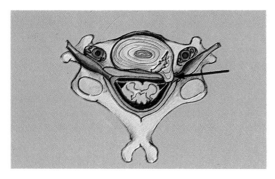

1.18, 1.19 *A central displacement (above) impinges on the dura mater, whereas a lateral protrusion can compress the nerve root sheath (below). This small shift of a few millimetres has a dramatic effect both on the area of perceived pain and on the type of signs/symptoms.*

Diagnostic skills

Diagnosis is a skill and clearly the physician learns from experience. Nevertheless, satisfactory results are soon achieved. It is well to remember that the object of the physical examination is to find the movement that elicits the pain of which the patient complains, rather than some other nebulous symptom of which she was previously unaware. Nor is it sufficient for a movement to prove painful; it must actually increase the patient's pain. During examination the patient is questioned in a neutral manner, being asked whether a movement has any influence on (rather than aggravating) his symptoms.

The examination for any given joint should always be performed in its entirety and in the same order – first the history, then the passive movements and finally the resisted movements. Only by sticking to a standard sequence will the physician be sure to leave nothing out and only by leaving nothing out are true findings feasible. A correct diagnosis is achieved not from evidence furnished by one painful movement but by careful detection of a consistent pattern.

Corroboration or disproof of the diagnosis may often be obtained by induction of local anaesthesia – a 1:200 solution of procaine is recommended. Following infiltration, the patient is asked to repeat whichever movement was found to be most painful. If the pain has gone, the anaesthetic was injected into the correct site. No other form of confirmation is comparably effective.

Slight pains often make for problems. It is sometimes wise to ask the patient to return a week later, by which time she may be either better or worse, in the latter case permitting a more conclusive examination.

Very severe pain may render clinical examination impossible on account of an excess of physical signs. Justifiable fear of pain may prevent the patient from moving; every movement may provoke intense exacerbation. In these cases history must be given its full weight, with gross signs viewed in light of the fact that only a limited number of disorders engender agonizing pain.

Double lesions are a source of confusion, with signs pointing, for example, to a lesion of both infraspinatus and supraspinatus, or to a lesion of both the shoulder and cervical spine. In such cases it is best to tackle one lesion at a time, beginning with the more common, tractable or painful. After one lesion has cleared up, the second will be easier to identify.

Psychogenic pain is no rarity, but detection is seldom difficult as the patient is ignorant of the principles of referred pain and the way the supposed lesion should behave. A host of contradictions with no coherent picture swiftly become apparent during the history and physical appraisal. The more thorough and systematic the questioning and examination, the more inconsistencies come to light.

The examiner should be on his guard against dismissing symptoms of hypersensitive patients as psychogenic. Malingerers, being pain-free and thus unaware of what should and should not hurt, are apt to produce a standard painful response across a broad spectrum of tests, in contrast to the neurotic who is likely to be most vociferous on the most painful movement.

Imaging techniques

Although of great assistance, in the broad run of cases the use of more sophisticated diagnostic techniques will neither be required nor justified. Where appropriate, they constitute an excellent adjunct to the clinical process but, as with X-rays, care must be taken not to attribute the patient's symptoms to all defects and disorders shown.

Computer assisted tomography

CT retains its place because of good bone imaging. It also shows certain elements of the soft tissues. CT is a cross-sectional imaging technique; reformatting the anatomical information in other planes is not very satisfactory and the production of three-dimensional images tends to be complicated and costly. A lateral or central disc herniation will be displayed, but as with any technique, experience is required to interpret the results. There are indications that patients who have had disc lesions displayed on CT and who become pain-free may still show protrusions on follow-up examination.

Magnetic resonance imaging

MRI is probably the best imaging technique for showing soft tissues in detail. It is useful both for detecting tissue abnormality and for accurate localization, including for example the precise tendon affected. Importantly, it can image in any plane. Although expensive in capital terms, MRI is an out-patient procedure increasingly acceptable as an alternative to arthroscopy, which is invasive and carries well-recognized morbidity. Unlike CT, MRI produces no ionizing radiation and for this reason alone is preferable.

The cruciate ligaments of well-paid sportsmen are a current focus of interest, with MRI providing generally accurate corroboration of disorders long diagnosed by clinicians. Other tears of ligaments and tendinitis may also be displayed, demonstrating lesions previously invisible to any imaging technique. At present, diffuse disorders such as capsulitis will often not be registered.

MRI shows disc protrusions and is particularly useful in excluding the difficult central cervical protrusions. It also displays the abnormal synovium of rheumatoid arthritis. The advent of the contrast medium gadolinium DTPA has opened up the potential to explore joint disease more fully, as any inflammatory disease is likely to be hypervascular.

Clearly, statistical work corroborating MRI findings with the results of clinical diagnosis is now an important possibility.

Arthroscopy and arthrography

Arthroscopy is rarely of value in inflammatory conditions and, although useful for lesions of the meniscus and Baker's cyst at the knee, has been superseded by MRI in the accurate diagnosis of cruciate ligament lesions. It is increasingly and successfully employed in the shoulder and, less frequently, in the wrist, hip, elbow and ankle.

At the wrist, arthrography has not yet been replaced by MRI. At the knee, its function is now partially superseded; results at the shoulder remain valuable. Both arthrography and arthroscopy have lost recent ground to MRI, and the latter's diagnostic role may still be overplayed.

Bone scintigraphy (technetium^{99m} phosphate compounds)

A highly sensitive but very non-specific technique. Sportsmen may produce stress fractures and early bone changes which are visible on bone scan before they are noted on X-ray. A blood-pool image will indicate blood flow and a three-hour scan, bony activity. A combination of images enables assessment of soft-tissue lesions, fractures, shin splints or avascular necrosis. A bone scan provides indications of increased activity suggesting pathology.

Diagnostic ultrasound

Useful for superficial tissues, provided they are of sufficient bulk and the signal not obscured by bone. Haematoma may be successfully monitored; lesions of the tendo Achillis, quadriceps expansion and patellar tendons can be demonstrated comparatively.

CHAPTER TWO

PRINCIPLES OF TREATMENT

Only after an exact diagnosis has been made is it possible to prescribe specific treatment, which must be:

(1) Administered to the specific site of the lesion diagnosed.
(2) Of a kind to exert a beneficial effect on the lesion.

Once the lesion is pain-free, it is important to provide advice and/or management to avoid recurrence.

It follows that for soft-tissue lesions the non-specific remedies such as heat, cold, water, generalized exercises, ointment, bandages, diffuse massage and analgesics are, with insignificant exceptions, palliative rather than curative.

The object of scientific treatment is recovery and, accordingly, the criterion is not whether the patient has received a course of therapy but whether the treatment has yielded any amelioration.

Thus the patient is continually reassessed to see if range has improved and pain diminished. If not, either the diagnosis or the treatment has been misconceived.

The requisite therapeutic skills are readily acquired and can be easily learned and applied. Virtually no special equipment is needed.

Joints other than the spine
Disorders
The salient disorders are discussed below and the appropriate treatments dealt with in the immediately ensuing section.

Muscles
Strain in a muscle causes a few fibres to part. The resultant scar tissue mats the fibres together not just longitudinally but also transversely and these microscopic adhesions generate pain when the muscle broadens on contraction (*Figure 2.1*). The painful adhesions can be broken up by deep massage (*Figure 2.2*).

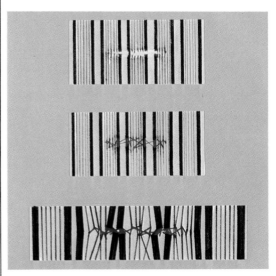

2.1 *Minor muscular tears. The formation of intramuscular scarring (top and centre) can painfully limit full broadening on contraction (bottom).*

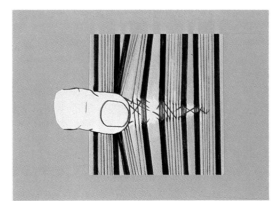

2.2 *Deep transverse massage. The muscle fibres are teased apart.*

19

Aborting muscular adhesions

If the tear lies clear of the tendon and in the belly of the muscle, inner range static contractions accompanied by an induction of local anaesthesia may also play their part in speeding recovery immediately after injury. The object is to broaden the muscles without straining the longitudinal scarring. The local anaesthesia allows for normal movement of the uninjured part of the muscle, with any stretching contraindicated until the structure is pain-free on resisted testing. Off-weight exercises encourage the formation of a supple scar that quickly becomes painless.

The nearer towards the tendon the scar lies, the less likely injection will succeed. The tactic is effective only during the first few days (at most) following injury and is strongly recommended, notably for sports injuries where the patient tends to seek immediate professional advice. The outstanding conditions to which this approach applies are lesions of the gastrocnemius, hamstrings and quadriceps. The pectoralis major, latissimus dorsi and trapezius also benefit. Resisted exercises are best avoided until recovery is well established but, for athletes, isometric exercises within pain-free range may be started early. Isokinetic work can follow soon after, but isotonic and pleomorphic work must be graded in when recovery is well established, using a 'ladder' principle of introducing new movement skills that require a gradually increasing amount of work for the damaged tissue. Different sports and different muscles follow different procedures.

Tendons

Strain on a tendon tears a few fibres and each subsequent muscle contraction is apt to renew the rupture in the healing breach. The result is an inflamed scar. Either the inflammation or the scar itself can be disposed of, the former by an injection of steroid suspension and the latter by deep massage. The injection is faster and less painful, but massage lowers the incidence of recurrence as the scar itself is effectively abolished and the repair process is not inhibited as with steroids.

The joint capsule

The joint capsule may become inflamed whether through traumatic or inflammatory arthritis.

In inflammatory cases without irretrievable damage to the joint, an intra-articular injection of steroid suspension can be relied on to bring immediate relief lasting many months, provided weight-bearing or over-use is avoided.

Traumatic arthritis at the shoulder, elbow, radio-ulnar joint and foot also respond well to steroid therapy. At the shoulder or hip, manipulative stretching may also be helpful.

Inflammatory arthritis strongly contraindicates manipulation.

Displacements

An intra-articular displacement will momentarily strain the capsule or ligaments about a joint. The loose body takes up intra-articular space and either distorts the capsule or enlarges the distance spanned by the ligaments. The displacement itself is insensitive as it is constructed of cartilage, a grossly aneural tissue.

The treatment is manipulative reduction to shift the displacement to a more favourable site. Loose bodies are found with varying frequency at most joints except the shoulder.

Ligaments

A ligament may be strained giving rise to painful stretching on further use. As healing proceeds, scar tissue may adhere the ligament to adjacent bone (*Figure 2.3*).

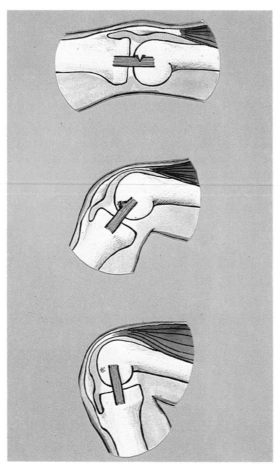

2.3 Ligamentous sprain. Following injury (top), adhesions bind the ligament down (centre). This formation can be prevented by transverse friction, but if untreated the adhesions must be manipulatively ruptured (bottom).

Treatment differs according to the site but consists of massage or an injection of steroid suspension. Infiltration clears up the inflammation. Massage physically moves the ligament in imitation of its normal behaviour, preventing the formation of adhesions which, if allowed to bind, must be manipulatively ruptured. This can also be helped by

TREATMENT AT THE PERIPHERAL JOINTS: SUMMARY

Disorder	Strained muscle	Strained tendon	Capsular inflammation	Intra-articular displacement	Ligamentous sprain	Tenosynovitis
Treatment	Deep massage and graded muscle rehabilitation	Deep massage *or* injection of steroid suspension as appropriate	*Traumatic:* injection of steroid suspension *or* manipulative stretching as appropriate *Rheumatoid:* injection of steroid suspension	Manipulative reduction	Deep massage and/or injection of steroid suspension as appropriate. Limit further stress by support where appropriate	Injection of steroid suspension *or* massage

massaging with a non-steroidal anti-inflammatory gel or, better still, by phonophoretic application.

The patient should not subject the ligament to undue stress until it is healed. Exceptionally, braces that allow joint movement but limit ligamentous stretch may be required.

Tenosynovitis
At the wrist and ankle this is a primary lesion of the gliding surfaces of the external aspect of the tendon. The sheath becomes roughened and inflamed from over-use and can be dealt with by an intra-synovial injection of steroid suspension or massage.

Treatments
Both deep massage and steroid injections are purely local in effect and assist only when administered to the lesion's precise site. No vestige of benefit accrues from treating healthy tissues nearby.

Deep massage
Deep massage, otherwise known as 'transverse friction', bears no relationship to conventional massage.

Reduced to its simplest, the operator's fingertip is placed on the exact site of the lesion (*Figure 2.4*) and rubbed hard *across* the direction of the fibres of the affected tissue. Sessions last for about 20 minutes and some discomfort may be caused for a few minutes before analgesia is induced, but this can be minimized by a gentle start.

The strength of the massage depends on the stage of the lesion. In acute cases it is given extremely gently and in chronic cases with greater vigour. Six to 12 treatments may be necessary, typically given every other day as otherwise the lesion would be too tender from the previous day's

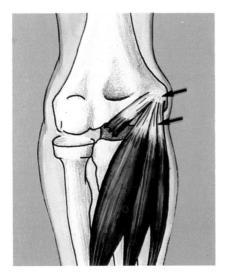

2.4 *Tendinitis, golfer's elbow. There are two sites; treatment to either must be given with scrupulous accuracy.*

encounter to tolerate adequate treatment. The key is that the therapeutic movement is confined to a very small spot (*Figures 2.5* and *2.6*).

In muscular lesions, the deep massage breaks down the adhesions formed by the scar tissue between individual muscle fibres. On the tendon, the scar is eroded by the abrasive action and, for ligamentous lesions, the formation of adhesions during the period of healing is prevented by moving the ligament over bone in imitation of its normal behaviour. With tenosynovitis it appears that the manual rolling of the tendon sheath to and fro against the tendon serves to smooth off the roughened surfaces.

The technique varies slightly for each condition, but the principles remain constant. First, the lesion must be brought within reach of the operator's finger. This entails positioning the patient carefully according to the dictates of applied anatomy. For instance, in supraspinatus tendinitis the patient's arm must be placed behind her back (*Figure 2.7*). This brings the tendon out from under the acromion which would otherwise shield the entire structure.

Second, the tissue to receive the massage should be appropriately tensioned. If a muscle is to be treated, it must be relaxed so the massage can penetrate deeply to tease the fibres apart (*Figure 2.8*), whereas a tendon without a sheath is simply put into the most accessible position. By contrast, with tenosynovitis the tendon must be tautened to form an

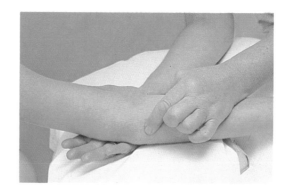

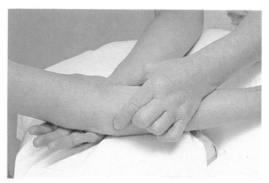

2.5, 2.6 *Massage, golfer's elbow. Note the movement of the index finger is of little more than 1 cm. It is the lesion itself that receives the friction.*

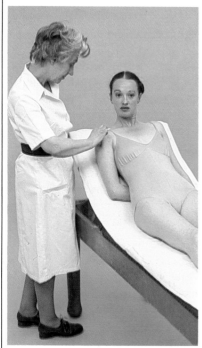

2.7 *Deep massage, supraspinatus. In this position the tendon is bent through a right angle and lies exposed in the sagittal plane.*

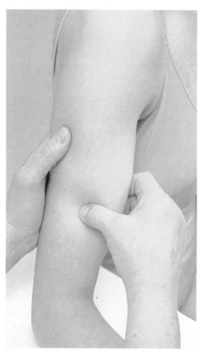

2.8 *Deep massage, the biceps belly. The patient must be told to stay relaxed. It is the substance, not the surface, of the muscle that needs treatment.*

immobile base against which to rub the tendon sheath (*Figure 2.9*). For a ligament, the joint may have to be taken as far as possible in one direction with the massage administered in that position and then taken in the other direction and the massage repeated.

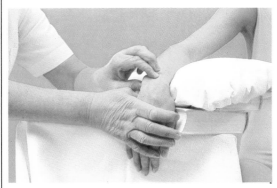

2.9 *Deep massage, extensor carpi radialis. The wrist is flexed over the pillow to tauten the tendon.*

Third, treatment is applied by the operator's fingertip(s). The technique is to move the whole hand, with the patient's skin and the operator's finger moving as one, otherwise a friction burn of the skin may occur. Some practitioners put a piece of tissue paper between fingertips and the lesion; this avoids the burn and absorbs sweat which might otherwise cause slippage. The friction must be *across* the fibres of the affected structure with sufficient amplitude of sweep to ensure that the frictional element (and not the pressure) is paramount. In general the finger, hand and forearm should comprise a straight line parallel to the movement imparted, with the distal interphalangeal

joint slightly flexed. In practice, however, there are many variations.

Thus two fingers may be needed for a large lesion, or more often one finger reinforces the other. The thumb is often used to supply counter-pressure so the finger can bear strongly on the lesion. For some disorders the massage is transmitted by alternate pronation and supination of the hand, thus rotating the digit. In others, the finger stays stationary while the limb is moved underneath it.

Occasionally, the lesion – typically in the belly of a muscle – must be squeezed between thumb and finger.

Finally, both operator and patient must adopt a position allowing sufficient leverage and comfort for the treatment to be kept up for 20 minutes at a time. The standard approach is shown for each lesion. But provided the massage itself is correctly administered, the operator may devise some variant or change position during a session to relieve fatigued muscles.

DEEP MASSAGE: SUMMARY

1. Administer to precise site of lesion
2. The digit is rubbed *across* structure undergoing treatment
3. Frictional element not pressure is paramount
4. Position the patient to:
   (a) render lesion accessible
   (b) put tissue under treatment into appropriate tension, e.g. muscles relaxed
5. Generally 6–12 sessions required, 20 minutes each on alternate days

   NB Precise procedure varies according to each lesion and the stage reached

Steroid therapy

Fibrous tissue appears capable of perpetuating an inflammation, originally traumatic, as the result of a habit continuing long after the cause has ceased to operate. But if this cycle of chronic inflammation is broken for only a couple of weeks, the scar becomes painless and usually remains so. This may be achieved by infiltration of steroid suspension at the exact site of the lesion.

Often the injections demand the utmost exactitude (see below) but none calls for more than routine asepsis. The treatment is thus eminently suited to outpatient/family medicine.

Steroid suspension

Injection of anti-inflammatory agents work, but only where they are put. A suspension of insoluble steroid is used. Hence its action is concentrated upon the cells with which it lies in contact and little systemic absorption occurs.

As a result, great precision in diagnosis and injection techniques must be maintained in order to deliver the

suspension to the correct spot. At tendinous sites (cf. capsular injections), delivery must be accurate to within a millimetre or so.

The following factors should be considered before undertaking an injection:

(1) In what tissue does the lesion lie?
(2) In what part of that tissue in a horizontal plane?
(3) In what part of that tissue in a vertical plane?
(4) How should the finger best be placed on the relevant structure to:
   (a) identify the tissue at fault?
   (b) in many cases feel the bubbles forming under the skin as the injection proceeds?
(5) Where should the needle be inserted; in what direction and how deeply?
(6) How long a needle is required and what size of syringe?
(7) How much suspension is required to infiltrate the whole affected area?

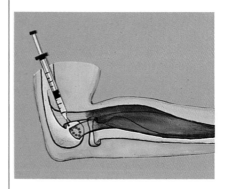 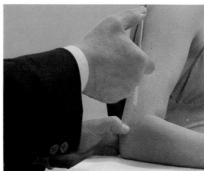

2.10, 2.11 *Injection, steroid suspension (tennis elbow). Delivery must be absolutely precise if the steroid is to abate the localised inflammation. Note infiltration to the cubic area of the lesion (left).*

If the steroid is placed or tracks into subcutaneous tissue (very rare), there is a risk of subcutaneous tissue atrophy, leaving thin white skin that recovers in two to three years. The patient should be warned prior to the injection.

Injection into a joint can be contrasted with injection into a tendon or ligament. The intra-articular injection is, on the whole, simpler but whatever the site of the injection the patient is instructed not to exert her limb for the week following infiltration. This gives the anti-inflammatory effect of the hormone the most favourable environment in which to act. No matter how well the patient may appear to herself to be, too early violent exercise could lead to relapse or ligament and tendon rupture.

Intra-articular injections
The infiltration is made as soon as the needle has passed through the capsule and the point lies intra-articularly. The suspension then distributes itself throughout the inside of the joint. Traction applied by an assistant is useful at the small joints of the fingers or toes where only 0.5–1 ml of steroid is required; at the larger joints the dosage ranges up to 5 ml.

An acute reaction, beneficial to chronic lesions, may be provoked for up to 48 hours.

Although the inflammatory arthritides have been shown to respond very favourably to intra-articular injections, it is the symptoms and not the cause that are abolished. Thus if relief is to be maintained, the injections must be repeated at whatever intervals prove necessary as part of an overall treatment policy linked with specific anti-rheumatic drug therapy. In practice the injections can often be semi-lastingly discontinued.

There is a limit to the number of intra-articular infiltrations that can be absorbed by a weight-bearing joint without running the risk of a steroid arthropathy.

In acute cases, where many joints are flaring at the same time, the treatment is impracticable and injection into unstable joints should likewise be avoided.

Ideally, synovial fluid aspirate should be examined for cells and crystals, and should be cultured prior to injection of steroid. This is particularly important if there is a preceding history of gastrointestinal or urogenital surgery.

But in the absence of suspicious signs, the synovial fluid aspirated at the time of the injection can be tested in the unlikely event of subsequent sepsis.

Occasionally an especially severe reaction occurs within a couple of hours of injection. This is too rapid a response to be due to injection and the cause is crystal-induced synovitis which lasts for up to 72 hours. This does not mitigate against a good eventual response and is best managed by the application of ice packs.

Tendinous injections
At the tendons a more precise approach is needed (*Figures 2.10* and *2.11*). Generally 1 ml steroid suspension is enough at a dilution of 10 mg/ml. This solution also suffices for capsular injections, but the dilution is vital for short tendons where rupture has been reported after using a strength of 40 mg/ml. However, such ruptures are more attributable to faulty technique.

A syringe with a thin needle must be employed and the entire suspension is never pumped into the same spot. Instead, a series of half-withdrawals and reinsertions are made with a dozen droplets or so injected into the three-dimensional area constituting the lesion. If part of the affected area is left out, the symptoms will persist. Normally, only one or two injections are required.

If the needle tip lies within a tendon it may be hard to press the plunger, and the needle should be withdrawn until it lies within the peritendon where injection pressure is slight.

The anti-inflammatory effect takes 12–48 hours to establish itself, before which a local irritant effect is manifest. Thus injection into, say, a tendon may create such discomfort that the patient is hardly able to use the part for a day or two. Then the anti-inflammatory effect comes into play and the symptoms are relieved with dramatic speed.

Athletes or dancers must follow carefully graded exercises during rehabilitation and must not return to full activity until this procedure has been followed or re-flare may result. In any case, stress to the tendon must be avoided for at least two weeks, or longer if there is any degenerative aetiology.

The injection of steroids into tendons has aroused controversy in connection with the possibility of rupture. It has been shown that post-injection weakness lasts about three weeks. But macroscopic and microscopic tendon changes suggest steroids have no effect on the structure of

STEROID INJECTIONS: SUMMARY

Capsular Injections					
Strength	**Equipment**	**Delivery**	**After-effects**	**After-care**	**Caution**
10 mg/ml	Syringe with thinnest possible needle	Relatively simple. Anywhere inside capsule	Little pain following injection, symptoms rapidly abate	Avoid or minimize use of limb for a week	Avoid repeated injections to weight bearing joints
Non-capsular Injections					
As above	As above	Relatively difficult. Precisely into exact cubic extent of the lesion, injected in droplets all over affected area	Pain for 1–2 days following infiltration, thereafter symptoms rapidly abate	As above	Follow individual procedures as set out in text

the tendon itself, but probably have a marked beneficial impact on the painful peritendinous adhesions and inflammation. It may be that the diminution of pain and inflammation brought about by the injection permits the imposition of loads ordinarily heavy enough to produce a rupture.

Ligamentous injections

Ligaments respond exceptionally well to deep massage. Although injections can be similarly effective, infiltration of the weight-bearing joints must be approached with extreme caution as the tendinous caveats (see above) apply with increased force. Nevertheless, for ankle strains in the acute phase injection is the treatment of choice, and at otherwise inaccessible locations – e.g. the cruciates at the knee – is the only practicable remedy.

Steroid therapy and deep massage

As a rule, steroid injections do not help muscle or musculotendinous lesions; these respond better to deep massage.

Further generalizations about the selection of treatment for the tendons and ligaments are difficult. Some lesions respond better to massage, others to injection; the preference for each is set out in the text. For some disorders, both remedies work equally well but they are alternatives not to be adopted at the same time.

Steroid infiltration's principal advantage is its rapid success; 6–12 sessions of painful deep massage may be needed to secure an equivalent result. But unlike massage, steroids provoke quite a strong reaction lasting one or two days. There is also a tendency to a higher rate of recurrence because the scar, although the inflammation in it has been inhibited for the time being, has not been removed. This consideration will weigh particularly with athletes, dancers and manual workers.

Deep massage may also be indicated in cases of diagnostic uncertainty, where the exact site of the lesion cannot be satisfactorily defined. Each of the operator's fingers is about 1 cm wide and the amplitude of sweep at least 2 cm. Hence the margin of diagnostic error is greater than for 1 ml of steroid suspension.

Manipulation

To manipulate means to move by hand. In orthopaedic medicine the technique is used in three distinct situations: capsular contracture, adhesions and displacements. In each classification, the movement is undertaken with different intent and therefore in a different way.

Manipulative stretching to counter capsular contracture is a slow, steady movement carried out over a number of sessions. Manipulative rupture of adhesions consists of a sharp jerk. Both techniques are of narrow application, the latter employed at the knee and ankle and the former only at the shoulder and hip. They are dealt with at the appropriate stages in the text.

Manipulative reduction

Manipulative reduction of a displacement is an important tactic, regularly called for at the peripheral joints as well as the spine. Its reputation notwithstanding, the treatment is straightforward, logical and safe and although much is gained from experience, competence and proficient results are soon achieved. Manipulation should be part of the standard armamentarium of the family physician or operator.

The basic principles are simple (*Figure 2.12*) and hardly vary from joint to joint. First, the manipulator exerts strong traction on the affected joint, distracting the joint surfaces and allowing the loose fragment space to move.

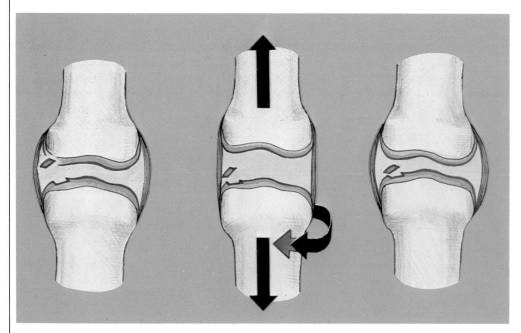

2.12 *The principle of manipulative reduction (diagrammatic). Manipulation can return a displaced intra-articular structure (left) towards its bed (right) by applying strong traction while rotating and/or extending the joint (centre). The patient is re-examined after each manoeuvre. Partial improvement shown.*

Second, the joint is rotated during continuing traction in an endeavour to shift the displacement.

Third, the patient is re-examined to see if the loose body now lies in a more favourable position. This is readily ascertained as, if it does, the patient's pain will have eased and/or her range increased. As these improvements are immediately apparent, the manipulator asks the patient to repeat the previously limited movements, observes whether range has improved and asks if the pain has altered.

If a particular manipulation has helped, it is repeated. If not, some variation is resorted to that imposes a different strain on the joint. This may mean no more than rotating the limb in the other direction. Alternatively, it may be a more elaborate refinement entailing adoption of a different posture by both patient and operator to apply a different leverage to magnify or alter the forces brought to bear. The methods for each joint and the standard progressions are displayed in the relevant chapters.

Three points are worth stressing. First, manipulation may be a vigorous business but it is never an uncontrolled wrench. It is a strict step-by-step process (*Figures 2.13–2.15*). To start with, manual traction is applied. Then the

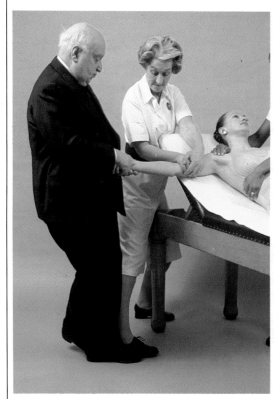

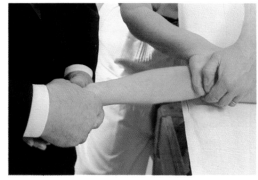

2.14

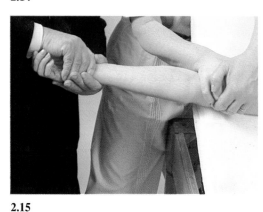

2.13, 2.14, 2.15 *Manipulative reduction in practice, for a loose body in the elbow. The operator leans back to separate the joint surfaces (Figure 2.13) and extends the patient's arm during repeated pronation and supination (Figures 2.14 and 2.15).*

operator takes the joint to the starting position for the manipulation. For instance, at the elbow the forearm is swung towards extension. At the cervical spine the neck is rotated until the tissue resistance that heralds the end of range. At the knee the tibia is rotated during increasing extension.

Finally, the operator applies his over-pressure: a small-amplitude, high-velocity thrust. Thus at the elbow, as the end of range is reached a small jerk secures additional extension and full rotation. At the neck, rotation is accentuated by a sharp twist of a few degrees. At the knee, a final thrust is given towards extension and rotation.

Second, the distraction must be maintained throughout the manipulation, particularly at the moment of the final thrust when the inexperienced can submit to a tendency to release the distracting force.

Third, re-examination after each manoeuvre is indispensable. Without it, the operator has no idea what progress has been made and thus what manipulation to attempt next. To report on any alteration in her condition, the patient must be conscious; anaesthesia is therefore highly unwise and in any case is not required (except occasionally at the knee for a meniscus) as manipulation is not painful.

The objective of manipulation is the restoration of full painless range and accordingly treatment is discontinued once maximum benefit has accrued. This is soon achieved as

manipulation works quickly or not at all. Most success will be registered during the first or second session, and many patients are quite well after the first. It is rare that a fourth treatment produces further improvement. A manipulative session typically lasts anywhere between ten and twenty minutes, depending on result and tolerance. Elderly patients are manipulated with equal vigour but for a shorter span.

Oscillatory techniques, described in detail by Maitland, may help in certain acutely painful situations where stronger techniques could be inappropriate or difficult.

Arthroscopy can be used in cases of failed reduction to confirm the diagnosis and suggest appropriate treatment.

MANIPULATION: GENERAL SUMMARY

---

1. Purpose: to reduce a displacement
2. Technique:
   (a) apply and maintain manual traction
   (b) for peripheral joints, take joint to extreme of range during repeated rotations
   (c) apply over-pressure
   (d) re-examine patient

NB Precise procedure varies from joint to joint. At the spine, the joint is taken to the extreme of comfortable range before delivery of a single over-pressure

---

Treatment at the spine

Disorders at the spine fall neatly into two categories. A number of relatively rare conditions occur such as inflammatory spondylitis, metastases, myeloma, chordoma, fracture, tuberculosis and Paget's disease. These nearly all cause radiological or systemic changes, and none is within the scope of the orthopaedic physician who should, nevertheless, diagnose each case correctly. But a substantial proportion of patients suffer from minor radiotranslucent displacements of disc material.

Additionally, other minor mechanical lesions of the posterior ligaments or muscular lesions (rare except at the thoracic spine) can sometimes occur.

The loose body can exert pressure either on the dura mater to give rise to extrasegmental referred pain, or on the dural investment of the nerve roots to produce segmentally referred pain. The disc lesion may consist of either a cartilaginous fragment or part of the nucleus pulposus.

TREATMENT OF AN INTERVERTEBRAL DISC LESION: SUMMARY

Cervical Displacement	Thoracic Displacement	Lumbar Displacement
Manipulative reduction	Manipulative reduction To forestall relapse: Sclerosants	Manipulative reduction if cartilaginous Traction if nuclear Epidural local anaesthesia if irreducible To forestall relapse: 1. Posture 2. Corset 3. Sclerosants Only a tiny proportion of cases go to operation

Note that signs or symptoms may strongly contraindicate manipulation or traction

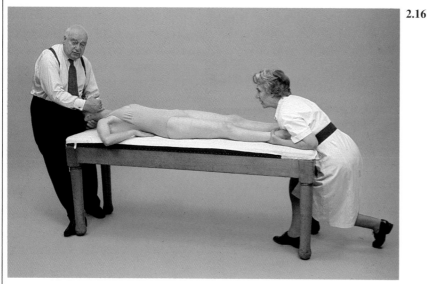
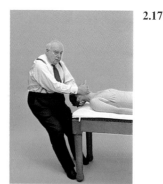
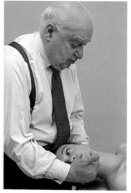

2.16, 2.17, 2.18 *Typical cervical manipulation. Nearly all cervical displacements respond to manipulation during traction. The neck is taken towards the extreme of comfortable range and then twisted a little further.*

Principal treatments

A small cartilaginous displacement at any spinal level can usually be reduced by manipulation (*Figures 2.16–2.18*). The principles are the same as for manipulation at the peripheral joints.

Manual traction is applied, except at the lumbar spine where it is ineffective. The joints are rotated and the patient is then re-examined. The rotation affects all the joints along any given extent and the treatment is thus to some degree non-specific. But the strain will be borne by the blocked joint (i.e. the joint with the displacement) as it is there the movement is restricted. For further background information the reader is referred to page 153.

A small lumbar displacement of nuclear material can usually be reduced by a course of sustained traction (*Figure 2.19*). Even on modern friction-free couches the distracting force is normally in the range of 20–50 kg. Sessions are daily for half an hour and the course lasts for two to three weeks.

The pain from a large lumbar disc lesion can ordinarily be abolished or permanently mitigated by desensitization of the dura mater and its sleeve. Accordingly a solution of 50 ml procaine is injected into the sacral hiatus (*Figure 2.20*).

Again, these treatments are easily mastered and often afford immediate relief. Additionally, sclerosant injections, the sinuvertebral nerve block and postural education all play a part in conservative management.

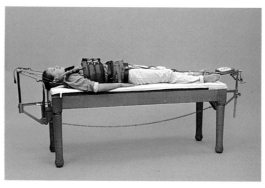

2.19 *Lumbar traction. Distraction of the vertebrae can suck a nuclear protrusion back into place. The treatment is useless if the pull is intermittent or too light.*

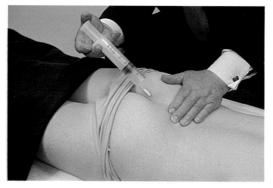

2.20 *Caudal epidural injection. The dura mater and lumbar nerve roots are bathed in anaesthetic, often resulting in permanent alleviation of pain*

Orthopaedic medicine

Equipment

A firm adjustable-height couch is a distinct advantage, especially one which can be fitted with 'Cyriax horns' and a 'lean-back bar' which together obviate the need for an assistant during cervical manipulation. Alternatively, two fixed-height couches, of about 15 and 30 inches respectively, may be used.

Imaginative use of the 'seat belts' commonly seen in physiotherapy departments circumvents the need for assistants in many peripheral manipulations.

The relative merits of add-on apparatus and purpose-built traction couches are discussed on page 223.

For operators contemplating steroid phonophoresis a therapeutic ultrasonic unit is necessary, as is steroid gel, obtainable only on prescription. In each case the patient's medical practitioner must be consulted. Doctors, in turn, will require supplies of local anaesthetic and steroid suspension for injection.

Application

Such resources are universally available within the existing medical framework. There is no shortage of patients.

Orthopaedic, sports and industrial medicine

Sports medicine is a speciality in its own right, encompassing a broad spectrum of knowledge. But since trauma to soft tissue (whether or not accompanied by fracture) may be assumed to form a component of a sports injury, orthopaedic medicine has a central and undiminished role to play in the diagnostic and curative process.

By no means are all soft-tissue lesions sports injuries, but most sports injuries are soft-tissue lesions. The issue is not whether the patient was playing sport when he suffered injury but what injury he suffered, and this is established in the same way whether a road accident or athletics was the cause.

Similarly, a primary endeavour of industrial medicine is preventative, establishing statistically the incidence of mechanical lesions and the likely causative work procedure which can then be modified. This valuable work is distinct from the complementary skills of diagnosis and treatment and thus for full patient care a double approach is required – one to minimize incidence and the other to diagnose and treat lesions which have nevertheless arisen.

In both sports and industrial medicine, repetition of the precipitating factor is a strong likelihood and thus a high degree of end-cure is essential.

Structure of this book

As spinal lesions frequently generate symptoms in the upper or lower limbs, a thorough understanding of the spine is indispensable before the peripheral joints are fully comprehensible. However, to avoid an accumulation of introductory material, the immediately ensuing chapters are devoted to the upper and lower limbs, while consideration of the spine is held back to Chapters 10 *et seq*. Diligent readers may care to reverse this order.

One chapter is devoted to each joint. In the appendices will be found:

(1) An illustration of each dermatome.
(2) A list of the capsular patterns.
(3) A summary of the examination and findings at each joint, together with treatment(s) for each condition.
(4) A consolidated tabulation of the causes of pins and needles in the upper and lower limbs.

PART TWO

THE PERIPHERAL JOINTS

CHAPTER THREE

THE SHOULDER

The shoulder is the most rewarding and straightforward joint to deal with in the whole body and the finding of a limited or painful movement regularly means exactly what it should on anatomical grounds. The mechanism of arm elevation is not always appreciated but has important diagnostic implications.

Lesions of the joint and soft tissues are easily treated; once relieved, they seldom recur.

Referred pain

Nearly all shoulder structures are derived from the C5 segment. Pain will be felt within the C5 dermatome (*Figure 3.1*) which includes neither the scapular area nor any part of the hand. The point of the shoulder is within the C4 dermatome (*Figure 3.2*) – the acromioclavicular joint refers to pain in this area.

The commonest cause of unilateral scapular pain is a cervical disc lesion giving rise to extrasegmental reference. With a cervical lesion the neck movements prove painful.

A lateral disc protrusion impinging on the C5, C6, C7 – the most common – or C8 nerve root produces root pain felt down the arm in the relevant dermatome (see page 178).

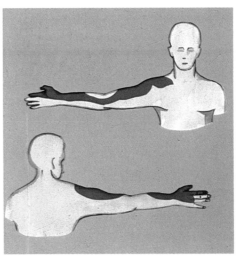

3.1 *The C5 dermatome.*

History

History will suggest whether a cervical or shoulder lesion is involved. Once established that the source of pain lies at the shoulder, history is relatively unrewarding – the ache is apt to be felt at the same place whatever the disorder. But the patient's age, site of pain, whether or not other joints were affected and whether there was any trauma must be ascertained.

Three further enquiries are made if the capsular pattern is found. Does the pain reach the elbow? Does the arm ache all the time, even when held still? Can the patient sleep on that side at night?

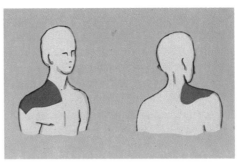

3.2 *The C4 dermatome.*

Examination

A brief preliminary examination consisting of the active, passive and resisted cervical movements will exculpate the neck. Further, active shoulder girdle elevation tests for the acromioclavicular joint and the rare cases of scapular/thoracic restriction (which may be serious). Resisted shoulder girdle elevation tests the integrity of the C2, C3 and C4 roots.

Involvement of the acromioclavicular joint may complicate the normal clarity of findings, since it is apt to produce pain at the end of range of most or all passive movements (the so-called 'muddle pattern'). If this occurs, a diagnostic injection into the joint should clarify matters.

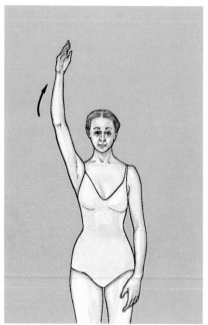

3.3 *Active elevation.*

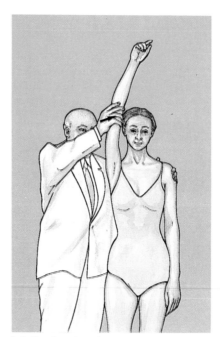

3.4 *Passive elevation.*

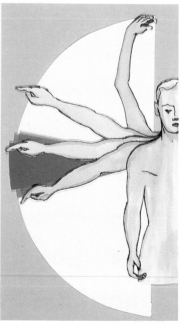

3.5 *A painful arc. The pain ceases on either side of the horizontal. It is an accessory sign.*

Active and passive movements

Once the lesion has been confined to the shoulder, the patient undergoes a routine of 12 shoulder movements. Examination should not be stopped until all have been tested, particularly since double lesions are an occasional feature and bursitis frequently causes pain on several passive or resisted movements.

The first step is active elevation (*Figure 3.3*), a composite movement testing the patient's willingness to use the arm.

Next, the patient's arm is elevated passively as far as it will go (*Figure 3.4*). Possibilities are full range, limited range, pain or no pain. The end-feel is gauged; the normal joint produces an unmistakable slightly elastic feel at extreme elevation. Osteoarthrosis is accompanied by a hard end-feel. Range of passive movement is compared with the range attained on the previous active movement.

Limitation and pain on the passive elevation is part of

the capsular pattern. Pain at full elevation can be a localizing sign in infraspinatus or supraspinatus tendinitis.

The patient then actively elevates her arm again and is asked to state at what moment (if any) the pain starts and whether it ceases on further elevation. A painful arc (*Figure 3.5*) is a secondary localizing sign normally indicating that the lesion lies in a pinchable position between the acromion and the tuberosities. Elevation beyond the painful arc may have to be accomplished in defiance of the patient's inclination (or by routing it through the sagittal plane) to verify that the pain does in fact cease.

Pseudo painful arcs occur in two sets of circumstances. First, where muscular effort causes transient compression of a cervical mechanical lesion, and secondly, where a lax shoulder joint capsule allows upward subluxation of the head of the humerus during the initial phases of elevation; reduction occurs with a painful click at 90° of elevation.

Next, the exact amount of glenohumeral range is established by testing passive abduction. The examiner fixes the lower angle of the scapula with his thumb, applying the heel of his hand to the patient's mid-thorax (*Figure 3.6*).

The patient's elbow is lifted upwards with the examiner's other hand until the scapula is felt to rotate as it produces the next stage of elevation. In a normal joint this starts when the arm reaches the horizontal. It is at this point that the glenohumeral movement has attained its full extent and the examiner's thumb starts to shift (*Figure 3.7*).

The two other passive movements for the joint are lateral rotation (*Figure 3.8*) and medial rotation (*Figure 3.9*). The capsular pattern is characterized by limitation of all three passive movements in a fixed proportion (see page 37).

Pathology at the acromioclavicular joint also results in pain at the end-range of all three passive movements (but in a non-capsular pattern of limitation) and its involvement can be confirmed by checking whether passive horizontal adduction hurts as well.

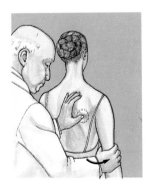 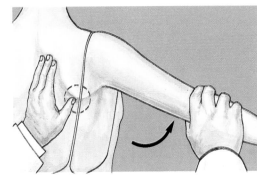

3.6, 3.7 *Passive elevation. The physician places his thumb on the angle of the shoulder blade and can thus detect the point at which scapular rotation commences.*

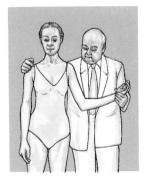 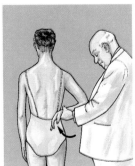

3.8 *Passive lateral rotation*   **3.9** *Passive medial rotation*

The mechanism of arm elevation

The first 90° of passive abduction take place at the glenohumeral joint. The scapula does not move appreciably in this phase.

The next 60° of elevation result from rotation of the scapula. Even if the shoulder is ankylosed, 60° of passive abduction are possible since 60° of arm elevation always consist of scapular rotation.

During the last 30° the scapula is stationary. The movement again takes place at the glenohumeral joint as a result of adduction of the humerus (*Figure 3.10*).

Diagnostic implications
The range of passive elevation possible at the shoulder is thus the 60° of scapular rotation always attainable plus the amount of glenohumeral movement whether occurring at the first or third stage of elevation.

The range of passive elevation must come to the amount of glenohumeral movement plus 60°

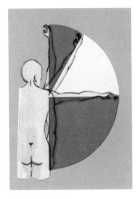 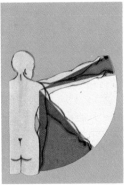

3.10 *Full passive arm elevation. Only the first 90° and the last 30° take place at the glenohumeral joint.*

3.11, 3.12 *Arm elevation, restricted. Sixty degrees always consist of scapular rotation irrespective of how much passive elevation is attainable. This makes neurosis easy to detect.*

(*Figure 3.11*). Thus if the patient alleges that elevation beyond the horizontal is not possible, it follows that her scapula should start to rotate at about 30° (*Figure 3.12*); if, in fact, her scapular rotation does not begin until 90°, the diagnosis is of neurosis or malingering, since there must

always be at least a further 60° of passive elevation after commencement of scapular rotation. The examiner will therefore mentally compare and contrast the amount of glenohumeral abduction with the degree of elevation achieved by the patient on the first active movement.

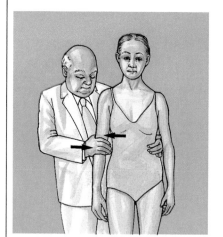

3.13 *Resisted abduction.*

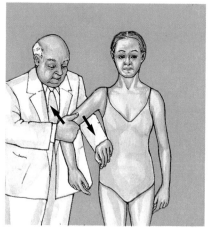

3.14 *Resisted adduction.*

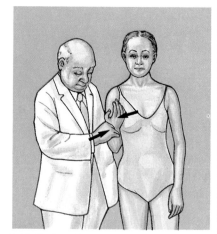

3.15 *Resisted lateral rotation.*

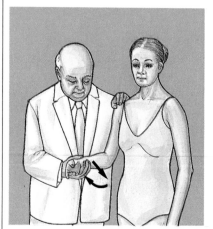

3.16 *Resisted medial rotation.*

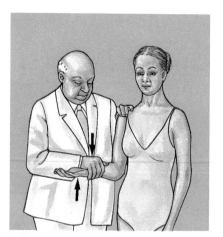

3.17 *Resisted elbow flexion.*

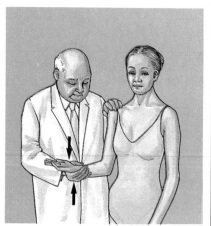

3.18 *Resisted elbow extension.*

Resisted movements

The resisted movements follow, evaluating contractile structures. To prevent ambiguity or false-positive findings, the actively resisting hand must be properly positioned to exclude involvement of other muscle groups. Attention must also be paid to stabilization of the patient by the appropriate counter-pressure during each resisted movement.

Pain indicates a lesion to the muscle or tendon. A finding of weakness alone is generally attributable either to a neuritis or, more likely, a cervical root palsy.

Resisted abduction tests the deltoid (rarely affected) and supraspinatus, commonly injured at one of four sites. The movement is resisted at or above the patient's elbow while counter-pressure is applied at the far side of the patient's trunk (*Figure 3.13*)

preventing other muscle groups coming into play.

Resisted adduction (*Figure 3.14*) tests the pectoralis major, the latissimus dorsi and both the teres; lesions to any of these are rare. Counter-pressure, this time at the hip, ensures muscle activity is limited to the shoulder joint.

Next, lateral rotation is resisted (*Figure 3.15*). Pain on this movement alone implies a lesion of the infraspinatus. Very occasionally, both resisted lateral rotation and resisted adduction hurt, showing the teres minor to be at fault. The patient's tendency to abduct the arm while rotating it outwards must be prevented.

Medial rotation is resisted with the patient keeping her elbow at her side (*Figure 3.16*). This principally tests the subscapularis. In theory the pectoralis major, teres major or

latissimus dorsi may be involved but in practice they are seldom injured.

Two movements follow for muscles which, although controlling the elbow, arise above the glenohumeral joint. Resisted elbow flexion (*Figure 3.17*) assesses the biceps, frequently affected at one of five sites. Resisted supination of the hand may be combined with the elbow flexion to stress this muscle even further.

Lastly, elbow extension – resisted at the forearm, not wrist – puts strain on the triceps, rarely at fault (*Figure 3.18*). In fact any pain from this last movement will normally be felt within the C5 dermatome and thus cannot emanate from the triceps (C7 derivation). Symptoms are generally attributable to upward pressure of the humerus against the tissues under the acromion (i.e. patients with a painful arc).

Findings

Capsular lesions

About a dozen separate disorders are characterized by limitation of movement in the capsular pattern, but the three commonest monoarthritides are traumatic arthritis, algodystrophy and osteoarthrosis. This last is often painless of itself, although the joint's heightened sensitivity makes it more liable to a superimposed traumatic arthritis; crepitus is palpable.

The capsular pattern is designated by a hard end-feel and limitation of all three passive movements in fixed proportions. Limitation of medial rotation (*Figure 3.20*) is slight; the patient cannot fully put her arm behind her back. The restriction of glenohumeral abduction (*Figure 3.21*) is

more pronounced, but it is impairment of lateral rotation (*Figure 3.19*) that is most marked. In a case of medium severity, medial rotation would be limited by some 10–15°, glenohumeral abduction by about 45° and lateral rotation by 60–70°. In a very mild attack, medial rotation is full but painful and the other limitations amount to between 10° and 30° and some 45°, respectively.

If arthritis in the elderly (60+) is accompanied by trophic changes and marked limitation of movement in the wrist and hand, the shoulder–hand syndrome is present. This is a variety of monarticular rheumatoid arthritis from which recovery is uncertain.

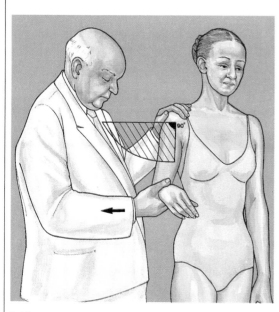

3.19

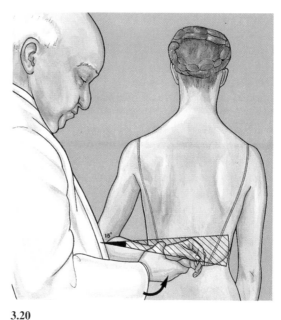

3.20

3.19, 3.20, 3.21 *The capsular pattern of arthritis. The shaded angles show the degree of limitation which – whatever the condition's severity – is always greatest in lateral rotation (Figure 3.19) and least on medial rotation (Figure 3.20) with elevation (Figure 3.21) in betweeen. The drawings depict typical limitation in a severe case.*

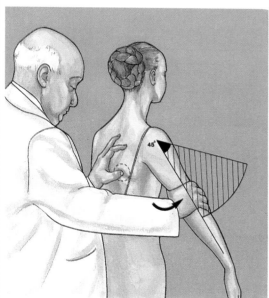

3.21

Traumatic arthritis

The patient is aged 45 or over. The causative trauma is often slight and the pain only starts a week later when it gradually spreads down the arm. If untreated, pain and limitation fill out together, reaching their maximum after about three months with symptoms extending to the wrist.

The pain wears off as it recedes up the arm over the next four months, but full range will not return for a year from onset.

Treatment differs according to the stage the disorder has reached.

Stages 1 and 3

These are relatively non-irritable phases: there is neither pain at rest, nor beyond the elbow, and the patient can lie on the affected side.

Following administration of short-wave diathermy or other appropriate modality as an analgesic, the joint is repeatedly stretched (*Figure 3.22*) towards the extreme of attainable elevation. Counter-pressure is maintained at the patient's sternum (*Figure 3.23*) to prevent spinal extension. Each stretch is gentle but firm, and not released until pain rather than discomfort is engendered.

An elastic end-feel at the joint is a good prognostic indicator. So too is abatement of pain within moments of each stretch. Conversely, if pain lingers for a minute or more after each stretch, or movement is abruptly halted by pain and spasm, injection or capsular distraction are substituted.

The patient is asked to note the duration of treatment soreness, the optimal period being two hours. If less than two hours of soreness is reported the joint should, at the next visit, be stretched more firmly. But if the treatment reaction lingers for considerably longer, this again indicates that injection or distraction should be substituted.

Immobilization arthritis can be avoided by daily use of the joint, but if stiffness has already set in, the treatment is stretching as above.

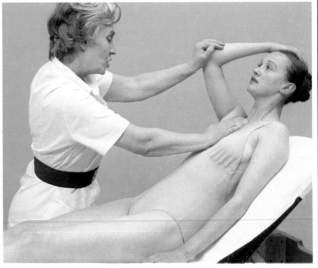

3.22 *Stretching the shoulder joint is called for in all cases of recent capsular trauma.*

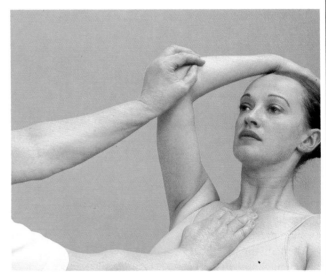

3.23 *Elevation is forced by upwards pressure against the patient's elbow. Active exercises in every direction follow each treatment, and the patient is encouraged to maintain the new range of movement.*

Stage 2

If untreated for the first month, the joint becomes too irritable to be stretched, a stage reached when all the following hold true:

(1) The pain has spread below the elbow.
(2) The arm is painful even at rest.
(3) The patient cannot lie on her bad side at night.

If only one or two of these indicators are present, stretching may be tried cautiously, but treatment must be stopped at once if there is any adverse response.

Treatment during the second stage consists of an injection of steroid suspension 2 ml using a 5 cm needle. The patient lies prone with her forearm under her stomach, thus turning the articular surface of the humerus posteriorly. The index finger of the operator's free hand is placed on the tip of the coracoid process with the thumb at the angle of the acromion and the spine of the scapula. An imaginary line linking the finger and thumb crosses the glenoid cavity (*Figure 3.24*).

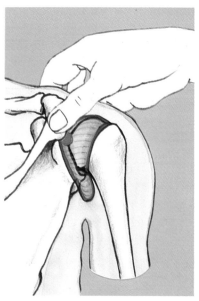

3.25 *The injection is given when impingement against cartilage is felt.*

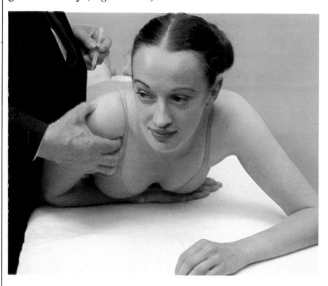

3.24 *Capsular injection. The glenoid cavity lies between the operator's thumb and index finger.*

The needle punctures the skin by the operator's thumb and is aimed just lateral to the tip of his index finger (*Figure 3.25* and *3.26*).

The joint capsule offers clear and distinctive resistance at about 4 cm. When impingement against cartilage is felt, the needle is withdrawn minimally by 0.5 mm and the injection given.

Alternatively the needle can be manoeuvred, usually slightly medially, to pierce the capsule so the tip lies between the glenoid and humeral head. This posterior approach has the advantage over the anterior in that the joint is held in medial rotation, the least restricted range. This is more comfortable for the patient.

The constant pain goes in 36 hours and the injection is repeated after a week. Further injections are given at increasing intervals to forestall return of pain; that is, just *before* relapse. Two is the lowest and eight the highest number of injections. Range of movement does not start to come back until after the first two.

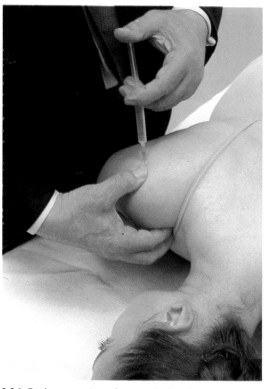

3.26 *Both traumatic and monarticular rheumatoid arthritis respond well to intra-articular steroid suspension.*

Alternatively, in the second stage, the joint can be distracted. First the patient is positioned with her arm in slight flexion and medial rotation, so each aspect of the joint capsule is relaxed.

Active treatment in the second phase consists of gentle endeavours to pull the head of the humerus away from the glenoid cup (*Figure 3.27*). There must be no abduction, which is prevented by exerting counter-pressure via a rolled towel at the patient's elbow. This ensures the whole upper arm is moved away from the thorax while remaining parallel to the axis of the patient's body. The pressure is directed outwards, with the hand slotted into the axilla (*Figure 3.28*). Pressure is intermittent and only minimal distraction, for example, 1 cm, can be coaxed from the joint. Sessions last half an hour, initially daily, and in a severe case the muscles will not relax until the second or third treatment, with no distraction attained at the first. As pain abates over succeeding sessions, greater distraction is employed until in due course the end-feel becomes elastic. Then the joint may be stretched in the ordinary way.

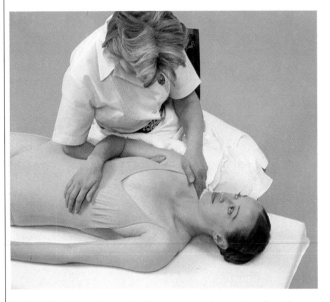
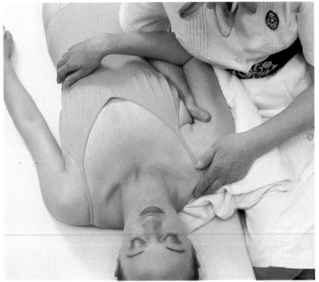

3.27, 3.28 *Distraction techniques are an alternative when the joint is too irritable for stretching. The hand in the axilla does all the work, and the patient's humerus is always kept parallel to her body.*

Stage 3
Recovery can be expedited by stretching, using the technique described above. The three diagnostic indicators will be absent. Normally this phase sets in some three months plus after onset, and thereafter stretching can lop up to several months off recovery time which might otherwise run to a full year.

Algodystrophic arthritis
The patient is aged between 30 and 70, more commonly between 45 and 60, and has sometimes sustained a stroke or myocardial infarction. There is no trauma. Over a span of three months, pain spreads down the arm to the forearm and wrist; the ache is constant with marked limitation in the capsular pattern. Spontaneous recovery takes up to two years, and limitation persists after the ache has gone. Sometimes there is recurrence at the other shoulder.

Steroid suspension 2 ml is injected into the joint using the technique for traumatic arthritis. The pain disappears by the next day. The injection is repeated weekly at first and thereafter at widening intervals, but in any event before the onset of pain. Six to 12 injections are the rule.

Monoarthritis
This may occur with psoriasis, ankylosing spondylitis, systemic lupus erythematosus or crystal arthropathy. Local injection may complement systemic therapy.

Non-capsular lesions

Acute subdeltoid bursitis

This uncommon condition limits passive movement but not in the capsular pattern. Without injury, the whole bursa (*Figure 3.29*) becomes acutely inflamed and in the course of two or three days the patient loses almost all capacity to abduct the arm. Pain may radiate as far as the wrist. Other passive movements retain very nearly full range, resisted movements are painless (except in the hyperacute stage when everything hurts), and the painful arc appears only as the condition abates because initially arm elevation is impossible. The patient recovers spontaneously within 4–6 weeks and there is often a history of previous attacks, particularly in cases with small areas of calcification (visible on the X-ray) which can be dissolved by local anaesthetic.

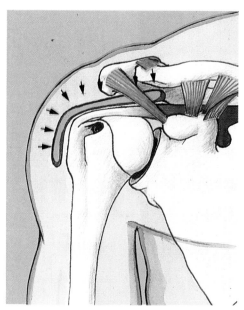

3.29 *The whole extent of the bursa is extremely tender and often thickened. A large portion of the lesion may lie in the restricted space under the acromial arch.*

Stage 1

The acute pain lasts 7–10 days and injection is only worth while in this period. Palpation outlines the extent of the tender area, but it should be remembered that part of the bursa is shielded by the acromion.

A strong analgesic is injected as a preliminary measure before the accessible extent of the bursa receives a cluster of little infiltrations (*Figure 3.30*) of steroid suspension 5 ml (5 cm needle).

Then the site and angle of insertion are altered; a further injection of steroid suspension 5 ml is given to the subacromial extent of the bursa (*Figure 3.31*) by similar multiple insertions. The point of the acromion is located by the thumb, and the needle slides under it so the approach is horizontal (*Figure 3.32*). By the next day the patient is sore but mobile. A second injection may be required a few days later.

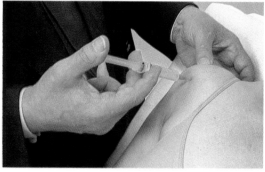

3.30 *Steroid suspension 5ml is injected throughout the directly accessible extent.*

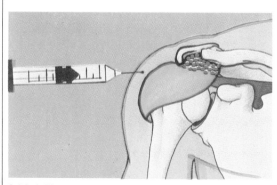

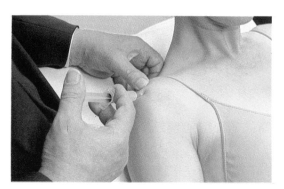

3.31, 3.32 *Another 5ml is directed into the part of the bursa under the acromion.*

Stage 2
After the first week the patient is on the mend and there is little point in injecting. Instead a figure-of-eight bandage (*Figure 3.33*) is needed at night to stop the arm drifting into painful range. Non-steroid anti-inflammatory agents provide a worthwhile alternative at either stage.

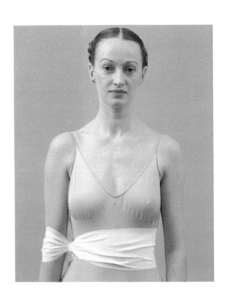

3.33 *Acute bursitis recovers spontaneously in six weeks. After the first phase, only a nocturnal bandage is needed.*

Chronic subdeltoid bursitis

Chronic subacromial or subdeltoid bursitis is not a later phase of the acute form, but a completely separate clinical entity which may continue indefinitely. Only a limited part of the bursa is affected and, again, calcium deposits may lead to recurrence.

The condition is hard to distinguish from minor tendinitis. It may give rise to only a painful arc, or may additionally give pain on several resisted movements or pain (or even slight limitation) on some passive movements. Occasionally a case is encountered where the findings vary from day to day. The impingement sign – taking the abducted arm into internal rotation – may reproduce the pain, but often a painful arc is the only

symptom. Sometimes the patient presents only with a history which, in sports, would typically comprise being able to throw overarm or bowl but not throw side-arm.

The sensitive spot is sought by palpation and, if found, injected. If the tender extent cannot be located, the inflammation must lie under the acromion and a likely area is infiltrated. A solution of 0.5% procaine 5–10 ml (depending on the size of the lesion) is injected in droplets all over the inflamed area. A couple of infiltrations into the correct spot are usually curative. If not, steroid suspension is added.

Persistent recurrent impingement may require surgery to the coraco-acromial ligament.

Subluxation

A recurrent transient anterior subluxation may occur in sportsmen without apparent trauma. The X-ray will be negative and the patient complains of a dead arm, or pins and needles following violent exercise such as serving at tennis or throwing – symptoms which disappear in a few minutes. It is a forceful hyperextension injury in the decelerating phase.

The shoulder should be laterally rotated and abducted to about 90°. Pressure on the posterior aspect of the humerus

at this stage, forcing the head out of the glenoid cavity, almost invariably produces apprehension suggestive of the diagnosis.

Recurrent subluxation should be treated with shoulder girdle muscle rehabilitation and rest from provoking activities, but may require surgery. In swimmers there is a possibility of a posterior dislocation, seen clinically from above, which may be confirmed by X-rays appropriately angled to reveal the condition.

Differential diagnosis

Other causes of limitation of passive movements – all rare except (6) – in the non-capsular pattern include:

(1) Pulmonary neoplasm: muscle spasm restricts elevation beyond the horizontal. The scapula is mobile and there is full range of movement at the shoulder joint.
(2) Capsular adhesion: localized capsular scarring. Treatment is by stretching.
(3) Subcoracoid bursitis: isolated limitation of lateral

rotation. Steroid suspension 2 ml should be injected.
(4) Contracture of the costocoracoid fascia: gradually intensifying pectoroscapular pain, slight limitation of elevation of scapula. No treatment avails.
(5) Fracture of the first rib: the pain is brought on by neck and scapular movements. Active elevation of the arm is limited but passive elevation is full. An X-ray is diagnostic.
(6) Psychogenic pain.

Contractile structures

Tendinous lesions abound at the shoulder. Although active range may often be limited by pain, passive movement is full. One resisted movement brings on the pain. In all cases, except the musculotendinous junction of the supraspinatus and glenoid origin of the biceps, the tendinitis responds to either massage or steroid injection.

Often localizing signs indicate the exact site of the lesion in the tendon. Usually, disorders are brought on by over-use or repeated strain rather than a single causative strain.

Recurrence is rare and responds to further injection or massage. In sportsmen, strength may be maintained by carefully graded isometrics to the arc–muscle complex.

Supraspinatus tendinitis

This is the commonest tendinous lesion at the shoulder, and is marked by painful resisted abduction. Often it shows no tendency to spontaneous recovery. The lesion can lie at any one of four different sites (*Figure 3.34 – 3.36*) readily differentiated by the presence or absence of a painful arc and/or pain on full elevation. The musculotendinous site is treated by massage; the other three by either massage or injection of steroid suspension.

Calcification shows on the X-ray and contraindicates massage. Five ml 2% procaine is then exchanged for the steroid infiltration, with rest in a sling and non-steroid anti-inflammatory agents if acute.

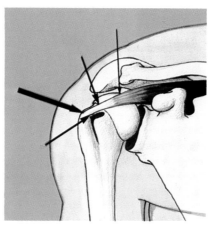

3.34 *Supraspinatus tendinitis. The lesion may lie at one of four sites and these are often clear-cut distinguishing signs confirming the diagnosis.*

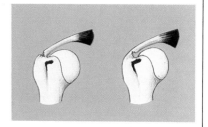

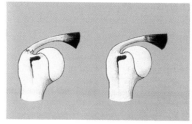

3.35, 3.36 *The four sites, marked red. Superior or inferior aspects, tenoperiosted junction (above); both together, or the musculotendinous junction (below).*

The tenoperiosteal site
Painful resisted abduction accompanied by a painful arc shows the lesion lies in a pinchable position between the acromion and the greater tuberosity, at the superficial aspect of the tenoperiosteal junction.

Momentary pain is caused as the inflamed area squeezes under the acromial arch on arm elevation (*Figure 3.37*) and if the arc is more pronounced when the arm is raised palm-upwards, the lesion lies at the tenoperiosteal junction's anterior aspect. If palm-downwards is the more painful, this points to the posterior aspect of the tendinous insertion.

Treatment is by either massage or injection, but either way the same obstacle must be overcome: the tendon in its horizontal course is shielded from above by the acromion.

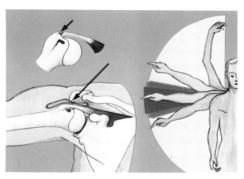

3.37 *The tenoperiosteal site (arrowed) gives rise to a painful arc. After the arm attains the horizontal, the head of the humerus starts to drop slightly in the glenoid cavity and gains additional clearance.*

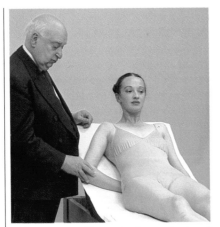

3.38 *Injection. The patient's arm is placed right behind her back.*

The lesion is accessible if the patient puts her arm behind her back with the elbow bent.

The medial rotation of the shoulder brings the greater tuberosity forwards, and adduction of the shoulder as the arm moves across behind the back further exposes the tendon which can now be felt just lateral to the bicipital groove, rising almost vertically from the tuberosity (*Figure 3.38*).

The needle is thrust downwards and the lesion infiltrated with steroid suspension 1 ml (*Figures 3.39 and 3.40*). No resistance is felt until the tendon is reached, and provided the needle lies correctly it encounters tough tendinous resistance as the injection proceeds.

About 20 droplets are distributed throughout the extent of the lesion by a series of half-withdrawals and reinsertions; the tendon is about 1.5 cm wide. Normally one or two injections are curative.

For massage, the patient's position is similar, with her arm behind her back (*Figures 3.41 and 3.42*). Sessions

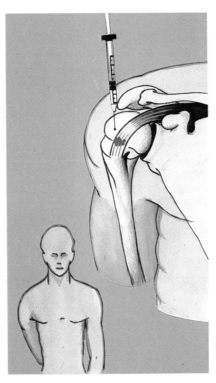

3.39 *In this position the tendon passes forwards over the head of the humerus. This makes it emerge from under the acromion.*

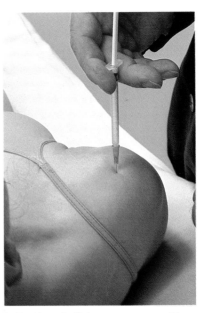

3.40 *About half the cases are cured by one injection. Most of the rest get well with two or three.*

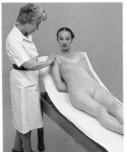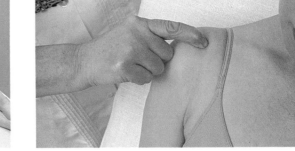

3.41, 3.42 *Massage is the alternative. On average the patient is better in a month.*

last 20 minutes twice weekly for two to five weeks. Counter-pressure is supplied by the thumb on the deltoid and the greatest strength is hardly

enough to break up the scar tissue. The amplitude of sweep is 2 cm with the fingers moving horizontally across the near-vertical tendon.

The tenoperiosteal junction, deep aspect

Painful resisted abduction linked with pain on full passive elevation shows the lesion is where the greater tuberosity and the glenoid rim pinch the tendon at the deep aspect of the tenoperiosteal junction (*Figure 3.43*).

Both massage and injection follow the technique for the superficial lesion except:

(1) The needle must penetrate more deeply.

(2) Recovery by massage is slower because the thickness of the tendon intervenes between the operator's finger and the lesion.

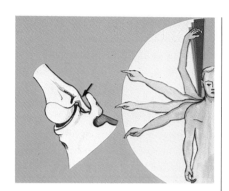

3.43 *Full passive elevation hurts if the scar lies deeply at the distal end (arrowed) of the tendon.*

The distal end of the tendon

Painful resisted abduction accompanied by both a painful arc and pain on full elevation indicates that the lesion occupies both the superficial and deep aspect of the tendon – that is, it runs right through (*Figure 3.44*).

Again both injection and massage are effective. The injection must reach both aspects of the tendon.

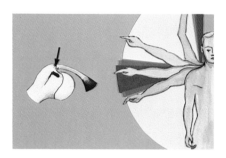

3.44 *If both signs are found, the distal end of the tendon (arrowed) is clearly traversed by the lesion.*

The musculotendinous junction

If resisted abduction hurts with neither a painful arc nor pain on full elevation, attention is drawn to the proximal end of the tendon (*Figure 3.45*). Palpation with the arm supported horizontally may locate the tenderness deep within the angle formed by the clavicle and the spine of the scapula, but diagnosis at this site (lacking the corroboration of localizing signs) should be verified by local anaesthesia. Massage is effective.

With the arm dependent, the lesion is completely shielded by the acromion. But if the patient sits with her arm supported horizontally, the musculotendinous junction slides proximally within reach.

The operator stands behind and to one side of the patient (*Figure 3.47*). The reinforced middle finger is pressed deeply into the angle formed by the spine of the scapula and the back of the outer part of the clavicle, while friction is imparted by rotating the forearm to and fro (*Figures 3.47* and *3.48*). At most, eight 15-minute treatments on alternate days should suffice.

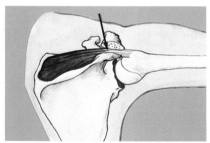

3.45 *Musculotendinous junction (arrowed). Diagnosis at this site may have to be verified by local anaesthesia.*

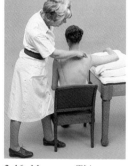

3.46 *Massage. This posture brings the lesion just within reach.*

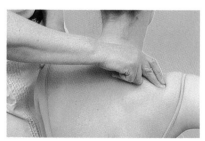
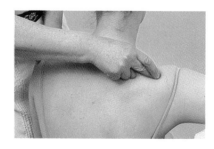

3.47, 3.48 *The forearm is rotated. Cure generally results after four treatments.*

The infraspinatus

Pain on resisted lateral rotation incriminates the infraspinatus, but localizing signs for the various sites (*Figure 3.49*) are not so plain. A painful arc suggests the lesion lies at the superficial aspect of the distal end of the tendon, and pain on full elevation focuses attention on the deep aspect of the distal end. In default of these signs, the body of the tendon (not the musculotendinous junction) is likely to contain the lesion and the point of maximum tenderness is sought. The lesion is rather difficult to pinpoint and if in doubt local anaesthetic is used diagnostically.

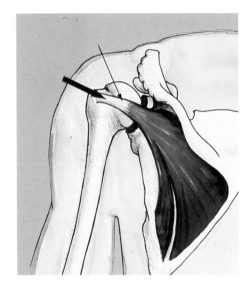

3.49 *The sites. The painful scar lies either close to or at the insertion of the tendon into the greater tuberosity.*

For injection or massage the patient lies prone, propped up on her elbows. This retracts the scapula and uncovers the head of the humerus. The patient's arm is in flexion and slight lateral rotation; then it is put into slight adduction (*Figure 3.50*), drawing the humeral tuberosity out from under the acromion.

This ensures the infraspinatus is easily found just below the most lateral extent of the spine of the scapula as it runs towards the head of the humerus.

The injection of 1 ml steroid (*Figure 3.51*) is delivered in 20 droplets to the affected area both deeply and superficially. A back-up injection may subsequently be required.

The massage position is identical. While the fingers supply counter-pressure, the thumb is alternately abducted and adducted across the lesion (*Figure 3.52*) for 20 minutes at a time every other day. Recovery can be anticipated in about three weeks.

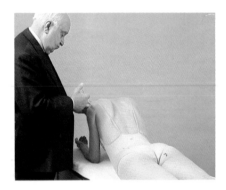

3.50 *Injection. This position draws the tendon well out from under the acromion.*

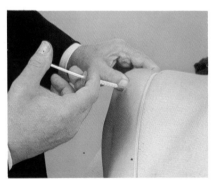

3.51 *Most cases are well after one or two injections*

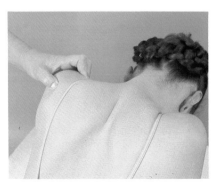

3.52 *Massage. The main difficulty is to ensure the treatment is given to the exact spot.*

The subscapularis

Pain on resisted medial rotation can be ascribed to the subscapularis, but in the unlikely event that resisted adduction also hurts, one of the other members of the group – the pectoralis major, latissimus dorsi or teres major – is to blame. There are two sites for a lesion to the subscapularis (*Figure 3.53*), both at the insertion into the humerus. Of all tendinous lesions at the shoulder, this is probably the most difficult to locate as the tendon is wafer-thin, lies deeply and the site is usually tender even in the uninjured.

A painful arc suggests that the tendon is injured at its upper half. But if full passive adduction of the arm across the front of the chest hurts, then the lesion is at the lower half of its insertion along the shaft of the humerus, where it is pinched against the point of the coracoid.

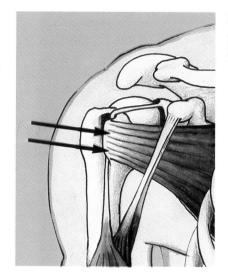

3.53 *The tendon is affected at the insertion into bone. There are two sites.*

For injection of steroid suspension 1 ml, the patient lies with hand on thigh so the bicipital groove faces directly anteriorly. To palpate, the thumb is laid on the head of the humerus and guided laterally until it encounters the bicipital groove, identification of which is facilitated by an assistant rotating the patient's arm. This shifts the two edges under the clinician's stationary thumb (*Figure 3.54*).

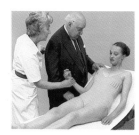

3.54 *Identification of the bicipital groove.*

The subscapularis is immediately medial to the inner edge of the groove. The tendon is extremely thin and feels as hard as the bone it overlies. The point of maximum tenderness is sought. As the needle proceeds it can be felt to pierce tendon and then hit bone. The tendon is infiltrated with about 20 droplets at points 0.5–1 cm medial to the edge of the groove (*Figure 3.55*). Results are good – one injection suffices.

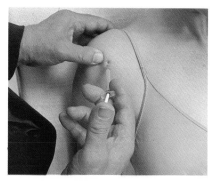

3.55 *Steroid suspension is extremely successful.*

For massage, the operator locates the tendon and hooks the thumb round the medial edge of the upper part of the deltoid. The belly is drawn laterally, letting the short head of the biceps slip under the finger so the thumb can connect directly with the subscapular tendon (*Figure 3.56*) without the intervening mass of deltoid belly.

The thumb is then moved vertically up and down while counter-pressure is maintained by the fingers at the back of the shoulder. The therapy is very painful, so treatment is limited to two sessions a week. Recovery takes about a month.

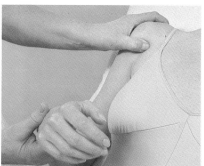

3.56 *Massage is the alternative, but no more than two-thirds of patients achieve full relief. The treatment is very painful.*

The biceps

There are five common sites (*Figure 3.57*), although occasionally the coracoid origin of the short head may be at fault. The two at the lower extent are dealt with as elbow structures on page 56. Trouble at the short head is very rare indeed.

Two movements are painful – resisted elbow flexion and resisted supination, which may be combined to increase the stress on the tendon. But if resisted supination does not hurt, the brachialis (rarely affected) is at fault.

The lesion may be at either the glenoid origin or the upper part of the tendon recessed in the bicipital groove. This latter site is accessible to palpation with the pain at the front of the upper arm.

By contrast, the glenoid origin is sheltered by the acromion and the coracoid, and pain is confined to the front of the shoulder.

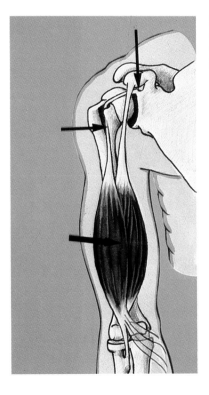

3.57 *There are three upper sites (arrowed). Only when the forearm is held supinated will a bicipital lesion cause pain on resisted flexion.*

The glenoid origin

Massage is impossible. For injection (*Figure 3.58*) the patient is in the half-lying position, the arm fully abducted and gripped by an assistant at about 45° short of full lateral rotation. This ensures the bicipital groove is level with the anterior edge of the acromion.

The left thumb is placed at the gap between the tuberosities either side of the tendon and the needle thrust in 1 cm distally (*Figure 3.59*).

As the tip passes backwards and medially between the two tuberosities, it runs into tendinous resistance at a depth of about 3 cm (*Figure 3.60*) and steroid suspension 2 ml is discharged in 20 droplets. As a rule, one injection is curative.

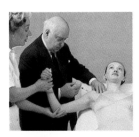

3.58 *Injection. The patient's arm is fully abducted and in lateral rotation. At this rare site, resisted adduction is sometimes the only movement that hurts.*

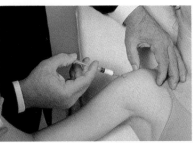

3.59 *The injection is difficult technically as the point of entry is distant from the lesion. The position of the patient's arm is critical.*

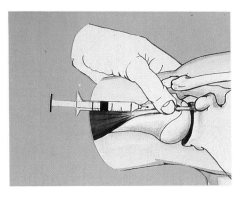

3.60 *Correctly placed infiltration is curative.*

The bicipital groove

The tendon is nearly always affected at its upper extent but the operator must palpate along its course to find exactly the right spot. Massage then succeeds so quickly, even in cases that have lasted years, that injection is hardly worth while. The biceps tendon is identified in the groove of the humerus and the fingers pressed down hard on the lesion. The humerus is then rotated to and fro using the patient's flexed forearm as a lever (*Figure 3.61* and *3.62*). If massage is kept up in this way for some 20 minutes on alternate days, the patient should be well in two weeks.

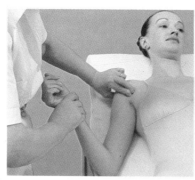 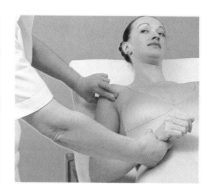

3.61, 3.62 *Massage, by rotating the tendon under the pad of the stationary index finger. An alternative approach is to move the thumb over the tendon.*

The belly

Normally the lesion lies deeply about half-way down the belly and can be located by pinching the deep aspect of the muscle between fingers and thumb, although in awkward cases local anaesthesia furnishes useful corroborative evidence. Palpation from in front is no help as the lesion does not lie anteriorly.

The treatment is massage. The tender area is squeezed between fingers and thumb, the pressure maintained while friction is imparted by pulling the whole hand vigorously to and fro by a good inch (*Figure 3.63* and *3.64*).

Sessions last 20 minutes on alternate days for two weeks. Steroids do less well.

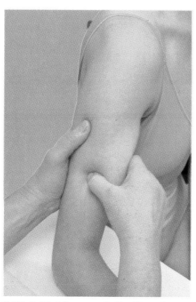 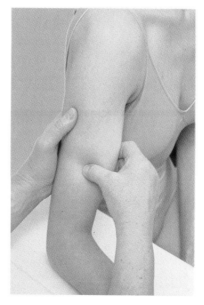

3.63, 3.64 *Massage, belly. Note the amount of pull. Only very chronic cases prove intractable.*

Painless weakness

Painless weakness in the arm may result from:

(1) A cervical root palsy with impaired conduction (see pages 177–179).
(2) Rupture, usually of the supraspinatus. The painful arc can be abolished by injection of local anaesthetic to the frayed ends of the tendon.
(3) Neuritides:
    (a) The long thoracic nerve of Bell to the serratus anterior results in 40° limitation of elevation and marked winging of the scapula.
    (b) Neuritis of the spinal accessory nerve to the upper fibres of the trapezius results in 10° painless limitation of active elevation.
    (c) Suprascapular neuritis is marked by very weak resisted lateral rotation and weak abduction.

In all three cases the pain lasts for three weeks and muscle power returns in four to eight months. Treatment does not accelerate spontaneous recovery.

(4) Neuralgic amyotrophy results in profound weakness involving muscle groups supplied by more than one nerve root. The condition is self-limiting.
(5) Polymyositis.

Painful weakness

Malignant deposits in the acromion may give rise to a painful arc plus pain on resisted action of any muscle attached to the acromion together with local bony tenderness.

The acromioclavicular joint

Because the joint is principally derived from C4 it rarely refers pain appreciably; the patient points to the spot. Exceptionally, the deepest capsular fibres may suffer injury, giving a painful arc and some C5 reference.

Acromioclavicular lesions are characterized by pain at the passive extremes of scapular and arm movement, but passive horizontal adduction is the most painful movement. There is no limitation. Osteoarthrosis with much the same symptoms can occur, and calcification and osteophytes may also form within the ligaments. Subluxation of the joint may result in stripping of the attachment of some anterior fibres of the deltoid muscle. In due course the neighbouring fibres may require strengthening in order to achieve full function.

The condition is usually traumatic and prevalent among athletes after a fall on the shoulder. Spontaneous recovery normally takes one or two months but the symptoms, whether traumatic, post-traumatic or osteoarthritic, may be eliminated in 24 hours by an injection of steroid suspension. Alternatively, massage alleviates the discomfort in a few weeks but the treatment is only successful if the superior ligament alone is affected.

For injection (*Figure 3.65*), the lateral edge of the acromion is identified. Two centimetres medial to this line is the gap between the acromion and clavicle, a tiny joint line which may be more readily located by maintaining the patient's arm in full lateral rotation with her elbow at her side.

The physician palpates for tenderness. Steroid suspension 1 ml suffices if just the inferior ligament needs infiltration, but if the superior ligament is to be tackled as well, the dosage is 2 ml.

The needle is thrust vertically downwards (*Figure 3.66*). Should bone be encountered at a depth of less than 1 cm, the tip does not rest intra-articularly and is adjusted until it slips in to about 2 cm. The deep ligament is infiltrated by 5 or 10 drops distributed fanwise and the superior ligament is similarly injected along each side of the joint line.

Occasionally the trapezoid and conoid ligaments may be strained. These respond to local injection of steroid around the superior surface of the coracoid process.

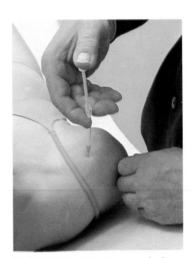

3.65 *Injection. One to two ml of steroid suspension get rid of the post-traumatic inflammatory reaction. The injection is viewed from above.*

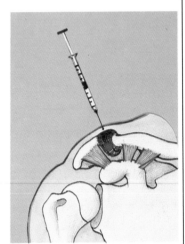

3.66 *Both the superior and inferior ligaments are injected. The joint line is tiny and difficult to palpate.*

The sternoclavicular joint

Pain is felt locally at the front of the base of the neck and, rarely, may be referred posteriorly or cephalically as far as the ear. The condition is nearly always traumatic. Both active and passive scapular elevation and elevation of the arm are painful. Passive neck extension and resisted neck flexion hurt too. This combination of pain on both neck and scapular movement directs attention towards the sternoclavicular joint, which proves tender. Symptoms tend to continue indefinitely if untreated, but may be cleared up by infiltration (*Figure 3.67*) of steroid suspension 1–2 ml. The point of entry is between the clavicle and sternum; the injection is made intra-articularly (*Figure 3.68*).

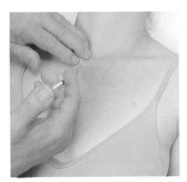

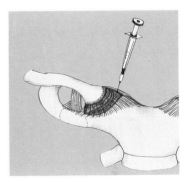

3.67, 3.68 *The joint responds so well to steroid suspension that other methods of treatment are not worth considering.*

CHAPTER FOUR

THE ELBOW

Although the elbow is anatomically complicated, lesions are relatively simple to identify. As at the shoulder, history is of little diagnostic assistance but clinical findings are clear-cut and easy to interpret.

Symptoms can of course be referred from the shoulder or neck, but the patient generally distinguishes pain of local origin since the reference of pain is slight.

The concept of end-feel is well demonstrated at this joint. In the normal elbow, extension gives a hard bone-to-bone feel, flexion the soft 'tissue approximation' and rotations the leathery capsular end-feel. Deviations from this norm suggest pathology.

Referred pain

The front of the elbow is within the C5 and C6 dermatomes (*Figures 4.1* and *4.2*), so symptoms may arise from the shoulder or cervical nerve roots. The posterior aspect of the joint is C7 (*Figure 4.3*). Referred pain is characterized by its indefinite edge.

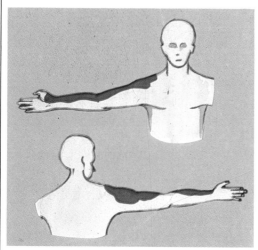

4.1 *The C5 dermatome*

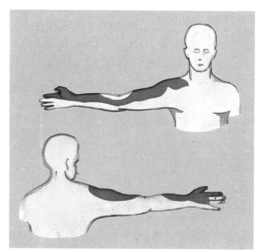

4.2 *Note the C6 dermatome includes part of the hand.*

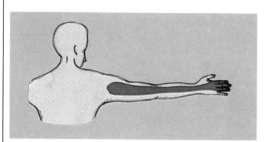

4.3 *The most likely cause of a C7 pain is a C6 disc lesion.*

Examination

A careful history and preliminary examination of the neck, shoulder girdle and shoulder excludes pain referred to the elbow. The functional examination involves 10 tests.

Passive movements

The primary movements are passive flexion (*Figure 4.4*) and passive extension (*Figure 4.5*). Early arthritis is marked by limitation in the capsular pattern of these two movements and, at a later stage, limitation of pronation and supination. A soft end-feel on extension suggests a loose body, a hard end-feel on flexion indicates arthritis.

Passive pronation (*Figure 4.6*) and supination (*Figure 4.7*) test the superior radio-ulnar joint; the elbow is held semi-flexed to avoid rotation at the shoulder. Painful limitation may arise in severe arthritis of the elbow; again the end-feel would be hard. Pain on passive pronation can be caused by a lesion of the biceps tendon at the tuberosity (see page 57).

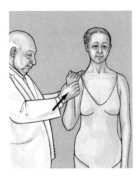
4.4 *Passive flexion.*

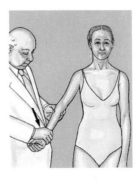
4.5 *Passive extension.*

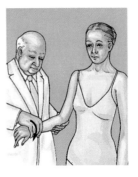
4.6 *Passive pronation.*

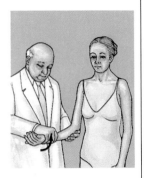
4.7 *Passive supination.*

Resisted movements

Resisted actions follow to assess the contractile structures. The resistance is applied to the lower forearm, not the wrist, to preclude the latter's involvement.

Pain on resisted flexion (*Figure 4.8*) incriminates the biceps (common) or brachialis (rare).

Theoretically, pain on resisted extension (*Figure 4.9*) suggests a lesion of the triceps (rare). But the pain is more likely to be produced at the shoulder as a result of the humerus impinging on the underside of the acromion in cases of subdeltoid bursitis.

Resisted pronation (*Figure 4.10*) puts strain on the pronator teres. But usually any pain on this movement is an accessory sign for a golfer's elbow.

Resisted supination (*Figure 4.11*) tests the supinator brevis (rare) and biceps (common), where a lesion also produces pain on resisted flexion.

For both resisted wrist movements, the elbow joint is held in full extension. Pain on resisted wrist flexion (*Figure 4.12*) points to a golfer's elbow.

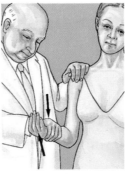
4.8 *Resisted flexion.*

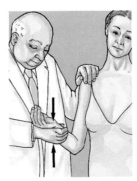
4.9 *Resisted extension.*

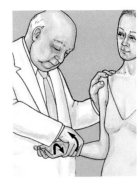
4.10 *Resisted pronation.*

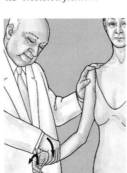
4.11 *Resisted supination.*

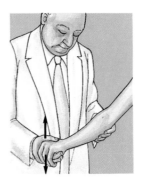
4.12 *Resisted wrist flexion.*

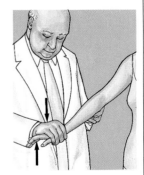
4.13 *Resisted wrist extension.*

Pain on resisted wrist extension (*Figure 4.13*) is normally due to a lesion of the extensores carpi radialis – a tennis elbow.

Findings

Capsular lesions

Both traumatic and inflammatory arthritis are common and respond well to treatment by steroid infiltration. Osteoarthrosis requires no treatment, being almost entirely without symptoms unless over-use has superimposed a traumatic arthritis.

The capsular pattern is greater limitation of flexion than of extension. Thirty degrees limitation of flexion (*Figure 4.14*) would correspond to about 10° restriction of extension (*Figure 4.15*), although occasionally the limitation is about equal. As arthritis is initially confined to an isolated affection of the humero-ulnar joint, the rotations stay free. But in advanced cases both pronation and supination are slightly limited (*Figure 4.16*), a finding most easily made by comparison with the good arm.

Palpation may reveal warmth and synovial thickening. Fluid may be present; aspiration will determine whether it is blood (aspirate *stat.*) or clear, in which case the cause must be found and dealt with.

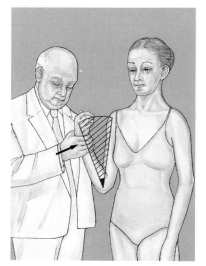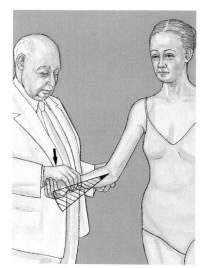

4.14, 4.15 *The capsular pattern is rather variable, but the limitation (shown hatched) of flexion is usually greater than of extension.*

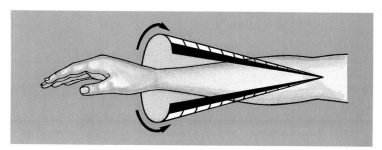

4.16 *In severe cases, the rotations may become limited.*

Myositis ossificans: caution

It is widely held that myositis ossificans results from improper treatment of traumatic arthritis at the elbow. Therefore forced movement towards extension in such cases is most ill-advised and must be avoided for fear of medicolegal consequences.

The only conditions at the elbow calling for manipulaton are a loose body blocking extension, sometimes an epicondylar tennis elbow and, provided bony trauma has been excluded, a pulled or pushed elbow in children (for which Mills's manipulation – see page 59 – was originally devised).

Arthritis

Arthritis, whether traumatic or inflammatory, can be effectively treated by an injection of steroid suspension 2 ml. In inflammatory cases the injection is repeated as symptoms warrant, but although pain is stopped, range of movement is not much enhanced.

With traumatic arthritis, any blood is aspirated before the first injection and a follow-up injection is required two weeks later. The arm is kept in a sling for the first few days. If rotation is painful in recent/acute traumatic arthritis, the head of the radius is almost certainly chipped, in which case an X-ray is diagnostic.

Some sports, such as badminton, are prone to produce a traumatic capsular lesion which must be treated before any accompanying tendinous lesion.

For injection, the patient lies prone with her arm fully supinated and in full extension by her side. The groove between the humerus and head of the radius can easily be felt posteriorly (*Figure 4.17*).

The needle is accurately introduced into the gap (*Figure 4.18*). At 2.5 cm the tip must repose intra-articularly and steroid suspension 2 ml is injected (*Figure 4.19*). With traumatic (but not rheumatoid) arthritis the arm is kept in a sling for about a week.

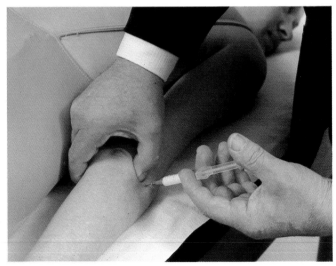

4.17 *The needle is inserted at the interval between the humerus and radius.*

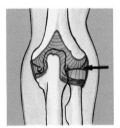

4.18 *The crack between capitellum and the head of the radius is identified.*

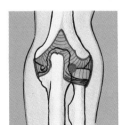

4.19 *All that is required is two injections, a week apart, into the joint. Point of delivery is marked.*

Rest in increasing flexion in a collar-and-cuff bandage is a slower but nevertheless effective remedy for traumatic arthritis. The elbow is supported in maximum attainable flexion and the bandage adjusted upwards each day as range towards flexion returns (*Figures 4.20* and *4.21*).

Support in full flexion must be maintained for about two weeks before the bandage can be lengthened in stages to allow extension. Enough range is gained in about six weeks for the patient to progress to an ordinary sling.

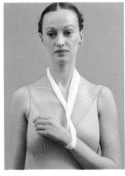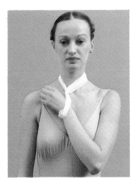

4.20, 4.21 *Rest in flexion. The bandage is shortened in stages until attainment of full flexion.*

Non-capsular lesions

Displacements

A displaced loose body blocks the joint, preventing either full extension or full flexion, but not both. In adolescence, osteochondritis dissicans leads to exfoliation of a fragment of bone covered by cartilage. Attacks of internal derangement follow, marked by sudden twinges at irregular intervals and abrupt fixation abating in the course of some days. Osteoarthrosis is a likely outcome giving little pain but limitation on extension. Further, the loose body will grow so it should be taken out, a procedure greatly facilitated by development in arthroscopic technique. Often there are several fragments. Manipulative reduction – strongly contraindicated by traumatic arthritis – is the short-term measure.

In adults, an impacted loose body causes a constant ache, intermittent attacks or pain whenever the elbow is moved.

Osteoarthrosis may well be accompanied by a loose body; the history is indicative. A middle-aged or elderly patient describes a slight long-standing ache in the elbow (the osteoarthrosis), punctuated by attacks developing over some hours and subsiding even more gradually (the displacement), during which time the elbow loses most of its movement.

The displacement may be lodged either:

(1) Between humerus, ulnar and radial head. This limits extension.
(2) Between the coronoid process and anterior aspect of the humerus. This restricts flexion; the end-feel is springy.

Manipulation is effective only if the displacement limits extension and, if the attacks are not too frequent, is all that need be done. But if flexion is blocked, treatment is removal of the loose body or nothing.

The manipulator needs two assistants. One anchors the patient's trunk; the other secures the patient's humerus to the couch and positions her forward foot as a pivotal point for the manipulator (*Figure 4.22*).

He grips the patient's lower forearm with her elbow semi-flexed – in as much extension as is painless – and applies traction by lifting his rear foot from the ground and leaning backwards, bracing his other foot against that of the assistant (*Figure 4.23*).

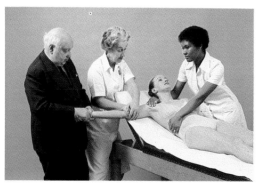
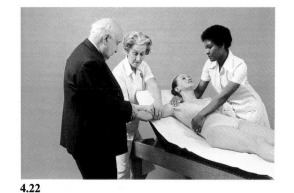
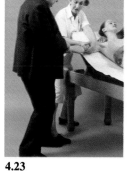

4.22 **4.23**

The manipulator then pivots round the assistant's foot, swinging the patient's elbow towards further extension; as he turns, he takes the arm as far as it will go and then forces extension a couple of degrees further (*Figures 4.24* and *4.25*). Throughout he repeatedly pronates (*Figure 4.26*) and supinates the patient's forearm, giving a final jerk (*Figure 4.27*) towards whichever rotation is found by trial and error to be most beneficial. Full extension should not be sought at first.

The patient is reappraised and the manipulation repeated as necessary up to, say, five times in a single session.

Since the elbow may remain in the site of traumatic arthritis consequent upon the original subluxation, the joint does not recover full range immediately. If arthritis persists, injection is required.

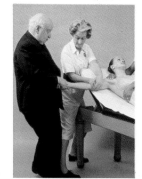

4.24 **4.25**

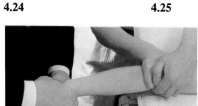
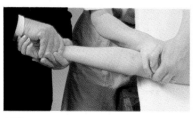

4.26 **4.27**

4.22–27 *Reduction of a loose body is only practicable if extension is limited. The elbow is swung towards extension. Meanwhile the patient's forearm is repeatedly rotated.*

Contractile structures

There are three main structures to be considered. The biceps is dealt with below; the tennis and golfer's elbow are described on pages 58–62.

Occasionally the triceps (painful resisted extension – see page 62) or supinator brevis (painful resisted supination without painful resisted flexion) are strained. A few sessions of deep massage are quickly curative.

Myositis ossificans has been associated with lesions of the brachialis near the joint following fractures of the distal end of the humerus. Accordingly before embarking on any active treatment to this structure, a month or so is allowed to elapse and an X-ray is taken.

The biceps

There are five sites. The three at the upper extent are treated as part of the shoulder on page 48 and the other two (*Figure 4.28*) discussed here. They are only a couple of centimetres apart, but as one is situated in the lowest extent of the belly it responds only to massage. In either case, two resisted movements are painful – elbow flexion and supination. If resisted supination does not hurt, suspicion falls on the brachialis (rare).

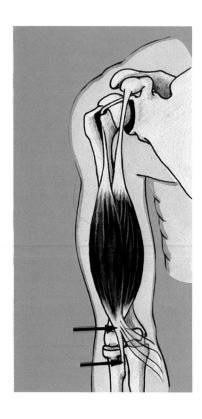

4.28 *The two sites. There is a distinct localising sign at the tenoperiosteal junction.*

The lower musculotendinous junction
The lesion, which may continue indefinitely at this site in the absence of treatment, is readily delineated by palpation for tenderness. Steroid suspension is ineffective. The treatment is massage, imparted by placing the finger and thumb in opposition behind the structure, and pinching them together while the hand is drawn anteriorly across the structure (*Figures 4.29* and *4.30*).

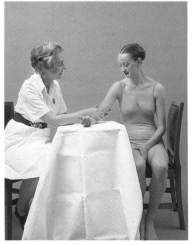
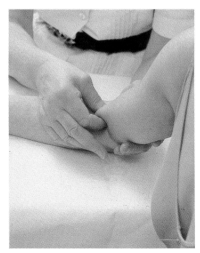

4.29, 4.30 *Deep friction, group and detail. There is no alternative to proper massage; without it, the pain may persist indefinitely.*

The lower tenoperiosteal junction
Here the complaint is of pain starting at the centre of the front of the elbow and radiating down as far as the wrist. The localizing sign is full passive pronation which also hurts as the lesion is caught between the radial tuberosity and the shaft of the ulna. No particular tenderness is found.

Treatment by injection (*Figure 4.31*) is preferable to massage. The patient lies prone with her elbow arranged in extension and full pronation. In this position the tubercle and insertion of the tendon are both rotated backwards and thus accessible to a posterior approach. The groove between the head of the radius and capitellum is identified posteriorly.

The needle is steered vertically downwards 2 cm distal to the groove until it penetrates the tendon just before hitting bone. Steroid suspension 2 ml is delivered in a series of droplets (*Figure 4.32*). Up to three injections may be required at fortnightly intervals.

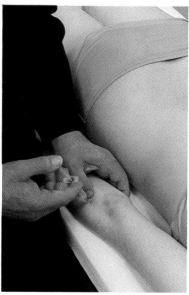

4.31 *The free hand identifies the groove. It is difficult to infiltrate the scar accurately in the absence of tenderness.*

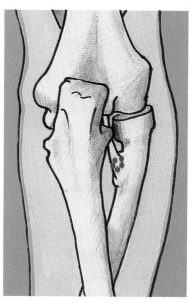

4.32 *A series of droplets are injected at the insertion into the tuberosity.*

For massage (*Figure 4.33*), the operator sits facing the patient. The tip of the flexed thumb is applied anteriorly to the radial tuberosity and the counter-pressure supplied by the fingers at the back of the forearm. With the other hand the patient's forearm is alternately supinated and half-pronated (*Figure 4.34*); the tendon can be felt to slip to and fro under the stationary thumb. Sessions are painful and last 20 minutes twice a week, with recovery in a week or two.

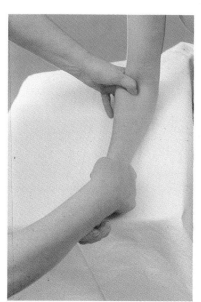

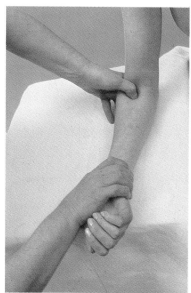

4.33, 4.34 *The massage is imparted by repeatedly rotating the patients' arm between full supination and half-pronation, which is the point at which the tuberosity goes out of reach.*

Lateral epicondylitis ('tennis elbow')

A lesion of the extensores carpi radialis longus and brevis is popularly known as a tennis elbow, although only about 5% of cases actually occur in tennis players. Any exercise involving repeated and forcible wrist extension can provoke the condition. Resisted wrist extension with the elbow in full extension is the painful movement and hurts at the elbow; usually pain is referred along the back of the forearm as far as the wrist and dorsum of the hand. At the moment of strain the patient feels nothing. Some days later an ache comes on and within two weeks the symptoms are fully developed indicating that it is not the minor tear in the tendon that causes pain so much as the repeated parting and resultant chronic inflammation of the healing surfaces during subsequent daily use. Sudden paralysing twinges are not uncommon. The patient is nearly always over 25 and generally between 40 and 60.

There are four sites (*Figure 4.35*), each responsive to a different treatment. The physician palpates, but will disregard associated tenderness often found at the posterior half of the lateral humeral epicondyle. Likewise, pressing the muscle bellies against the radius is normally painful so they are palpated from the side and not from above.

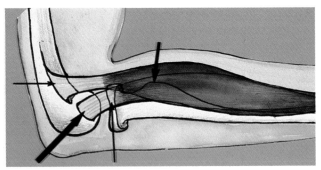

4.35 *The four sites. Ninety per cent of cases occur at the anterior aspect of the lateral humeral epicondyle.*

A tennis elbow must be distinguished from radial nerve entrapment which it resembles (see page 62).

It seems that impingement of the active extensor tendon on the annular ligament and/or any outpouching of the synovial membrane reproduces many of the symptoms of the tennis elbow, including pain on resisted movement. But the pain is felt posteriorly over the radiohumeral joint and the condition, otherwise unresponsive to treatment, responds well to a local injection into the joint.

The epicondyle

About nine lesions out of ten lie at the tenoperiosteal junction at its origin from the lateral epicondyle. At the other sites there is no spontaneous recovery; here the patient is better in one year, or two if she is over 60. Pain on resisted extension is so pronounced that the patient usually winces and lets her hand go.

A progression of three treatments is available.

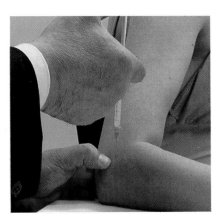

4.36 *Steroid suspension only helps at the epicondylar site. Subject to standard caveats, the process can be repeated on subsequent relapses.*

Injection

Steroid suspension 1ml is injected in droplets (*Figure 4.36*). The patient sits with her elbow supported in mid-flexion and fully supinated while the precise extent of the lesion is ascertained.

The 2cm needle is aimed vertically downwards until it touches bone. A droplet is injected here and then the entire cubic extent of the lesion infiltrated by a series of half-withdrawals and reinsertions (*Figure 4.37*). As the tendon is about as thick as the little finger, great care is taken to cover the area both deeply and superficially with multiple

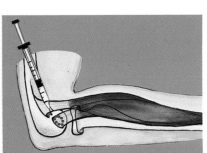

4.37 *The exact cubic limits – a three-dimensional area – of the lesion are infiltrated by a series of punctures.*

punctures. The operator's thumb can monitor each droplet as it goes in.

The injection is painful for a day and *must* be repeated within two weeks unless *all* symptoms, even on exertion, have been abolished. The patient avoids all activity of the arm for a week. Failure or repeated relapse are treated by a combination of massage and Mills's manipulation.

Massage and Mills's manipulation
The object here is to pull apart the two surfaces joined by the painful scar so the rest of the tendon takes the strain instead. In due course, this fresh tear is bridged by new fibrous tissue under no tension. This can be tried first if there is no one to give the injection.

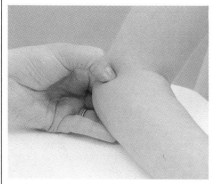

4.38 *First analgesia is produced by deep massage with the forearm in full supination.*

First the patient receives strong, deep friction (*Figure 4.38*) for 15 minutes to engender hyperaemia. Counter-pressure is afforded by the fingers at the medial side of the joint while the thumb crosses to and fro over the tendon.

Mills's manipulation immediately follows the preliminary massage while hyperaemia is at its height. The operator takes up position behind the seated patient who lifts her arm to a right angle, internally rotates her shoulder and pronates her forearm (*Figure 4.39*).

The operator clamps the patient's wrist into fullest flexion and rests the other hand lightly on the patient's flexed elbow (*Figure 4.40*).

The elbow is then snapped smartly into full extension (*Figure 4.41*).

Provided that full wrist flexion has been maintained, sharp strain falls on the extensor carpi radialis tendon – the muscle spans both the elbow and wrist. Thus it is only fully stretched when the elbow is in extension and the wrist in flexion.

The manipulation is extremely painful momentarily. It is repeated twice a week – once on each visit – for a month or more. If traumatic arthritis supervenes, inadequate maintenance of flexion at the wrist is the probable cause; strain has been taken by the joint and not the tendon. The ensuing session must be deferred pending subsidence of the arthritis.

Mills's manipulation is dangerous if full extension is not attainable and strongly contraindicated by signs of capsular disorder.

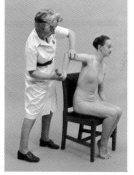
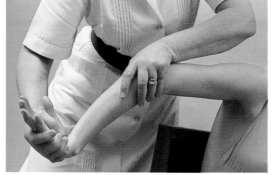
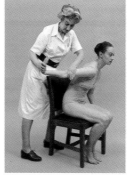

4.39, 4.40, 4.41 *Mills's manipulation may succeed at the epicondyle should injection fail, but the procedure is valueless unless the patient's wrist is fixed in fullest flexion throughout. The patient must be both relaxed and unsuspecting, lest tensing of the arm prevents achieving full extension, only the last millimetres of which are therapeutic.*

Tenotomy
If Mills's manipulation fails, an injection of sclerosant solution 1 ml (P2G, see page 195) may provoke dense adhesions to engulf the scar. Alternatively, tenotomy can produce good results (*Figure 4.42*) by dividing the tendon across its full width down to the bony epicondyle.

Procaine 2 ml is first injected to both the overlying skin and tendon and Mills's manipulation immediately follows the tenotomy. If this approach does not work of itself, steroid infiltration should now succeed.

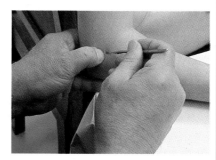

4.42 *Tenotomy is reserved for obstinate cases.*

The bellies

The tender spot is deep to the brachioradialis muscle and level with the neck of the radius. About 10% of tennis elbows occur here. The great difficulty is to find the right point and infiltrate it thoroughly. Palpation for tenderness is conducted by squeezing the belly between finger and thumb and although the whole arm may be tender there will always be a localized area of extreme tenderness.

For injection (*Figure 4.43*), the elbow is bent to a right angle and 10 ml 0.5% procaine injected, the fingers pinching up the lesion.

Delivery commences when the tip of the needle (5 cm) lies between the operator's fingertips, and as it continues the needle is half-withdrawn and repeatedly reinserted at different angles and depths to saturate the entire lesion at and around the point of maximum sensitivity (*Figure 4.44*). If the correct spot is found, resisted extension proves painless a few minutes later. Two or three well-placed injections afford lasting relief even after years of pain. The results of massage are disappointing.

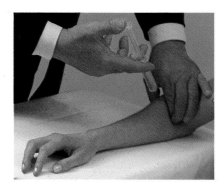

4.43 *The fingers feel the belly expand as the fluid is forced in.*

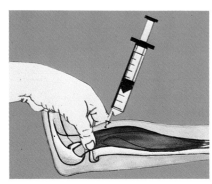

4.44 *Local anaesthesia produces permanent cure even in longstanding cases.*

The tendinous and supracondylar sites

The sprain may lie either at the body of the tendon by the head of the radius or at the origin of the extensor carpi radialis longus at the supracondylar edge. A lesion at either site is very rare but responds swiftly to massage. Steroids do not work.

For the supracondylar variety (*Figure 4.45*), the massage is imparted by drawing the thumb proximally and distally. The pressure must be directed onto the anterior aspect of the supracondylar ridge. The fingers apply the counter-pressure while the patient's hand is clasped in supination.

For the tendinous variety (*Figure 4.46*), massage is given by drawing the thumb to and fro across the tendon. The forearm is half-extended and nearly fully pronated. In this position the tendon is directly over the head of the radius which provides a firm basis against which to massage.

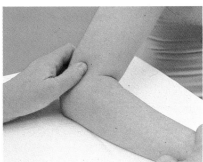
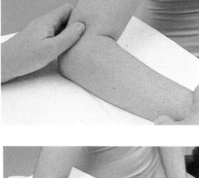

4.45 *Massage, supracondylar site. This is the easiest tennis elbow to relieve.*

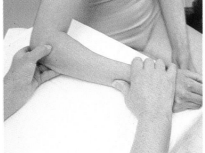

4.46 *Massage, tendinous site. Four to eight sessions suffice.*

Lateral epicondylitis ('golfer's elbow')

Less common and less disabling than a tennis elbow, this is a lesion of the common flexor tendon at the medial epicondyle. Resisted wrist flexion is painful, although painful resisted pronation may be the only finding in the early stages.

Pain is felt clearly at the inner side of the elbow and does not radiate far, seldom straying beyond the ulnar side of the mid-forearm. The patient is normally aged 40–60.

There are two sites, only 5 mm apart (*Figure 4.47*). But they must be differentiated and injection may not work at the musculotendinous junction.

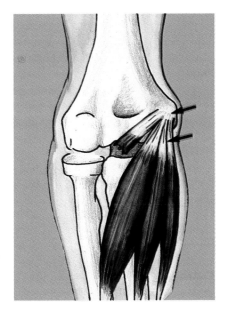

4.47 *The two sites. Wrist flexion should be tested with the elbow in extension.*

The tenoperiosteal site

Here the lesion responds to either massage or steroid infiltration. For injection (*Figure 4.48*), the most tender point is located by the thumb and the entire cubic extent of the lesion infiltrated with steroid suspension in a series of droplets (*Figure 4.49*). One or two injections normally suffice. In the event of failure, massage should succeed.

For massage (*Figure 4.50*), the elbow is supported in full extension and supination – this provides a firm, bony foundation against which to rub the tendon. The thumb applies counter-pressure on the outer side of the arm, and finger movement is not vertical but almost horizontal following the contour of the epicondyle. The very strongest friction is scarcely powerful enough. Sessions last 15 minutes on alternate days and secure relief in a month or less.

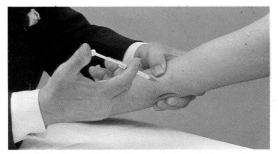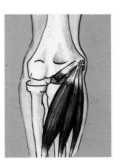

4.48, 4.49 *Some 20 droplets are injected all over the affected area of tendon. The tip of the needle is against bone.*

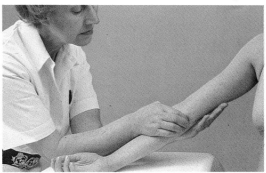

4.50 *Massage is an alternative. The motive force is flexion and extension of the physiotherapist's wrist.*

The musculotendinous site
The lesion lies about a quarter of an inch distal to the medial epicondyle, just below the previous site. Again the patient's arm is held in extension and supination over a firm support (*Figure 4.51*).

The thumb applies counter-pressure; strong friction is required. Considerable pain is provoked but recovery in four to eight sessions is the rule.

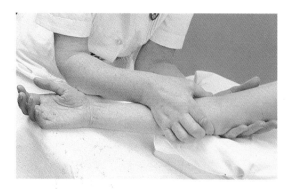

4.51 *Massage is both tiring and painful, but there is no alternative.*

Triceps

Training with weights can produce a lesion of the triceps which, if suspected, should also be tested in the 'triceps curl' position. Deep massage (musculotendinous junction) or injection (tendon/tenoperiosteal junction) are rapidly effective. Weakness may be attributable to either a radical palsy or seventh root palsy.

Radial nerve entrapment

Although not a true lateral epicondylitis, this unusual condition mimics the symptomatology. But typically there is a history of night pain (with or without accompanying weakness), often referred distally from the posterior interosseous supply to the wrist and hand.

The radial nerve is entrapped either around the radial head or through the interosseous fascia, and is tender to palpation.

Electromyographic studies can help with diagnosis, and surgery may be required to release the trapped nerve.

Pronator teres

This is a rare cause of pain in the forearm with point tenderness over the anterior surface of the flexor muscles. Resisted pronation may produce the pain as may flexor digitorum sublimis (i.e. pressure on the terminal phalanx). The condition is thought to be due to interosseous nerve entrapment and, although it can respond to local steroids over the tender area, may require surgical exploration.

Olecranon fossa impingement

This is caused by forced extension of the elbow when, for instance, throwing. Both passive and active extension hurt, and resisted extension may or may not be painful depending on whether there is accompanying triceps tendinitis.

The condition responds well to local steroid injection into the impinged area within the olecranon fossa.

Other symptoms

Weakness of the resisted movements may be caused by a cervical root palsy (see pages 177–179).

In Volkmann's ischaemic contracture, finger extension is impossible without wrist flexion (an example of the constant length phenomenon).

Lesions of the brachialis, triceps or supinator brevis are rare. All three can be cleared up by massage; in addition, the tendon of the triceps responds to steroid infiltration 1 ml.

Paraesthesia at the fourth and fifth fingers may result from interference with the ulnar nerve; friction against bone at the medial humeral condyle is responsible. Such frictional neuritis commonly – and confusingly – accompanies the increase in elbow use associated with capsulitis at the shoulder. An injection of steroid suspension 1 ml not into but along the nerve can afford lasting relief, but postural strain must be forestalled by avoidance of prolonged flexion. If this fails, transposition of the ulnar nerve is curative.

The reader is referred to Appendix II for a summary of the causes of pins and needles in the fingers.

CHAPTER FIVE

THE WRIST AND HAND

Lesions at the wrist and fingers are most often due to injury or inflammatory arthritis, although they may be induced by over-use. Symptoms of local origin are not referred appreciably and the patient can normally tell from where the pain comes.

A more misleading referred phenomenon is pins and needles, which seldom arise from a local stimulus.

The C5 dermatome extends to the radial side of the wrist. The distal extent of the sixth, seventh and eighth cervical dermatomes covers the hand and fingers. Cervical discs (most commonly at C6) compressing a nerve root can cause pain, paraesthesia and weakness in this region, whereas the carpal tunnel and thoracic outlet syndromes may account for painless pins and needles.

Examination follows the standard principles of assessment of function by passive and resisted movements. But at the wrist many joints have to be handled simultaneously, so the final diagnosis may depend on palpation for tenderness. Lesions of the radio-ulnar joint are rare, but must not be overlooked.

Inspection

After a careful history, the joints are inspected in good light. Many conditions may readily be discernible, including:

(1) Heberden's and Bouchard's nodes in osteoarthrosis. These may be mimicked by rheumatoid nodules.
(2) A tender, red and swollen joint suggests septic or (rare) gouty arthritis.
(3) Swollen and tender joints (usually involving sym-metrical joints bilaterally but sparing the terminal inter-phalangeal joints) suggest rheumatoid arthritis. In advanced cases typical deformities occur. The terminal interphalangeal joints are often affected in the sero-negative arthropathies and there may be psoriatic nail changes. The terminal interphalangeal joints are also involved in Still's disease.

(4) Skin contracture occurs in scleroderma.
(5) Atrophic changes in which the skin is smooth, shiny and thin occur in Sudeck's atrophy and the shoulder/hand syndrome.
(6) Localized swelling may represent effusions into tendon sheaths. A firm round lump suggests a ganglion.

Wasting of the thenar eminence suggests the carpal tunnel syndrome. Wasting of the abductor pollicis alone is nearly always attributable to either the carpal tunnel syndrome or pressure on the nerve trunk by a cervical rib. This latter may also cause disappearance of the pulse on scapular elevation. Crepitus is one of the classical signs of tenosynovitis, common only at the abductor and extensor tendons of the thumb where they curl round the wrist.

Examination

The radio-ulnar joint

The first two tests are passive pronation (*Figure 5.1*) and passive supination (*Figure 5.2*) to evaluate the capsule of the inferior radio-ulnar joint. The grip is above the wrist to stop any strain reaching the carpal joints.

Alternatively, the first metacarpus, carpal bones and radius may be fixed with one hand while the other glides the ulna in an anterior-posterior motion or adds rotation to the ulnar bone.

Pain or limitation should be treated by mobilization of the joint or injection (see page 66). Tenderness in an adolescent gymnast over the anterior surface of the radius, sometimes bilateral, is suggestive of an epiphyseal stress fracture and must be X-rayed.

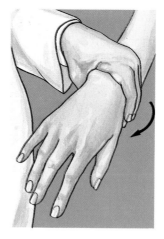 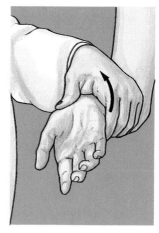

5.1 *Passive pronation.* **5.2** *Passive supination.*

The wrist

The wrist joint is now examined by four passive movements. Passive wrist flexion (*Figure 5.3*) and passive extension (*Figure 5.4*) both test the capsule, but passive flexion also stretches the ligaments at the dorsum of the wrist.

Passive radial deviation (*Figure 5.5*) puts strain on the ulnar collateral ligament; conversely, passive ulnar deviation (*Figure 5.6*) tensions the radial collateral ligament, rarely affected.

The same four actions are now repeated against resistance to assess the contractile structures. Resisted wrist flexion (*Figure 5.7*) tests the flexor tendons of both the wrist and fingers. Lesions of either are unusual. Similarly, resisted wrist extension (*Figure 5.8*) tensions the extensor tendons of both the wrist and theoretically the fingers.

Resisted ulnar deviation (*Figure 5.9*) assesses the ulnar deviators.

Pain on resisted radial deviation (*Figure 5.10*) can be ascribed to the radial deviators, which can be differentiated by holding the wrist in extension or flexion.

5.3, 5.4, 5.5, 5.6 *Passive wrist movements. Flexion, extension, radial and ulnar deviation (left to right).*

5.7, 5.8, 5.9, 5,10 *Resisted wrist movements. Flexion, extension, ulnar and radial deviation (left to right).*

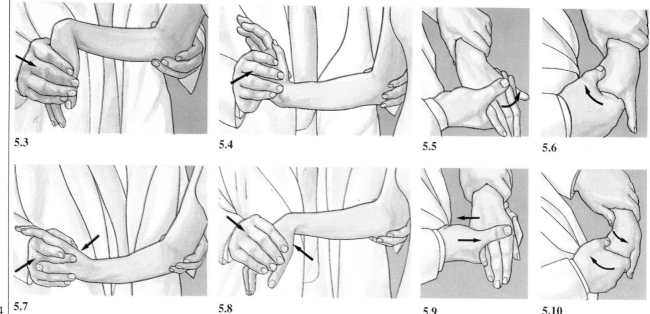

5.3   5.4   5.5   5.6

5.7   5.8   5.9   5.10

The thumb

The thumb can give rise to pain felt at the wrist. Only one passive movement is necessary: extension combined with adduction (*Figure 5.11*) which stretches the anterior aspect of the capsule. This always hurts in arthritis of the trapezio-first-metacarpal joint.

Resisted thumb movements come next. Painful resisted extension (*Figure 5.12*) is nearly always associated with pain on resisted abduction which tests the abductor longus and extensor pollicis brevis.

Resisted thumb flexion (*Figure 5.13*) puts strain on the flexor pollicis longus.

Resisted abduction (*Figure 5.14*) tensions the abductor longus and extensor brevis which are often at fault.

Resisted adduction (*Figure 5.15*) tests the adductor of the thumb, an unusual cause of trouble.

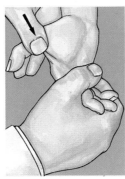

5.11 *Passive thumb extension.*

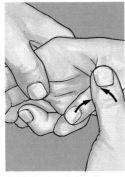

5.12 *Resisted thumb extension.*

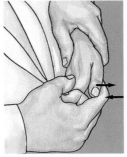

5.13 *Resisted thumb flexion.*

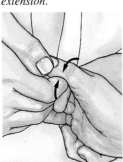

5.14 *Resisted thumb abduction.*

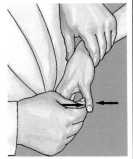

5.15 *Resisted thumb adduction.*

The fingers

The intrinsic muscles of the fingers are examined by resisted finger abduction (*Figure 5.16*) and adduction (*Figure 5.17*). A strained interosseous muscle can produce pain felt at the wrist if the proximal part of the muscle is affected. The first interosseous strain may appear in squash players who force the index finger too far down the racket handle.

Resisted extension and flexion of each finger checks the integrity of the flexor and extensor muscles in the palm and fingers, but for convenience all fingers may be assessed simultaneously (*Figure 5.18*).

Finally, passive flexion and extension can be treated for each joint of each digit. In arthritis both movements tend to be equally limited and painful. Again, all digital joints may be assessed together.

Throughout, the examiner listens and feels for crepitus, a sign of tenosynovitis or osteoarthrosis. Dupuytren's contracture leads to a fixed flexion deformity of the fingers, and a trigger thumb or finger causes

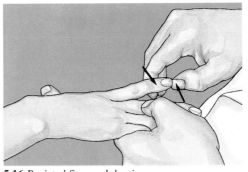

5.16 *Resisted finger abduction.*

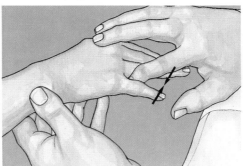

5.17 *Resisted finger adduction.*

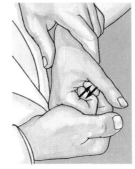

5.18 *Resisted finger extension.*

fixation in flexion of one or two digits which the patient can overcome by stretching out with her other hand.

The radio-ulnar joint

Lesions of the radio-ulnar joint are unusual and only set up pain at the wrist. The one common condition is arthritis. The capsular pattern is pain (but no limitation) on both passive rotations.

A single injection of steroid suspension 1 ml is effective unless the condition is rheumatoid, in which case repetition is called for as symptoms warrant. The joint also responds to mobilization.

For injection, the patient's forearm is fully pronated and the line of cleavage can be identified (*Figure 5.19*) by gliding the ulna anteriorly and posteriorly. A point is chosen on this line and the insertion made at the mid-point of the joint about 5 mm proximal to the ulna's sharp lower edge (*Figure 5.20*).

The needle is thrust down until it hits bone at about 1.5 cm and is then nudged into the joint. Use of a 2 cm needle prevents the tip emerging at the far side.

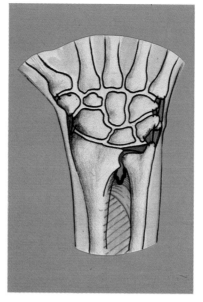
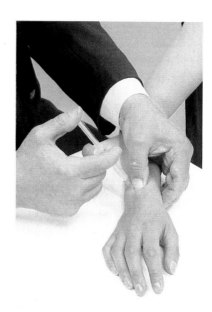

5.19, 5.20 *The joint (marked red) is seldom tender but it can be identified by moving the radius and ulna backwards and forwards on each other. The only effective conservative treatment is steroid suspension injected into the joint.*

The wrist

The capsular pattern (*Figure 5.21*) is denoted by roughly the same limitation of flexion as of extension, ultimately resulting in fixation in the mid-position. Both deviations are slightly limited.

(1) Traumatic arthritis results from a carpal fracture, generally of the scaphoid, since it spans the joint between the proximal and distal rows of carpal bones. The whole wrist is swollen, with both passive flexion and extension limited by muscle spasm. The radiograph may disclose no lesion for the first two weeks. A plaster cast should be applied immediately.

(2) Rheumatoid arthritis usually affects both wrists. In the acute stage the entire wrist is inflamed and swollen, limitation is very pronounced and rest in a back-slab may be the only option. In the sub-acute or chronic stage, the tender and swollen area is normally more easily defined and the entire extent of capsulo-ligamentous thickening can be infiltrated with steroid suspension 2 ml (*Figure 5.22*). The injection itself is painful, but results are worth while.

(3) Osteoarthrosis engenders little pain and no treatment has appreciable effect. The symptoms seldom merit arthrodesis.

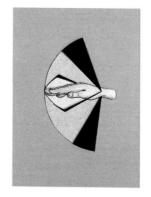

5.21 *The capsular pattern. Limitation of the deviations is minimal except in extreme cases.*

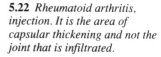

5.22 *Rheumatoid arthritis, injection. It is the area of capsular thickening and not the joint that is infiltrated.*

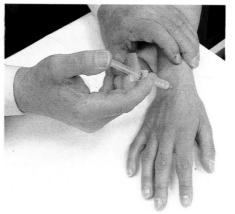

Carpal capitate subluxation

Passive extension is limited by 5° or 10°. Passive flexion is full and painful (*Figure 5.23*). Pain is localized to the dorsum of the wrist and on examination a bump is usually visible, particularly on flexion.

In difficult cases an X-ray may be necessary to exclude Keinboch's disease, un-united carpal fracture or an isolated osteoarthrosis, all of which give rise to similar findings. In cases of carpal capitate subluxation, the X-ray is uninformative, as the edge of the capitate bone merges with the others and cannot be separately visualized. But with the wrist held in flexion the projection can be seen and felt with ease and the strained ligaments about the capitate bone (*Figure 5.24*) are tender.

Manipulative reduction can readily be achieved during traction and is accomplished by separating the proximal from the distal row of bones and then gliding them anteroposteriorly.

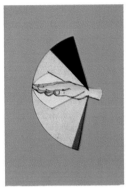

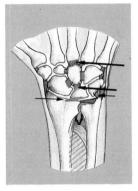

5.23 *Persistent subluxation. The sign that draws immediate attention is limitation of movement in one direction only.*

5.24 *With a carpitate subluxation, some or all of the ligaments tethering the capitate to its neighbours are tender.*

For the manipulation the patient half-lies. An assistant grips the patient's arm just above the elbow while the operator grasps the patient's forearm and hand and leans backwards, his foot braced against the assistant's foot (*Figure 5.25*).

One of the operator's thumbs lies just above and the other just below the wrist. Traction is obtained by pulling only with the hand distal to the wrist (*Figure 5.26*).

The operator's hands move vertically up and down in opposite directions while his little finger presses up against the patient's palm (*Figure 5.27*) emphasizing an anteroposterior glide that is devoid of both flexion and extension. The patient is reassessed and the process repeated if necessary.

One session usually affords full relief, and any residual symptoms from ligamentous strain can be cleared up by massage to the ligament. A variant of this manipulation involves the same position, except that the operator's upper hand is used to squeeze the wrist as hard as possible during traction. A little click is felt on reduction.

If a ligament has actually ruptured, the joint is unstable and manipulative reduction cannot last. Accordingly a sclerosant solution is injected at the point of rupture immediately following successful manipulation. The procedure is painful and not always successful. Usually the capitate-third-metacarpal ligament is involved.

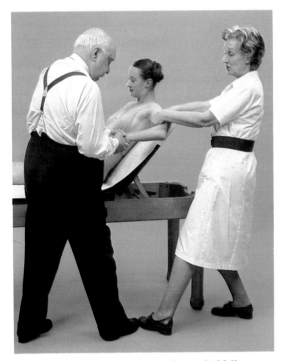

5.25 *Reduction is easy, and immediate relief follows even in cases that have lasted years.*

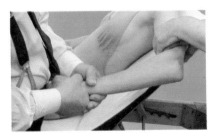

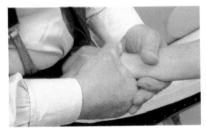

5.26, 5.27 *Traction is negated if the manipulator pulls towards himself with the hand lying above the patient's wrist. The operator's near hand glides the carpal joints up and down. Maximum upwards lift is shown in Figure 5.27.*

Ligamentous sprains

There are several sites; the commonest is sprain to the lunate-capitate ligament which, like the radial collateral ligament, responds to massage.

For treatment by friction, it will be remembered that the dorsal mid-carpal ligaments are arranged transversely and the dorsal radiocarpal and radiometacarpal ligaments run longitudinally. At the ulnar collateral ligament the only successful measure is injection.

The lunate-capitate ligament

Passive wrist flexion at the extreme of range is the one painful movement, with symptoms concentrated at the dorsum of the wrist. Sprain and/or adhesions may occur with or without accompanying capitate subluxation. If untreated the condition can drag on for years. Other ligaments (e.g. the radiolunate, capitate-third-metacarpal, ulnar-triquetral) may be affected at the same time and the examiner palpates for tenderness (see *Figure 5.24*).

Steroids are ineffective. Massage is the treatment of choice (*Figure 5.28*) both for strains and adhesions, but to ensure recovery *all* the sprained ligaments must be treated. Manipulative rupture, forced movements and so on are contraindicated.

The wrist is held fully flexed with one hand. The digital extensor tendons must be pushed aside so that the thumb can connect directly with the ligament to apply transverse friction (*Figure 5.29*).

Counter-pressure is maintained by the fingers at the front of the wrist. Full recovery is invariable, rapidly established after two to six sessions.

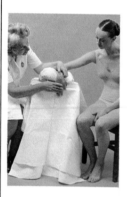
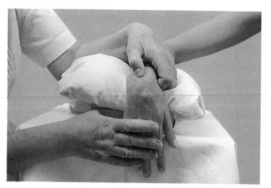

5.28, 5.29 *Massage. The tender spots lie superficially and are easily found if the wrist is kept flexed. The thumb moves to and fro over the ligament.*

The radial collateral ligament

Sprain of the radial collateral ligament is highly unusual. Although passive ulnar deviation is the only painful movement, hurting at the extreme of range, the disorder is often confused with tenovaginitis of the thumb.

Both infiltration of steroid 1 ml and massage are effective, although the latter measure requires several sessions.

The ulnar collateral ligament

This is sometimes the structure first affected in rheumatoid disease, and radiology may show an erosion at the base of the styloid.

Sprain to the ulnar collateral ligament (rare) may be the legacy of imperfect reduction of a Colles's fracture or fracture of the styloid process of the ulna. Of all the movements, only radial deviation hurts.

Spontaneous recovery takes a year, but injection of steroid suspension 1 ml into the tender area is rapidly curative. Massage does not work.

Pain on forced ulnar deviation caused by squeezing the triangular cartilage between ulna-triquetral and pisiform may confuse the clinician since the pain is over the ulnar side. But the condition is aggravated by compression rather than distraction, thus further distinguishing it from the ulnar collateral ligament.

The cause is often a backhand shot with dropped wrist and leading elbow. It is slow to respond to treatment, although local steroid may help.

The carpal tunnel syndrome

Pressure exerted at the distal part of the median nerve gives rise to well-defined pins and needles which are perceived at the anterior aspect of the radial three-and-a-half digits (i.e. excluding the little finger) of, usually, the right hand (*Figure 5.30*). The pins and needles are the first symptom, but in due course pain may be felt in the forearm and, classically, wakes the patient at night. The symptoms are increased by use of the hand and the condition should be distinguished from a cervical disc lesion and the thoracic outlet syndrome.

The symptoms may be evoked by:

(1) Pressing over the carpal tunnel while the patient flexes and extends her fingers.
(2) Keeping the wrist flexed for about a minute and then extending it abruptly.
(3) Tinel's test is positive in some 70% of cases.

There are numerous possible causes. Some are listed below:

(1) No apparent cause (about 50% of cases, typically in middle-aged women).
(2) Rheumatoid-type arthritis: consider division of the carpal ligament.
(3) Systemic conditions (e.g. acromegaly, pregnancy, contraceptive pills, myxoedema, diabetes).
(4) Repetitive trauma (e.g. scrubbing, chopping).
(5) Swelling on a digital flexor tendon: consider acupuncture of the swelling.
(6) Colles's fracture: await spontaneous recovery.
(7) Subluxation of the lunate bone.

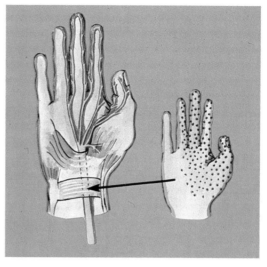

5.30 *Pins and needles. They are brought on by pressure on the nerve as it passes under the transverse carpal ligament, and are increased by use of the hand.*

There are various other contenders, many responding to steroid therapy. In any event (except with a carpal subluxation), steroid suspension should be injected diagnostically. Electromyography may confirm thenar weakness and delayed conduction. If the diagnosis is well founded, relief may last for some weeks and in some cases – about half the total, being those where no abnormality is palpable – the injection is curative.

For injection of steroid suspension 2 ml, the patient sits with her forearm supported in full supination and the wrist extended. The point of entry is about 4 cm proximal to the wrist (*Figure 5.31*) at the mid-line or just to the radial side of the palmaris longus.

The needle is angled almost horizontally and passes its full length into the carpal tunnel without piercing either the tendon or nerve. Injection of the latter results in a shower of pins and needles and the needle must be repositioned. The entire suspension is discharged under the transverse ligament (*Figure 5.32*).

Should the symptoms return after months or years, the injection is repeated as needs be.

Surgical tenotomy is indicated where injection fails or in cases of objective neurological deficit.

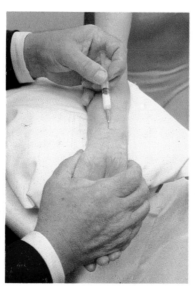
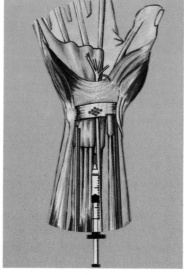

5.31, 5.32 *The diagnosis is confirmed by injection. Note the angle of entry; the needle travels parallel to the tendons and nerve.*

Contractile structures at the wrist

Malfunction may occur in either the flexor or extensor mechanism. The lesion may lie at the elbow (golfer's or tennis elbow – see *Chapter 4*) or at the wrist itself, but the patient is almost sure to know which end is affected. In most cases the lesion is at the insertion of the tendon into bone, but particularly at the thumb a tenosynovitis may be present.

Tendinous conditions of the forearm, wrist and hand account for many of the disorders currently banded together under the heading repetitive strain injury (RSI), recently the subject of much employee litigation.

Although this new nomenclature accurately characterizes the aetiology, it does not define either the pathology or structure affected. Nevertheless the conditions are no more difficult to diagnose or treat than formerly.

Resisted wrist extension

Pain felt at the wrist on resisted wrist extension incriminates the extensor tendons. Resisted radial and ulnar deviation ascertain whether the extensores carpi radialis or extensor carpi ulnaris are involved; in both cases the lesion is rare and tends to result from over-use. Either massage or injection is effective, unless the inflammation is rheumatoid in which case the wrist is palpably warm, swollen or nodular. Massage is then contraindicated. The long extensors can be excluded by testing extension with the fingers flexed.

The extensores carpi radialis

The lesion is somewhere in the distal inch of the tendons, frequently at their insertion into the bases of the second and third metacarpal bones (*Figure 5.33*). Palpation is conducted with the wrist gripped in full flexion – usually both radial extensor tendons are inflamed. Pain is accurately localized at the dorsum of the wrist. One injection of steroid suspension 1 ml delivered in droplets does the trick (*Figure 5.34*).

For the alternative treatment, massage, the wrist is held in full flexion to stretch the tendons *(Figure 5.35)* and one finger reinforced by another is rolled hard across the lesion. Twenty-minute sessions are given every other day and usually result in recovery in about two weeks.

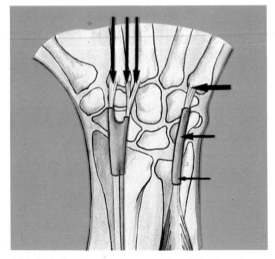

5.33 *Right wrist, posterior view. Possible sites of a lesion of the extensores carpi radialis (left) and ulnaris (right).*

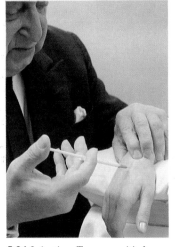

5.34 *Injection. Tenosynovitis here results from over-use.*

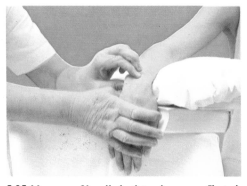

5.35 *Massage. Usually both tendons are affected, but the tender spot is easy to locate.*

The extensor carpi ulnaris

The lesion may be at one of three sites (see *Figure 5.33*). There is a localizing sign at the groove in the lower extent of the ulna, when pain is elicited at the extreme of passive supination of the forearm. The two other locations are between the ulna and triquetral or at the base of the fifth metacarpal bone. The wrist is palpated in full radial deviation.

An injection of steroid suspension 1 ml (*Figure 5.36*) delivered in droplets into the affected area is normally effective.

If treatment is by massage the wrist is maintained in flexion and radial deviation (*Figure 5.37*). This divides the base of the metacarpal bone from the cuneiform bone and the head of the ulna. One finger is placed squarely on the lesion and, using the thumb as a fulcrum, the wrist is flexed and extended across the tendon. Sessions take 20 minutes on alternate days, with recovery in about two weeks.

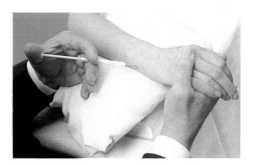

5.36 *Injection. The tender area is sought and infiltrated with the wrist in radial deviation.*

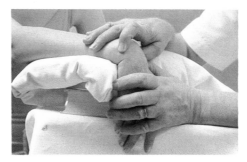

5.37 *Massage. The tendon is maintained on the stretch by wrist flexion.*

Resisted wrist flexion

The normal inference to be drawn from pain at the wrist on resisted flexion is a lesion of the flexor carpi radialis or flexor carpi ulnaris, although the flexor digitorum occasionally gives rise to symptoms at the wrist. Rheumatoid tenovaginitis can affect just one flexor tendon.

The flexor carpi ulnaris

For the flexor carpi ulnaris, the lesion is either proximal or distal to the pisiform bone (*Figure 5.38*); the site is palpated. The cause is normally a single over-strain. Both resisted wrist flexion and resisted ulnar deviation reproduce the familiar symptoms.

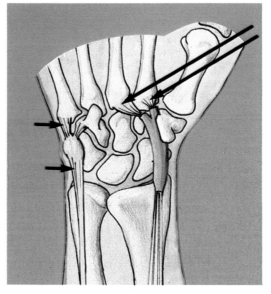

5.38 *Right wrist, anterior view. Possible sites of a lesion of he flexor carpi ulnaris (left) and radialis (right).*

Ulnar neuritis produced by local pressure at this point may be a differential diagnosis.

For the tendinitis, either injection or deep massage work well. Steroid suspension 1 ml is injected in droplets into the tendon (*Figure 5.39* and *5.40*).

For deep friction, the patient's wrist is held in extension (*Figure 5.41*). The massage demands great strength.

The operator lets the patient's little finger flex to relax the hypothenar muscles. Counter-pressure is applied at the dorsum of the wrist. The massage is delivered hard at the site of the tear for 20-minutes at a time with a 10-minute rest halfway through – sessions given twice weekly should achieve recovery in about a month. It is tiring work and it may be preferable to use the strength of the thumb.

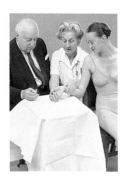
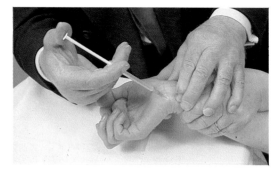
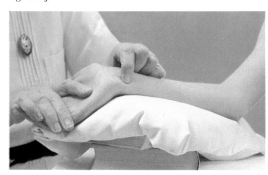

5.39, 5.40 *Injection. An assistant positions the patient's hands. Treatment by one or two infiltrations gives lasting relief.*

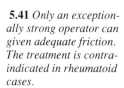

5.41 *Only an exceptionally strong operator can given adequate friction. The treatment is contra-indicated in rheumatoid cases.*

The flexor carpi radialis

The lesion is often found at the base of the second or third metacarpal bone (see *Figure 5.38*). The examiner palpates. Both injection (steroid suspension 1 ml) and massage are effective, provided that the wrist is maintained in full flexion for either treatment.

The flexor digitorum

The standard indicator for the flexor digitorum is pain on resisted finger flexion. Discomfort is felt either in the palm (see page 76) or in the lower forearm. In the latter case the painful area usually extends over some 4 cm and is due to a tenosynovitis, either rheumatoid in origin or an over-use phenomenon.

Both respond to injection of steroid suspension 2 ml (*Figure 5.42*). The patient sits with her forearm supinated, straightening her wrist and fingers to stretch the tendons. The needle slips in almost horizontally parallel to the tendon, and is pushed along until the tip rests level with the lesion. The entire suspension is deposited there.

For deep friction, three fingers are placed on the affected tendon with friction imparted by the operator drawing the whole forearm to and fro (*Figure 5.43*). The patient's hand is held in extension. Treatments last 20 minutes on alternate days and should confer relief in two weeks.

Massage must be avoided in rheumatoid cases, characterized by local warmth and/or nodules along the tendon.

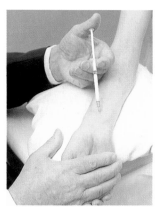

5.42 *Injection of steroid suspension is the only treatment if the condition is rheumatoid.*

5.43 *Massage, for non-rheumatoid cases. Lasting relief is secured in two weeks. The patient's wrist is in extension to stretch the tendons.*

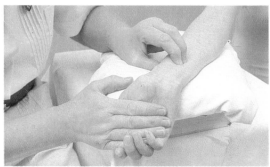

The thumb

Arthritis

The hallmark of arthritis of the trapezio-first-metacarpal joint is pain on passive backward movement during extension, because the anterior capsule is the most involved. Limitation is largely confined to abduction and in the final stage the joint is fixed in adduction. The pain is at the wrist.

Traumatic or rheumatoid arthritis can be relieved by injection of steroid suspension 1 ml, but in rheumatoid cases the injection must be repeated as required. Osteoarthrosis is discernible radiographically and steroid injection occasionally helps.

An assistant distracts the joint surfaces by pulling hard on the thumb and exerting counter-pressure with the other hand on the patient's upper forearm (*Figure 5.44*).

The base of the first metacarpal bone is identified dorsally and the needle directed through the gap at a slope of about 60° (*Figure 5.45*). If bone is encountered at about 1 cm, the needle does not lie inside the joint and the tip must be adjusted until resistance ceases at 1.5 cm.

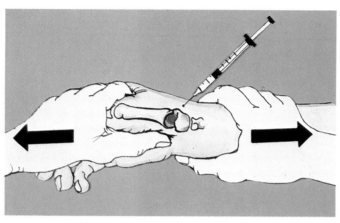

5.44 *Traction opens the joint space for the injection.*

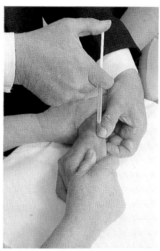

5.45 *Injection of 1 ml steroid suspension. Tenderness is most obvious at the front of the joint.*

Deep massage to the capsule on alternate days can treat either traumatic arthritis or early osteo-arthrosis. One hand hyperadducts the thumb in extension to bring the thenar joint into prominence (*Figure 5.46*).

The thumb of the operator's free hand imparts the transverse friction along the line of the joint. The outer aspect of the joint must also be massaged. Recovery takes two to three weeks.

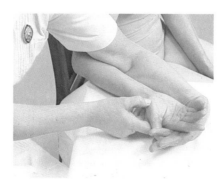

5.46 *Massage. Both traumatic arthritis and early osteoarthritis respond well to deep friction delivered by the operator's thumb.*

Contractile structures

The abductor longus and extensor brevis are often the seat of trouble; in either case, pain will be evoked both by resisted extension and resisted abduction, although passive movements may hurt as the inflamed tendon slides through the sheath. Because the ache is perceived by the patient as within the wrist joint, the condition is easy to mistake for a fractured scaphoid unless resisted thumb movements are tested. The tendinous lesion may lie at the lower forearm, in which case it is some two inches in extent and massage is the treatment of choice, although in sportsmen such as rowers, surgical splitting of the sheath may be needed to prevent recurrence. At and distal to the wrist an injection of steroid suspension is rapidly curative.

Lesions of the flexor pollicis longus tendon are very rare.

Pain in a racket player on resisted index and thumb extension suggests a grip fault. The grip should be tightened with the third, fourth and fifth fingers, and released between thumb and index finger. A correctly sized handle is important, and for each individual this will involve thickening or even thinning the grip to his or her requirements.

The abductor longus and extensor brevis pollicis (de Quervain's syndrome)

The cause is over-use or idiopathic. Tenosynovitis results (*Figure 5.47*).

Above the wrist all the tendons are affected simultaneously, normally where they curl round the shaft of the radius, and the pain is focused at the radial side of the lower forearm. Crepitus may be present, particularly in recent cases. Pain may occur on full passive supination if the lesion lies where the tendons lie in a groove at the lower end of the radius.

At or below the wrist the tendency is towards more diffuse symptoms referred to the thumb. The misleading associated tenderness of the styloid process of the radius should be ignored. The lesion may also occur at the insertion into the base of the first metacarpal.

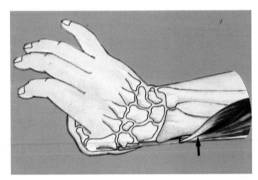

5.47 *The arrow marks the musculotendinous site, but often the lesion is an inch or two distal, inside the sheath itself.*

At the lower site, only infiltrating avails. For injection of steroid suspension 0.5–1 ml, the patient's thumb is fully flexed by an assistant with the wrist in full ulnar deviation and slight extension. This tightens the tendons and leaves the operator with both hands free (*Figure 5.48*).

The 2 cm needle is inserted at the base of the first metacarpal bone and thrust in horizontally while the tendon is pinched up with the free hand. This enables the point to penetrate the sheath and glide between it and the tendon. As the fluid is injected, a little sausage-type swelling is felt to expand along the tendon as far as the styloid process (*Figure 5.49*).

Rheumatoid tenovaginitis, which can be relieved by injection of steroid suspension 1 ml, sometimes affects the carpal extent of the abductor longus and extensor brevis pollicis tendons. The gross thickening of the tendon sheath contrasts with the slightness of the symptoms.

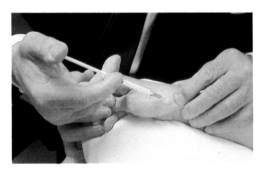

5.48

5.48 *At the lower site one, or at most two, injections cure. Spontaneous recovery takes three to four years.*

5.49 *The only difficulty is to place the injection correctly along the gliding surfaces between tendon and tendon sheath. Note the trail of solution delivered during withdrawal of the needle.*

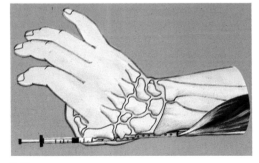

5.49

At the upper site, massage is the treatment of choice (*Figure 5.50*). One hand arranges the wrist in flexion. With the operative hand the fingers apply counter-pressure while the thumb is laid flat on and parallel to the affected tendons near the lower end of the radius.

Deep friction is imparted by alternate abduction and adduction of the thumb. Sessions last 20 minutes, during which the entire extent of the lesion is massaged. Treatment is given on alternate days and recovery ensues in about two weeks.

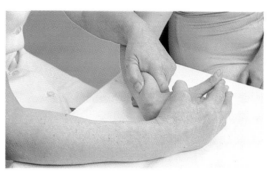

5.50 *The thumb delivers the deep friction. Neither crepitus, swelling nor an effusion contraindicate massage.*

The flexor pollicis longus tendon
Two conditions occur: tenosynovitis and a trigger thumb.

Tenosynovitis
Strain or over-use gives pain on resisted thumb flexion. There are two sites (*Figure 5.51*). If the lesion lies at the metacarpal extent under the thenar eminence, an injection of steroid suspension 1 ml is curative but massage usually disappoints. At the wrist, both massage and injection are successful but massage is often impracticable because of the lesion's proximity to the median nerve.

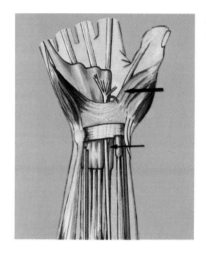

5.51 *Tenosynovitis. The two sites.*

Trigger thumb
If the patient cannot voluntarily straighten the thumb following flexion (or vice versa) a palpable swelling on the flexor pollicis tendon may be engaged in the tendon sheath. It lies just proximal to the head of the first metacarpal bone.

An injection of steroid suspension 1 ml into the swelling is often effective symptomatically (*Figure 5.52*). In the event of failure, the possibility of operation can be investigated.

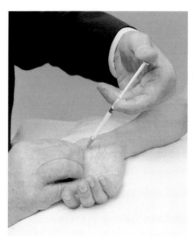

5.52 *Trigger thumb. The injection is made into the nodule.*

Weakness on resisted movements
Consider *inter alia*:

(1) C8 root palsy.
(2) Pressure on the posterior interosseous nerve.
(3) Tendon rupture.
(4) Ischaemic contracture.
(5) Cervical rib.

The hand

Capsular lesions

Arthritis may afflict any of the finger joints. The capsular pattern is equal limitation of flexion and extension with the rotations painful at the extreme of range rather than limited. The causes are:

(1) Rheumatoid arthritis – injection of steroid suspension 0.5–1 ml (if only a few joints are affected).

(2) Osteoarthrosis – normally symptomless.
(3) Traumatic arthritis – no treatment. Immobilization is contraindicated.

Local swelling from an unreduced dislocation is sometimes erroneously attributed to arthritis.

Contractile structures

These consist of the dorsal and palmar interosseous muscles and the flexor tendons.

The dorsal interossei are more often to blame than the palmar and give pain on resisted abduction. A lesion of the palmar interossei produces the symptoms on resisted adduction. Tenderness is sought between the metacarpal shafts, normally distally; in both cases the cause can be traumatic or occupational. The bellies and tendons respond to massage imparted by the fingers via rotation of the forearm (*Figure 5.53*) but not to steroid suspension. Two or three treatments of 15 minutes are enough, even in long-standing cases, although the tendons may take a good deal longer.

The long flexor tendons in the palm benefit from steroid suspension 1 ml but not massage.

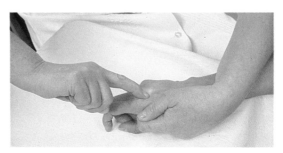

5.53 *The dorsal interossei resist every treatment except rotary friction.*

The flexor digitorum

Pain on resisted finger flexion incriminates the flexor digitorum. The trouble may be a tenosynovitis at the wrist (see page 72), but if the pain is felt at or below the wrist, either rheumatoid inflammation or a trigger finger is responsible.

For rheumatoid inflammation the injection (1–2 ml) is made by a series of droplets along the line of the tendons, about 5 cm in extent. The needle is inserted parallel to the tendon and slides forward along its surface as the injection proceeds.

A trigger finger may be caused by a swelling on any of the digital flexor tendons. The affected finger, usually the third or fourth, can no longer be extended voluntarily. In minor cases an injection of steroid suspension 1 ml into the swelling abolishes the symptoms (*Figure 5.54*).

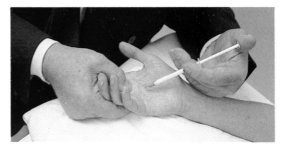

5.54 *Injection, trigger finger. Operation should be the last recourse.*

Pins and needles

The reader is referred to Appendix II for a summary of the various causes of paraesthesia.

CHAPTER SIX

THE SACROILIAC, BUTTOCK AND HIP

Most pain felt in the buttock is referred from the spine. Mechanical lesions of the sacroiliac joint are both rare and controversial, although inflammatory disease is not uncommon and its diagnosis important. In the buttock, serious disorders such as fractures, septic conditions and neoplasms occur and, although rare, must be distinguished from the confused signs and symptoms of sub-gluteal bursitis. At the hip a number of conditions occur including osteoarthrosis, displacements, muscular lesions and, in sportsmen, stress fractures giving rise to pain in the thigh. These must also be differentiated from symptoms referred from the lumbar spine.

Referred pain

Extrasegmental dural reference from a lumbar disc lesion may cause pain in the buttock, iliac fossa, groin, thigh or leg (*Figure 6.1*).

A posterolateral disc lesion impinging on the L3, L4, L5, S1 or S2 roots produces pain in the appropriate dermatome (*Figures 6.2–6.6*). The gluteal bursae are derived from the L4 and L5 segments, and the hip and psoas bursae predominantly from the L3 segment.

There is evidence accruing that the facet joints may produce dermatomal referred pain, but this is restricted to capsular lesions (rare). Thus with pain felt in the buttock and thigh, the first issue is whether the symptoms are of lumbar origin and a detailed history (together with examination of the lumbar movements if necessary) helps clarify the position. Once the spinal joints are excluded, the examination passes to the sacroiliac, buttock and hip.

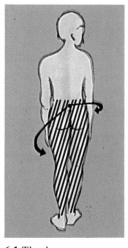

6.1 *The dura mater can refer pain anywhere within this region. The spine is the most likely cause of pain in the buttock.*

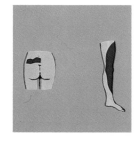

6.2 *Pain of lumbar origin can be felt in any of the areas illustrated. Pain from lesions of the sacroiliac, buttock and hip are limited to the L3, L4 and L5 dermatomes. The hip is an L3 structure, shown by Figure 6.2.*

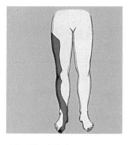

6.3 *The L4 dermatome.*

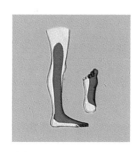

6.4 *The L5 dermatome.*

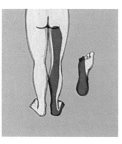

6.5 *The S1 dermatome.*

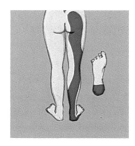

6.6 *The S2 dermatome.*

Examination

Passive movements

The patient lies supine. There are three methods of exerting tension on the sacroiliac joint(SIJ). For the first, the examiner presses downwards and laterally on the anterior superior spine of each ilium (*Figure 6.7*) thereby stretching the anterior ligaments. As these are lateral structures, the response to the stretch is positive only if unilateral gluteal or posterior crural pain is evoked.

Moreover, the downwards thrust causes some movement at the lumbar spine. Accordingly, in the event of a positive response the test should be repeated with the spine immobilized by the patient placing her forearm in the small of her back supporting the lumbar lordosis.

The posterior ligaments are assessed by forcing the uppermost part of the iliac crest downwards with the patient on her side (*Figure 6.8*). It is not so delicate a test as the previous measure.

Finally, the patient lies prone and downwards pressure is exerted on the sacrum (*Figure 6.9*). Again this stretches the anterior ligaments.

Attention now turns to the hip joint where the capsule is assessed by four passive movements, each repeated on the good side for comparison. But passive hip flexion (*Figure 6.10*) is an ambivalent test, being also part of the 'sign of the buttock' (see below). Additionally, it is painful at extreme of range in psoas bursitis and may cause movement at the lumbosacral joint.

Severe limitation of flexion accompanied by full rotations is a common finding in psychoneurosis but, owing to the diffuse and uncertain signs often encountered (as in e.g. bursitis), such a diagnosis should be considered only with caution.

Passive medial rotation (*Figure 6.11*) of the hip is tested. This is the most limited range with the capsular pattern, and in difficult cases there is another more sensitive test. The patient lies prone with knees bent to a right angle and the operator, standing at her feet, internally rotates the hips by pressing both feet apart and

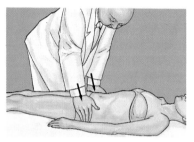

6.7 *SIJ stretch, anterior ligaments. The pelvis is not allowed to rock.*

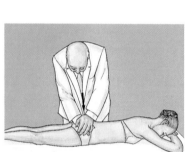

6.9 *SIJ stretch, anterior ligaments. Attempted forward luxation of the sacrum.*

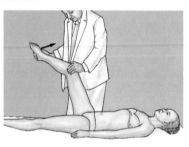

6.11 *Passive medial rotation of the hip.*

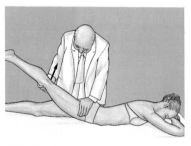

6.13 *Passive hip extension.*

downwards, noting any discrepancy in range between the two sides.

Passive lateral hip rotation (*Figure 6.12*) and passive extension (*Figure 6.13*) are tested. The end-feels are noted; in a healthy joint, flexion is halted by tissue approximation while the other three movements end with elasticity. Arthritis produces a hard end-feel.

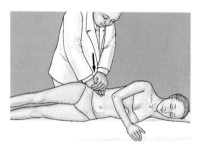

6.8 *SIJ stretch, posterior ligaments.*

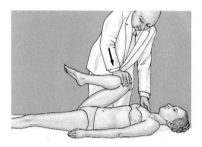

6.10 *Passive hip flexion.*

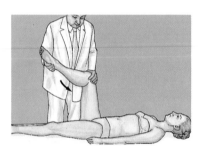

6.12 *Passive lateral rotation of the hip.*

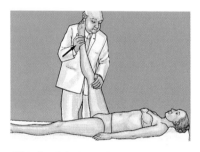

6.14 *Straight-leg raise.*

Straight-leg raise (*Figure 6.14*) stretches the dura mater via the sciatic nerve, and pain on straight-leg raise alone suggests involvement of the lumbar spine. But if the actual (rather than apparent) range of hip flexion with the knee bent is more limited and more painful, this dual finding points to a severe lesion at the buttock (the 'sign of the buttock' discussed later).

Resisted movements

Next the resisted actions are tested, but in practice only resisted hip adduction and flexion and resisted knee flexion and extension are tests for muscular lesions of the hip. Paradoxically, the other resisted movements are accessory signs in bursitis when a muscle contracts round or over an inflamed area of bursa.

In the absence of a major rupture, a lesion in a contractile structure will produce pain but not weakness on resisted movement.

Findings may also be made of:
(1) Pain and weakness.
(2) Painless weakness.

These possibilities are set out on page 91.

Resisted hip flexion (*Figure 6.15*) puts strain on the psoas and, to a lesser degree, the quadriceps.

The next four resisted movements – medial rotation, lateral rotation, extension and abduction (*Figures 6.16– 6.19*) – can compress the gluteal bursa, and pain on any or all of these may result from gluteal bursitis, as can painful passive abduction. The glutei themselves are practically never at fault.

But the next three resisted movements do assess contractile structures. Pain on resisted adduction (*Figure 6.20*) suggests a lesion of the adductors, known as rider's sprain. The knees are squeezed together. If abdominal pain is produced the possibility of traumatic osteitis pubis symphysis must be considered.

Resisted knee extension (*Figure 6.21*) with the patient prone tests the quadriceps. A lesion at the origin of the anterior inferior spine produces pain felt in or about the groin.

Finally, resisted knee flexion (*Figure 6.22*) tests the hamstrings and it is a lesion at the ischial origin which causes pain around the hip. Lesions at the lower extent of these last two structures are considered as part of the knee (see Chapter 7) where the pain will normally be felt.

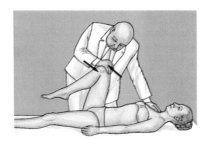

6.15 *Resisted hip flexion.*

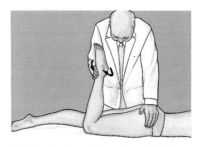

6.16 *Resisted medial rotation of the hip.*

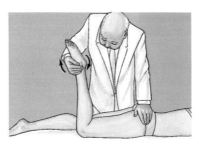

6.17 *Resisted lateral rotation of the hip.*

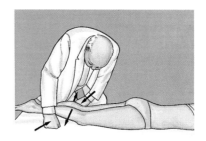

6.18 *Resisted hip abduction.*

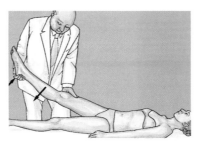

6.19 *Resisted hip extension.*

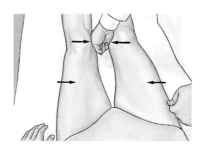

6.20 *Resisted hip adduction.*

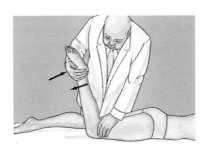

6.21 *Resisted knee extension.*

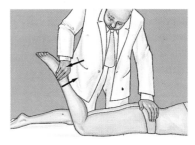

6.22 *Resisted knee flexion.*

The sacroiliac joint

Movement does occur at the sacroiliac joint. At the extreme of trunk flexion and extension, rotation takes place between the sacrum and the ilium. But it appears to be limited to 0.25mm. No muscles span the joints' interlocking articular surfaces, which are strongly bound together by the dense fibrous tissue of the interosseous and posterior sacroiliac ligaments. There is no intra-articular meniscus and, although a synovial plane joint, the articular surfaces are roughened with fibrous septa ensuring great stability.

Despite this anatomical arrangement, minor subluxation can occasionally be a cause of pain. The surrounding capsular ligaments may be sprained, most commonly in pregnancy but also as part of a more generalized lumbo-sacral chronic ligamentous insufficiency. The minor degrees of subluxation that occur during pregnancy are a result of the hormone relaxin and may also be found in hypermobile young females between the ages of 17 and 25.

Thus there exists a caucus of cases, where disc signs are hard to elucidate, which respond well to manipulation, most probably because reduction of an underlying subluxation reduces the strain on the ligaments. Thus where gluteal and dorsal thigh pain are accompanied by an apparent partial articular pattern at the lumbar spine in the absence of dural, neural and palpatory signs, three additional stretches are performed for the iliolumbar, sacrospinous and sacrotuberous ligaments. Of these, only the first are accessible to friction.

A positive result to any of these stretches indicates a subluxation, calling for manipulation. Failure in the case of the iliolumbar ligaments can be treated by transverse friction (usually at the lateral end) administered with the patient prone-lying with the pelvis elevated by a pillow. Three or four sessions are usually effective, with an immediate improvement on the first.

Manipulative techniques differ from the lumbar rotations and involve using the forearms (not the hands) as levers. The patient lies on her painless side facing the operator, and her upper shoulder is approximated to the couch by the forearm placed on the deltopectoral fossa whilst the pelvis on the upper side is drawn towards the operator with the other forearm. Further control is achieved by clamping the patient's painful-side fully flexed knee between the operator's thighs. The manipulation is delivered by a sharp thrust of the trunk as the patient's shoulder and pelvis are moved in opposite directions. The patient is re-examined.

The operator's arm position depends on whether the clinical examination established that the posterior iliac spine on the painful side was up or down relative to the painless side. In uncertain cases, the manipulation is mainly rotational by simply thrusting the painful-side hemi-pelvis forwards/towards the operator. But if discernibly out of alignment, the thrust is directional. If up, the operator's active arm is below the curve of the buttock, and the movement is towards distraction/rotation by rotating the pelvis. If down, the forearm is placed on the dorsal aspect of the iliac crest and the thrust is towards approximation with the buttock moved towards and the shoulder away from the operator. Further force can be achieved by increasing the leverage through the thigh.

This achieves an upward corrective thrust in the latter case and downwards in the former. In unresponsive cases, oscillatory mobilization may prove helpful. The patient again lies on her painless side. To move the posterior superior iliac spine down, the operator leans over the patient's buttock and the hand nearest the patient's head is placed over the anterior aspect of the iliac crest. The other forearm is placed below the curve of the buttock and the fingers can be interlinked while the patient's painful-side knee is fixed by the operator's inguinal fossa. The mobilizing action is applied by backward pressure of the upper hand and forwards pressure (i.e. towards the operator) of the lower forearm whilst additional pressure is transmitted through the patient's knee. Where the posterior superior iliac spine is lower on the painful side the process is adapted to achieve a reverse thrust.

Ankylosing spondylitis

Inflammatory sacroiliac arthritis only accounts for about 1 in 250 cases of low back pain. It occurs in the HLA–B27 group of disorders, and is commonly a presenting symptom in ankylosing spondylitis.

This occurs in young people, usually between the ages of 15 and 39, with an incidence twice as high in men as in women. Not being of mechanical origin, the onset is not associated with a mechanical cause and thus the pain comes and goes irrespective of exertion. The attack – in one, both or alternating sacroiliac joint – arise for no special reason and settle spontaneously. They respond well to non-steroid anti-inflammatory drugs. These, therefore, can to some extent be used as a diagnostic test. In difficult cases a lumbar disc lesion may be differentiated by a diagnostic injection of epidural local anaesthetic.

The ankylosing pain will be in one or other or both buttocks and may radiate down the leg in the S1 and S2 dermatomes, the sacroiliac ligaments being derived from these segments. During an attack one or more of the sacroiliac tests – although not normally the one for the posterior ligaments – are likely to be positive. It is therefore often possible to make a presumptive diagnosis before radiological changes are apparent and the erythrocyte sedimentation rate becomes raised.

Typically the process extends up the lumbar spine and beyond. The sacroiliac joints become ankylosed, at which stage they no longer give rise to pain.

Physiotherapy is directed at the patient's general state, not the sacroiliac joints. Non-steroid anti-inflammatory drugs can be used to control the condition symptomatically.

Osteitis condensans ilii and sacriliac osteoarthritis are purely radiological findings without practical significance.

The buttock

Major lesions

Major lesions of the buttock are indicated by an example of the constant length phenomenon, the so-called 'sign of the buttock', marked by:

(1) Slightly limited and painful straight-leg raise, coupled with
(2) Passive hip flexion with the knee flexed more limited and more painful than the straight-leg raise.

Greatly increased hip flexion should be attainable once the stretch on the sciatic nerve imposed by straight-leg raise is eased by flexing the knee. Thus if *apparent* range remains unchanged with, for example, the leg reaching the vertical in both cases, the *actual* range of hip flexion with the knee flexed is markedly the more limited of the two.

These findings show:

(1) The lesion does not involve the dura mater or nerve roots. If it did, straight-leg raise would be painful but passive hip flexion with the knee flexed would be painless.
(2) The lesion has nothing to do with the hip joint since, provided the hip rotations are full and painless, the capsular pattern for the hip is absent.

Provided always that sub-gluteal bursitis can be excluded, the lesion must involve structures other than the joint itself which are stretched on hip flexion. Disorders affecting these structures are likely to be serious, e.g. iliac metastases.

With a destructive lesion the end-feel is prematurely empty, that is, although the examiner can feel further range is attainable, severe pain makes further movement impracticable. Sometimes the resisted movements hurt since they alter the tensions in the buttock.

A radiograph and blood count are mandatory. Possibilities include:

Neoplasm at the upper femur.
Iliac neoplasm. Osteomyelitis of the upper femur.
Chronic septic sacroiliac arthritis.
Ischiorectal abscess.
Septic bursitis.
Rheumatic fever with bursitis.
Fractured sacrum.
Gluteal bursitis.

It will be remembered that pressure on any nerve root below L3 gives rise to buttock pain.

Minor lesions

A lesion in the buttock itself is suggested when a patient complains of pain in the buttock and examination of the lumbar and sacroiliac joints proves negative. The main symptom is usually pain brought on or increased by walking.

Diagnosis can be bewildering, not least because the significance of both passive and resisted movements is ambiguous. Thus full passive hip flexion can painfully squeeze the psoas bursa. Nor is a muscle lesion ordinarily the cause of pain on a resisted movement. For example, contraction of the gluteus medius on resisted abduction squeezes the gluteal bursa and is thus painful in gluteal bursitis (characterized, in common with psoas bursitis, by soft end-feel at the hip; arthritis gives a hard end-feel)

In fact muscle lesions in the buttock are almost unknown and the only resisted movements implying trouble in the muscle itself are:

(1) Lateral rotation – quadratus femoris (very uncommon).
(2) Resisted knee flexion – hamstrings (ischial tuberosity).

At the hip, resisted adduction is a test for rider's sprain (the adductor longus) and flexion for psoas strain. Knee extension tests the quadriceps.

Instability of the pelvic ring may produce changing patterns where the problem appears to range through the piriformis, psoas and sacrotuberous ligaments. Stabilizing the posterior lumbar ligaments with sclerosants (see page 231) may help.Occasionally a stress fracture of the inferior pubic ramus occurs in track and field athletes.

Psoas bursitis

Psoas bursitis is an uncommon cause of pain at the front of the upper thigh (L2 and L3 dermatomes). It appears gradually for no apparent reason and can go on for years, causing pain near the groin on walking. It may be seen particularly in sports that entail running with a flexed hip, such as field hockey or cross-country running over muddy terrain.

Passive adduction in flexion (*Figure 6.23*) is the most painful movement; this compresses the bursa. Passive lateral rotation usually hurts but medial rotation does not, and all resisted movements are painless except sometimes flexion with the hip in extension.

The symptoms resemble a loose body in the hip (see page 87), distinguished by its sudden twinges of intermittent pain.

Diagnosis is tentative and pursued simultaneously with treatment. A solution of 0.5% procaine 50 ml is injected using an 8 cm needle.

The clinician palpates for the femoral artery and the thumb is then moved laterally to locate the head of the femur (*Figure 6.24*); the bursa lies anteriorly. The needle is introduced well lateral to the mid-point of the inguinal ligament and 5 cm distal to it (*Figure 6.25*).

This approach gives a wide berth to the femoral artery and nerve. The needle proceeds medially (*Figure 6.26*) until striking bone near the junction of the head and neck of the femur. It is then retracted a few millimetres until it lies extra-articularly. By a series of small withdrawals and reinsertions, the

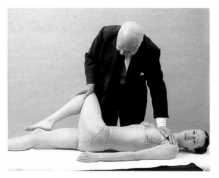

6.23 *The most painful movement in psoas bursitis.*

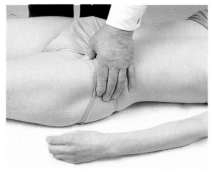

6.24 *The head of the femur lies immediately deep to the bursa.*

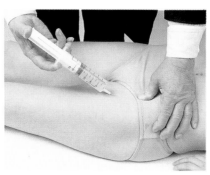

6.25 *The injection can be both diagnostic and therapeutic.*

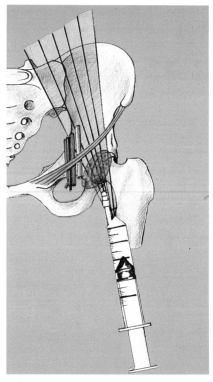

6.26 *Local anaesthetic is infiltrated when the needle lies just outside the articular capsule and several centimetres lateral to the artery. The bursa (shown blue) lies deep to the psoas ligaments.*

area between the hip joint and the psoas muscle is infiltrated. The cubic extent is about the size of a golf ball.

A correctly placed injection often has enduring therapeutic results. If benefit is still apparent after seven days, the injection is repeated two or three times at weekly intervals until the patient is well. If no lasting improvement is afforded, steroid suspension 5 ml is substituted.

Weakness and pain on testing the psoas are (when coupled with other inconsistencies) a common finding in psychoneurosis.

Sub-gluteal trochanteric bursitis

A more common cause of pain in this region is gluteal bursitis. As the bursa is derived from L4 and L5, symptoms are produced in the buttock and lateral aspect of the thigh. Onset is gradual, coming on for no particular reason and the symptoms persist for years, making walking uncomfortable.

As a rule, full passive hip flexion and full passive lateral hip rotation elicit the pain, although full passive abduction may squeeze the bursa painfully against the blade of the ilium. Resisted abduction can also pinch the lesion between the muscle fibres.

Treatment confirms the diagnosis.

The lateral approach

The patient lies prone. The operator uses his thumb to identify the upper edge of the greater trochanter (*Figure 6.27*) and the injection is delivered to the tender area immediately above its upper surface.

The solution is 0.5% procaine 50 ml and the needle is inserted horizontally just above the trochanter (*Figure 6.28*). Several injections may be needed before achieving the necessary accuracy in siting the fluid.

The probable depth of the lesion is 5–8 cm from the skin. The entire cubic extent of the lesion – approaching the size of a tennis ball – is infiltrated by a series of small withdrawals and reinsertions.

Results and follow-up procedure are as for the psoas bursa (see preceding page).

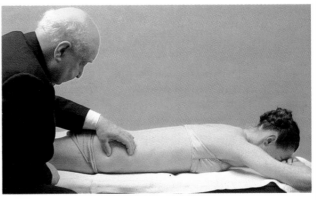

6.27 *Tenderness is sought in the area lying between the trochanter and the iliac crest.*

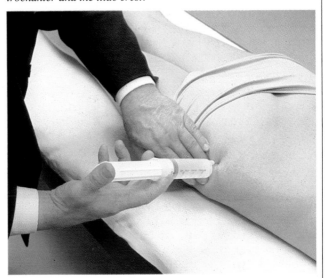

6.28 *The lesion lies deeply, but within a few minutes of a successful injection the previously painful movements stop hurting.*

The vertical approach

Pain on full passive abduction indicates the lesion is between the trochanter and ilium. It thus lies less deeply and may be more accurately located by a vertical approach. The patient lies prone on a low couch with her leg over the edge so it touches the floor; the upper surface of the greater trochanter can now be seen and felt as a horizontal plateau. The physician palpates deeply for the bone and also for tenderness (*Figure 6.29*).

The needle is inserted almost vertically (*Figure 6.30*) until the tip is felt to touch bone. It is then withdrawn by about 1cm and the cubic extent of the inflamed tissue saturated with 0.5% procaine 50ml.

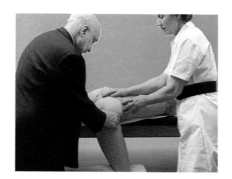

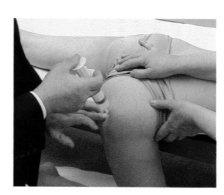

6.29, 6.30 *Injection, group and detail. This different position is adopted if the lesion lies close to the trochanter. If local anaesthetic does not give lasting relief, steroid suspension 5 ml can be used instead.*

Claudication in the buttock

This is an unusual cause of pain at mid-buttock. A severe ache (or sometimes numbness) is produced by walking for 100 yards or so. When the patient stands still the symptoms go, and on examination not one movement is found to hurt.

The condition is diagnosed by raising the patient's fully extended hip (*Figure 6.31*) and asking her to keep the lower limb off the couch for several minutes.

The result of this sustained gluteal contraction is the familiar pain in the buttock. The cause is muscular ischaemia and only operative recanalization of the artery is effective.

Two other conditions give rise to similar symptoms:
(1) The 'mushroom phenomenon' (producing pain when the patient is upright, irrespective of any walking).
(2) Spinal claudication resulting from stenosis (pins and needles in both legs on walking).

Three other causes of pain in the region of the buttock and hip are:
(1) Ischial bursitis or 'weaver's bottom' – local anaesthesia is induced at the site of tenderness at the tuberosity. Pain is felt on sitting down (cf. a nuclear disc protrusion – pain on getting up).

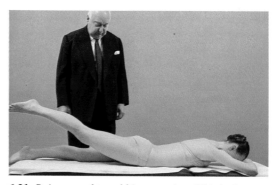

6.31 *Pain on prolonged hip extension. This is the only positive finding in claudication of the buttock.*

(2) Haemorrhagic psoas bursitis – 90° limitation of hip flexion. Following aspiration, the condition is treated as for psoas bursitis. Spontaneous cure takes 3–4 months.
(3) Tuberculous abscess – a large, symptomless, fluctuant lump arising from the sacroiliac joint. Rest in bed and anti-tuberculous drugs are prescribed.

The hip

The hip is largely of L3 derivation. Therefore pain originating at the hip may be felt in the upper buttock and the front of the thigh and knee, on occasions extending as far as the ankle. Pressure on the L3 nerve root can produce pain of identical distribution, but as often accompanied by pins and needles.

The hip itself is affected by arthritis, displacements and lesions to the contractile structures; bursitis has already been considered above. On the whole, diagnosis does not present great obstacles.

With sportsmen the possibility of stress fractures, notably at the neck of the femur, should always be considered if no clear clinical diagnostic pattern emerges. The history is of gradual onset of pain on exercise, especially on foot strike. No back signs are elicited and sometimes a muddled pattern from the hip accompanies the history. A technetium bone-scan may be required for early diagnosis, although the lesion may be visible on either the caudal or cranial aspect of the neck of the femur. The condition settles with rest.

Osteoarthrosis is common. Childhood disorders of the hip are nearly all serious.

Capsular lesions

Restriction of medial rotation is the most pronounced feature of the capsular pattern. It is accompanied by limitation of flexion and abduction linked with slight limitation of extension. External rotation remains full or nearly full, the opposite of the finding in a bursitis.

The end-feel will be hard, most notably on medial rotation which, in advanced cases, is restricted to the extent that the patient walks with the foot turned outwards.

Rheumatoid (rare), spondylitic and traumatic arthritis may all benefit from an injection of steroid suspension 5 ml (10 cm needle). In all three instances, the X-ray may be normal. With rheumatoid arthritis the other hip is the only other joint likely to be involved. Traumatic arthritis is distinguished by its history of injury.

To be absolutely certain of needle placement, radiological control may be helpful, but injection is perfectly feasible relying on the needle's end-feel. The easiest method is to lie the patient on her pain-free side. An assistant extends her hip, holding the leg off the couch in slight abduction (*Figure 6.32*).

The edge of the trochanter is identified and the needle introduced just above it (*Figure 6.33*).

The needle is thrust vertically downwards through the resistance of the thick capsule and then proceeds easily until the tip strikes the bone at the neck of the femur close to its junction with the head (*Figure 6.34*) and the injection delivered after a minimal withdrawal.

The injection itself is painful and quite severe discomfort may come back two hours later, persisting for several hours. The patient is advised to avoid weight-bearing for two days and to restrict activities for a fortnight. At the end of this period she is seen again and very often (particularly in rheumatoid cases) does not require a second injection. Too frequent reinjection should be avoided for fear of provoking a steroid arthropathy.

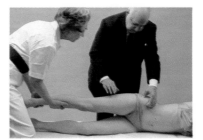

6.32 *The lateral approach is simplest, but the leg must be supported in slight abduction.*

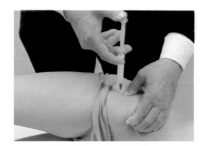

6.33 *Thumb and long finger span the greater trochanter. No large nerves or blood vessels are in the vicinity.*

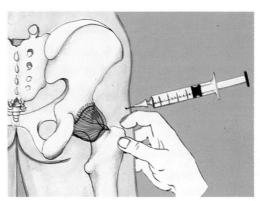

6.34 *Posterior view. Reaction to the injection is sufficiently painful to warrant an analgesic.*

Osteoarthrosis

In the early stages, stretching the capsule often produces relief for many months or years, but although the pain at night may be abolished, range is not improved. The more elastic the end-feel, the better the immediate prognosis. Treatment is repeated on return of the symptoms after some months' remission, probably with diminished success. Sessions are twice weekly for about a month.

First the joint is sedated by short-wave diathermy or other appropriate modality. The hip is then flexed as far as it will comfortably go, whereupon it is forced to further flexion by slowly increasing pressure applied at the knee (*Figure 6.35*). No jerk is given. This continues with breaks for some 5–10 minutes.

To force extension, the patient's good hip is then put into fullest possible flexion, thereby raising the bad thigh slightly off the couch. Maintaining pressure at the good knee, gentle repeated force is exerted downwards at the lower end of the bad thigh (*Figure 6.36*). With pauses for rest, the physiotherapist keeps this up for 5–10 minutes.

For the alternative method of forcing extension the patient lies prone. The stretching must be confined to the hip joint by preventing any stress reaching the spine, so one hand is used to press the pelvis down. The physiotherapist musters all her strength and gives repeated pulls upwards with her other hand (*Figure 6.37*).

When medial rotation is stretched the pelvis must not be allowed to tilt. The operative's hand holds the patient's ankle and, using the tibia as a lever, repeatedly stretches the hip into internal rotation (*Figure 6.38*).

Forcing lateral rotation is normally only required for dancers needing exceptional mobility.

When stretching ceases to benefit, surgery should be considered and indeed is always the likely outcome if the patient has an aplastic acetabulum or, conversely, those with protrusio acetabuli. Cases where the osteoarthritic degeneration is confined to the lateral edge of the femoral head have a relatively hopeful long-term prognosis.

A radiotranslucent loose body may form secondary to osteoarthrosis, in which case manipulative reduction is undertaken.

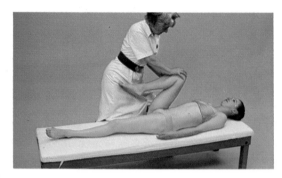

6.35 *Forcing hip flexion. Cases that do best with stretching have little erosion of articular cartilage superiorly.*

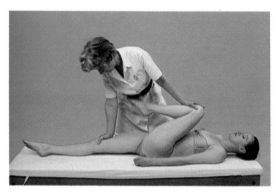

6.36 *Forcing extension. Full knee flexion of the good leg lifts the bad thigh off the couch. The physiotherapist has full control and an easier posture.*

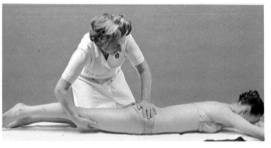

6.37 *Forcing extension — the alternative method.*

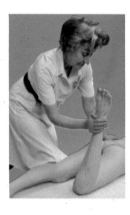

6.38 *Forced medial rotation. Too much pressure could fracture the neck of the femur.*

Displacements

A loose body at the hip is not always correctly identified, not least since the displacement is usually secondary to osteoarthrosis, and is most unlikely to contain an osseous nucleus. But the history is diagnostic, consisting of sudden twinges of pain shooting down the front of the thigh with the leg giving way, often temporarily immobilizing the patient. These attacks punctuate the minor ache from any osteoarthrosis (which is responsible for the capsular pattern).

The attacks of severe pain and inability to bear weight on the affected leg last for, at most, a minute whereas the chronic symptoms may persist and thus be present at the time of the patient's attendance. Generally there is some discomfort on full flexion and full lateral rotation.

The loose body must be shifted to some more favourable part of the joint by manipulative reduction. Most cases can be dealt with successfully, but although patients may have very long periods of freedom, recurrence is common and must be treated in the same way.

Manipulation – 1

The patient lies face upwards on a low couch. An assistant holds the patient's pelvis down to stop it being lifted by the traction of the operator, who stands on top of the couch grasping the leg at the ankle (*Figure 6.39*).

The manipulator leans back with all his weight and gradually steps off backwards (*Figures 6.40* and *6.41*). As he does so, the patient's leg is slowly extended during repeated rotation. The manoeuvre is concluded with a sharp jerk towards one extreme of rotation range (*Figure 6.42*). This final over-pressure is given in the direction found most beneficial and thus the patient is usually manipulated at least three times – once one way, then the other way and again in the most favourable direction. Re-examination follows each attempt, and if recovery is incomplete the operator moves on to the next method.

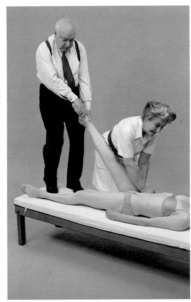

6.39

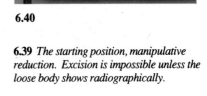

6.40

6.39 *The starting position, manipulative reduction. Excision is impossible unless the loose body shows radiographically.*

6.40, 6.41 *Mid-action. The hip is extended during rotation and traction. In Fig 6.41 the operator's right foot is shown suspended in mid-air during his descent.*

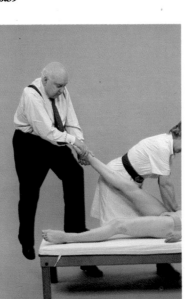

6.41

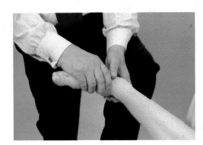

6.42 *The foot is used as a lever.*

Manipulation – 2

Usually the last movements to stop hurting are full flexion and full lateral rotation. If not rendered painless by the previous manipulation, a stronger rotation strain – best avoided with the frail or osteoporotic – can be applied (*Figure 6.43*).

The patient lies face upwards on a low couch. Her pelvis is anchored by an assistant while the operator places the crook of the patient's knee over his knee. He then plantiflexes his foot and presses down at the patient's ankle over the fulcrum of his thigh, thereby exerting traction on her hip (*Figure 6.44*).

A single smart rotation is then applied to the hip joint by using the tibia as a lever (*Figure 6.45*) during continuing traction. Preferably the manipulation is given in the direction previously found most beneficial. The patient is re-examined and the process repeated as necessary, say three or four times.

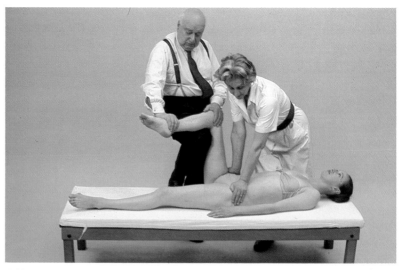

6.43 *The starting position. An assistant holds the patient's pelvis down onto the couch throughout the manoeuvre. Some two-thirds of loose bodies can be reduced by this and the previous method.*

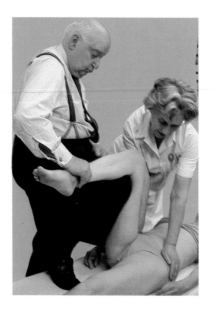 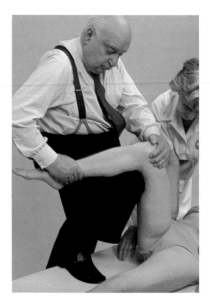

6.44 *To assume the starting position, the operator first hooks the patient's knee over his, and then applies traction by raising his heel.*

6.45 *The finishing position. The patient's lower leg is swung sharply round to push the hip into internal rotation during traction.*

Lesions of the hip joint in children

Bed-rest and immediate X-ray are obligatory if a child is found limping or complaining of even a slight ache in the thigh or knee when coupled with any limitation of movement at the hip joint. Many conditions are age-related and in some the capsular pattern is present. Possibilities include:

Congenital dislocation: age 1–5 years.

Pseudocoxalgia (Perthes' disease): age 5–10 years.
Tuberculosis of the hip: 1–10 years. Capsular pattern.
Slipped epiphysis: age 10–15 years.
Transitory arthritis: age 1–10 years. Capsular pattern.
Haemophilia: capsular pattern.
Trapped ligamentum teres.

Contractile structures

Athletes frequently strain the hamstrings. The psoas, adductor longus and rectus femoris do not give trouble so often. When several resisted hip movements hurt, the likelihood is gluteal bursitis (see page 83). Treatment of choice, whether for the belly or body of a tendon, is massage. Steroids are reserved for the tenoperiosteal junctions.

The psoas

Strain of the psoas is rare and responds well to massage. Injection is ineffective. As with the bursitis, the condition is linked with sprint drills, hill-running and running with a flexed hip. The painful movement is resisted flexion with the hip bent to a right angle, a test which excludes the action of the quadriceps.

Normally the lower part of the muscle is injured, with the site below the inguinal ligament just medial to the inner edge of the sartorius (*Figure 6.46*).

Transverse massage with the patient half-lying is administered twice a week with recovery in a few sessions (*Figure 6.47* and *6.48*).

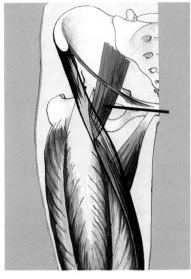

6.46 *The arrow marks the usual site.*

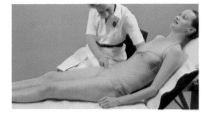
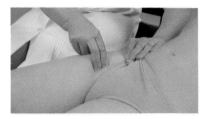

6.47, 6.48 *Massage, group and detail. The lesion responds well to deep friction. In half-lying, the muscle is relaxed.*

Adductor longus – rider's sprain

Resisted adduction of the hip is the painful movement, although sometimes full passive abduction also hurts. The condition is uncommon except in athletes, the strain is always traumatic and the lesion is more often at the musculotendinous than the tenoperiosteal junction. Treatment differs from site to site (*Figure 6.49*). Should the belly be affected (rare) it can be treated either by massage or local anaesthetic 20 ml.

Failure to respond should raise the possibility of traumatic osteitis pubis symphysis or conjoint tendon/crypto hernia where the fascia is continuous with that of the adductors. Surgery to the external ring may help.

At the tenoperiosteal junction either massage or steroid suspension 2 ml is effective. The patient half-lies and for injection the needle is inserted at the site of tenderness until its point reaches bone (*Figure 6.50*). The entire cubic extent of the tender area is infiltrated with a series of droplets.

Massage is the only effective treatment at the musculotendinous junction. The operator grasps the affected area between the thumb and fingers and friction is imparted by

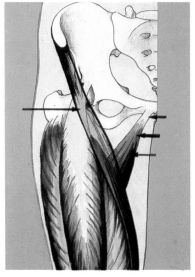

6.49 *Possible sites of a lesion of the adductor longus (right) and rectus femoris (left).*

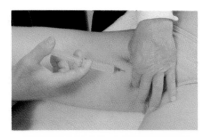
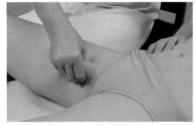

6.50 *Steroid suspension only works at the tenoperiosteal junction.*

6.51 *Massage is curative in all recent and most chronic cases.*

drawing the hand medially (*Figure 6.51*). Two 20-minute treatments a week should suffice, with recovery in three to four weeks.

The quadriceps

Athletes sometimes strain the quadriceps, often the rectus femoris tendon (see *Figure 6.49*), although the vasti may be individually injured calling for deep friction. Resisted extension of the knee is the primary painful movement, although full passive flexion or rotation may also pinch or stretch the tissue. Massage is the treatment of choice.

However, this area is prone to the formation of myositis ossificans and an avulsion fracture may occur in adolescence. Thus care with massage is required and gentle faradism or interferential may be helpful.

The patient half-lies to put the hip joint in flexion and relax overlying tissues. The rectus femoris tendon is about 8 cm below the anterior spine of the ilium and two fingers are laid firmly on the lesion with friction applied using the thumb for counter-pressure (*Figure 6.52*). Treatments lasting 20 minutes twice a week should ensure recovery in a month or less.

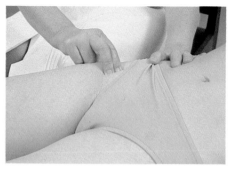

6.52 *Results of massage are uniformly good. The overlying sartorius must first be pushed aside.*

The hamstrings

These may be affected at the ischial origin, the belly or the knee (see page 110). Direct trauma or sudden strain may be responsible and the pain intensifies over 24 hours; the patient – usually an athlete – walks with a limp. Resisted flexion at the knee hurts at the back of the thigh and if a haematoma is present it should be aspirated *stat*. Quite often, resisted flexion of mid-range proves painless, and thus the muscle should be retested in inner and/or outer range.

At the ischial origin, steroid suspension is the treatment of choice. The tendon is identified and the tender area, which usually lies in the upper 5 cm, infiltrated throughout with steroid suspension 5 ml delivered in droplets when the tip touches bone (*Figure 6.53*). In sportsmen, the condition may take months to settle.

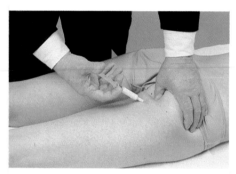

6.53 *Ischial origin, injection of steroid suspension.*

Massage is an uphill task because of the tendon's size and density. To render it palpable the hip must be supported in flexion (*Figures 6.54* and *6.55*). Two or three fingers exert strong transverse friction by flexion and extension of the wrist, emphasized by abduction of the shoulder. This can be extremely tiring, and it may be easier for the assistant to grasp the wrist of the operative hand, lean towards the patient's head and impart the friction by slight rotation of the thorax.

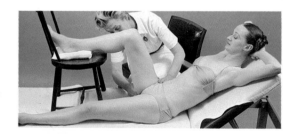

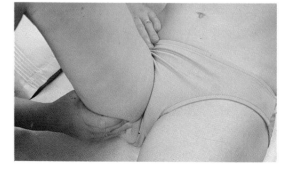

6.54, 6.55 *Massage, ischial origin, group and detail. Note support. The tendon must be kept taut. In chronic cases relief may take two months.*

If the lesion lies at the belly, local anaesthetic solution 50 ml is injected at first attendance to enable the muscle to move during a period of painlessness. This approach is worth while only during the first few days following injury.

On the next attendance, massage is administered. The knee is kept flexed to relax the muscle (*Figure 6.56*).

The deep friction is extremely tiring and given five minutes on, five minutes off, over half an hour. For the first week sessions are daily and thereafter taper off to alternate days. Treatment continues for a week after recovery to forestall recurrence.

The lesion is grasped between thumb and fingers of both hands and the fingers are flexed and extended while the hand is drawn upwards (*Figure 6.57*). Each session may be concluded by faradism to the affected part of the belly (again with the knee in flexion) to broaden out the muscles without stretching the healing fibres.

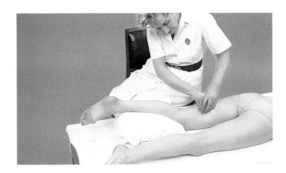

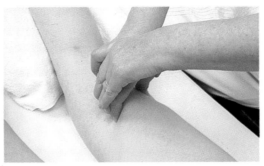

6.56, 6.57 *Massage, group and detail. This is a common injury of sprinters and footballers. Note the leg is supported in flexion.*

Other findings on resisted movements

Painful weakness
   Flexion – adolescent traction-fracture of the trochanter or the anterior superior spine of the ilium.
   Flexion – abdominal neoplasm infiltrating the psoas.
   Flexion – metastases at the upper femur.

Painless weakness
   Lumbar disc lesion if unilateral (common).
   Spinal neoplasm.
   Abduction – congenital dislocation of the hip.
   Hip flexion and knee extension – if bilateral, myopathy or myositis.

Coxalgia

Direct trauma to the coccyx can produce debilitating pain that may be relieved with a steroid infiltration to the sacro-coccygeal ligaments.

CHAPTER SEVEN

THE KNEE

An exact diagnosis can be made at the knee with considerable certainty and many conditions are easily curable. History is of critical diagnostic importance.

The knee's mechanical structure as a weight-bearing joint with long levers above and below means that the ligaments maintaining its integrity are particularly liable to strain(s), often multiple and almost invariably accompanied by secondary traumatic arthritis.

Indeed the characteristic response to injury is an acute synovitis denoted by the capsular pattern. Thus the phenomenon is frequently encountered as a secondary capsular pattern which will subside spontaneously when the primary lesion is treated.

Arthroscopy has brought new sophistication to the diagnosis and treatment of intra-articular disorders but, in the absence of any particular difficulty, routine examination meets the broad run of the clinician's case-load.

Knee pain is usually well localized and many of the tissues are accessible to palpation. Painless osteoarthrosis should be disregarded.

Referred pain

Pain referred to the knee is characterized by its indefinite extent. Although in theory the L4 and L5 dermatomes overlie this joint, in practice it is with L2 and L3 that the physician is primarily concerned (*Figure 7.1*). Tissues derived from the latter segment provide the more likely cause of referred symptoms, in particular from a disc lesion compressing the L3 root or, more often, osteoarthrosis of the hip.

Disorders of the knee itself very seldom produce posterior pain only. The back of the knee is covered by the S1 and S2 dermatomes (*Figure 7.2*). A fifth lumbar disc displacement exerting pressure on the first or second sacral nerve roots may be responsible for pain in this region, as may a lesion of the lower part of the hamstrings or of the upper part of the gastrocnemius.

Extrasegmentally referred pain of dural origin may also cause pain in the lower limb (*Figure 7.3*).

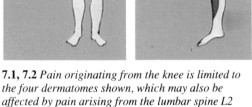

7.1, 7.2 *Pain originating from the knee is limited to the four dermatomes shown, which may also be affected by pain arising from the lumbar spine L2 (left) and L3 (right).*

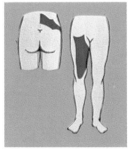

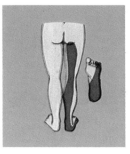

7.3, 7.4 *The dermatomes, posterior aspect. S1 (left); S2 (right).*

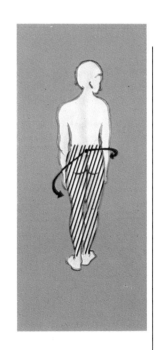

7.5 *Pain of dural origin can extend to the knee and beyond.*

History

Provided the lesion actually lies at the knee, the primary distinction is between disorders of inflammatory disease and those of traumatic origin. In the former case the cause may be, for example, rheumatoid arthritis, ankylosing spondylitis, Reiter's disease, psoriasis or lupus erythematosus.

In the event of injury the most detailed history is needed – for two reasons. First, the examiner must assess the exact strain imposed on the joint at the moment of trauma and the exact site of pain. Thus a valgus strain falls on the medial collateral ligament giving pain on the inner side of the knee.

Secondly, many disorders can be identified by their typical history and progression. A number of avenues should be explored. Did the knee give way? Could the patient get up and walk? Did the joint lock? If so, in flexion or extension? Did it unlock itself? Did the pain and disablement come on suddenly or over some hours? Was the pain momentary? Were there any twinges? Did any swelling come on rapidly? Or slowly? Is there any history of overload, e.g. pain during weight-training,

revealing a disorder not apparent during ordinary use?

Each disorder has its idiosyncratic course from which the diagnosis can often be made, before being confirmed by the physical examination.

The classic sports injury is a rotation strain during weight-bearing, by an athlete twisting his leg while his foot is directionally fixed by, for example, a spiked shoe or ski. If the knee is in extension at the moment of impact the force is transmitted distally, but in flexion it is the meniscus that takes the strain. The close interrelationship of the medial meniscus and the ligament means that injury strong enough to tear one will often affect the other. Thus multiple injuries are commonplace.

For example, a dislocation of the meniscus must entail damage to some of the fibres of its stabilizing coronary ligament, and may go on to attack the medial coronary ligament to which it is adherent. Similarly, O'Donoghue's triad involves the medial collateral ligament and the cruciate ligament (usually the anterior) as well as the medial cartilage. Thus if two of these signs are present, it is sound practice to check for the third.

Examination

Inspection

The joint should be examined for bruising, discoloration, swelling and wasting. Assessment of the legs will check whether the knee is influenced by anatomical abnormalities such as genu varus or valgus, tibial torsion or foot mechanics causing excess pronation or supination.

The patient lies and the joint is tested for fluid. The first method is the standard patellar tap (*Figure 7.6*). The more delicate and preferred test is to elicit fluctuati6n (*Figure 7.7*); with experience, blood and fluid can be differentiated. Blood fluctuates *en bloc* like a jelly, whereas fluid runs up and down piecemeal. One hand is placed flat above the patella and exerts downwards pressure. The movement of any fluid thereby induced forces apart the thumb and forefinger positioned either side of the patella. Blood fills the joint swiftly, fluid in the course of some hours, characteristically overnight. Blood is an irritant and must be aspirated immediately. That is the therapeutic measure. Aspiration of clear fluid is likely to be a waste of time unless further diagnostic analysis is required or the effusion is large; anything over 30 ml fluid may give rise to accelerated wasting of the quadriceps.

Heat is sought using the back of the hand, the more sensitive aspect (*Figure 7.8*). Warmth indicates the lesion is still in the active stage and localized heat may pinpoint its exact site.

Finally, the physician palpates for the synovial thickening indicative of the inflammatory arthritides. It may be felt by gently rolling the fingers upwards and downwards (*Figure 7.9*) at the reflexion of the membrane where it overlies each condyle of the femur (*Figure 7.10*). The sound knee is compared.

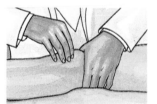
7.6 *The patellar tap.*

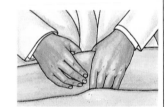
7.7 *Eliciting fluctuation.*

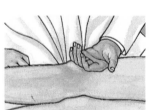
7.8 *Feeling for heat.*

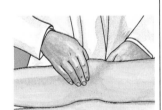
7.9

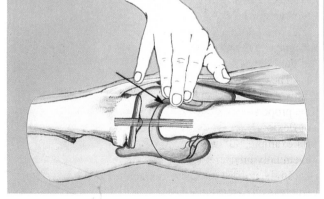
7.10

7.9 , 7.10 *Palpatating for a thickened synovial membrane*

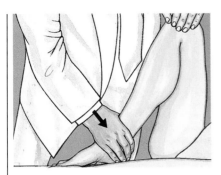

7.11 *Passive flexion.*

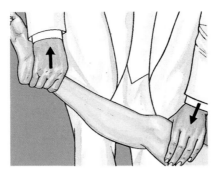

7.12 *Passive extension.*

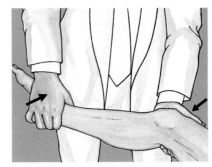

7.13 *Valgus strain. Note the knee is in extension.*

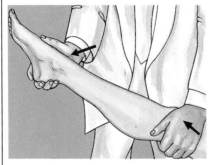

7.14 *Varus strain.*

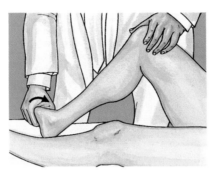

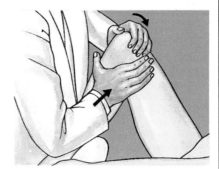

7.15, 7.16 *Passive lateral and medial rotations. Full rotation is not possible unless the knee is flexed, as extension tautens the ligaments.*

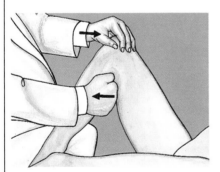

7.17 *Forwards shearing.*

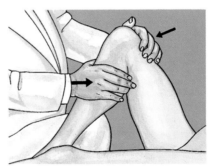

7.18 *Backwards shearing.*

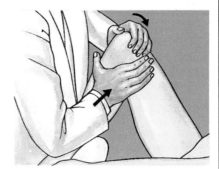

7.19 *Lateral shearing.*

Passive movements

Preliminary examination will, of course, have excluded the lumbar spine and hip as the source of pain.

First, the two primary passive movements of flexion (*Figure 7.11*) and extension (*Figure 7.12*) evaluate the state of the joint capsule.

The capsular pattern is greater limitation of flexion than of extension, with no restriction of either rotation (e.g. in the proportion of 5° limitation of extension, 70° limitation of flexion, both rotations full). It is only gross arthritis with, for example, 90° of limitation of flexion that may eventually interfere with the rotations.

In the normal joint, the end-feel on flexion is soft, whereas on extension it is fairly hard. Seven passive movements follow, testing the ligaments not only for pain but also for laxity. Pain indicates a sprain, and pain and laxity a severe strain. Painless laxity may denote a past

strain or, if it emerges as a major traumatic arthritis settles, a recent complete rupture. If abnormal laxity is detected by the systematic examination, a series of accessory tests are undertaken to ascertain whether surgical intervention is warranted.

Returning to the standard examination, first valgus strain (*Figure 7.13*) is applied with the joint in slight flexion, opening the inner side of the knee. Pain elicited by this test indicates a sprain of the medial collateral ligament, a frequent occurrence.

Varus strain (*Figure 7.14*) opens the outer side of the joint, testing the lateral collateral ligament, infrequently at fault.

Painful passive lateral rotation (*Figure 7.15*) incriminates the medial coronary ligament and is a secondary sign for the medial collateral ligament. Sprain to either coronary ligament is prone to occur in conjunction with damage to the relevant meniscus inflicted at the same time.

Passive medial rotation (*Figure 7.16*) is tested; pain on this movement suggests a lesion of the lateral coronary ligament.

Pain on forwards shearing implicates the anterior cruciate ligament; the knee is pushed away from, and the lower leg is pulled towards, the examiner who sits on the patient's forefoot to stabilize the leg (*Figure 7.17*).

However, the problem may arise of the patient using his hamstrings to protect the movement; Lachman's variation of this test positions the knee in 20° of flexion, thereby allowing the same anteroposterior glide but reducing anterior capsular tension.

Straining the tibia backwards on the femur (*Figure 7.18*) stretches the posterior cruciate ligament.

The tibia is pushed laterally on the femur (*Figure 7.19*). This is a secondary test for the posterior cruciate, although a cracked meniscus may be felt to subluxate momentarily.

Resisted movements

The patient lies on her stomach and four resisted movements assess the contractile structures.

Resisted flexion (*Figure 7.20*) tests the hamstrings. If this movement hurts, further tests establish from which member of the group the pain originates.

For resisted medial rotation (*Figure 7.21*) the patient attempts to turn her foot inwards. Pain on this movement, if accompanied by painful resisted flexion, suggests a lesion of the semimembranosus (rare), the semitendinosus or popliteus muscles (both very rare). But painful resisted lateral rotation (*Figure 7.22*), together with painful resisted flexion, shows the biceps to be at fault.

Resisted extension with the patient prone (*Figure 7.23*) tensions the quadriceps. If painless weakness is detected, a lesion of the nervous system, an L3 tumour, metastases, myopathy or myositis should be considered.

In conclusion the joint should be re-checked for possible warmth induced by the examination, a characteristic of an impacted loose body complicating osteoarthrosis.

In addition, since nearly all the relevant tissues lie superficially, palpation lends great accuracy to diagnosis and is thus conducted along the structure identified at fault by the clinical examination.

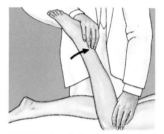

7.20 *Resisted flexion.*

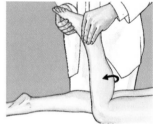

7.21 *Resisted medial rotation.*

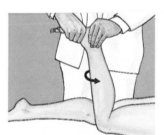

7.22 *Resisted lateral rotation*

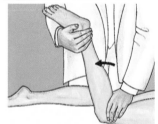

7.23 *Resisted extension.*

Findings

Capsular lesions

Capsular lesions are indicated by markedly more limitation of flexion than of extension (*Figure 7.24*). Except in advanced arthritis, both rotations remain free (*Figure 7.25*). The capsular pattern by itself indicates a capsular lesion, but if present in conjunction with other individual sign(s) designates a secondary traumatic arthritis.

The commonest primary capsular lesions are the inflammatory-type conditions signalled by warmth, fluid, synovial thickening and, in the earliest stages, full range. The patient complains of gradual onset of unprovoked swelling, at first painless. Then the knee starts to ache all over and in due course the capsular pattern supervenes but without any history of recent trauma. Pain and warmth are equal all over the joint.

Osteoarthritis is visible on the radiograph of nearly all middle-aged patients and of itself is often symptomless, although in advanced cases there may be constant aching; gross osteoarthrosis causes pain as soon as articular cartilage wears through. More likely, the cartilaginous attrition will result in one or more radiotranslucent loose bodies which may, if impacted, be manipulatively reduced (see page 105). Caution should thus be exercised against assuming the radiographic appearances are necessarily diagnostic of the condition of which the patient complains.

Fluid if aspirated is usually tested for cells, crystals and organisms.

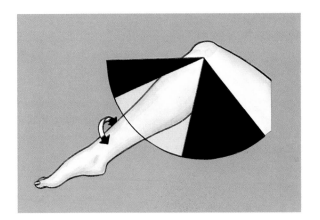

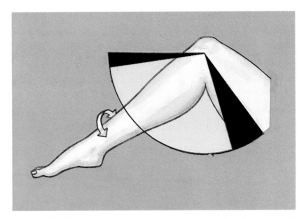

7.24, 7.25 *Capsular pattern in a severe case (top). In a mild case (bottom), note that the rotations remain free. The blocked areas denote the limitation of movement.*

Inflammatory arthropathies

For inflammatory arthropathies at any stage, the joint is injected. Two or three injections abolish the symptoms but do nothing to eliminate the cause; the treatment should therefore be repeated as the symptoms warrant, but sparingly, for fear of a steroid arthropathy.

The patient lies with her quadriceps relaxed and steroid suspension 2 ml without local anaesthetic is delivered into the joint. The point of insertion is just by the thumb where it is placed half-way down the edge of the patella (*Figure 7.26*) lifting it off the condyles.

This allows the 4 cm needle to slide in parallel to the posterior surface of the patella and the infiltration is made between the two condyles (*Figure 7.27*). Thereafter the patient should avoid weight-bearing for a day or so, and take things easy for two weeks. If no benefit results, a bolus of steroid can be introduced.

Inflammatory conditions
(1) Rheumatoid disease.
(2) Reactive arthritis.
(3) Seronegative arthritis and connective tissue disease.
(4) Gout.
(5) Crystal arthropathy.

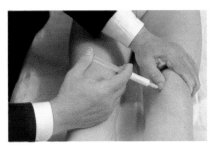

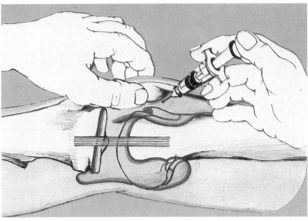

7.26, 7.27 *Injection, monarticular rheumatoid arthritis. The patient complains of gradual onset of unporvoked swelling; the injection must not be given more often than once every six months.*

Haemarthrosis

Intra-articular bleeding may be of either spontaneous or traumatic origin. The former occurs both in elderly patients, presumed to have suffered venous rupture, and haemophiliacs. Common traumatic causes are anterior cruciate rupture or sprain (some 70%), and direct contusion with or without fracture. Restriction of movement will in some cases total as much as 45° limitation of extension and 90° limitation of flexion.

The blood suddenly fills the capsule and in even a few minutes the joint can be distended to near bursting, a quite different progression from the slow effusion of capsular fluid.

Arthroscopic aspiration should take place as soon as possible with subsequent management depending on the lesion present; the aspirate is tested for cells, crystals and organisms.

Haemophiliacs must receive prior systemic attention.

Baker's cyst

This produces swelling in the upper calf in the absence of any injury; the patient complains of a sudden pain at the back of the knee and is discovered to have long-standing arthritis at the knee. The extravasation of fluid into the calf attendant on the bursting of a *large* Baker's cyst may seriously impede venous return, an outcome to be prevented by prior prophylactic aspiration (*Figure 7.28*).

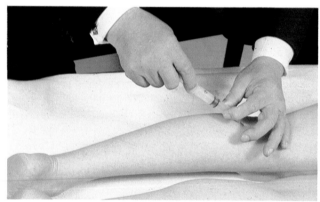

7.28 *A Baker's cyst impedes the venous return. A fluctuant swelling is aspirated via the calf, but if no fluctuation can be detected the fluid is tapped from the joint itself.*

Non-capsular lesions

Ligamentous lesions: general principles

Ligamentous sprains are very common, not least as sports injuries where twisting during weight-bearing gives rise to a meniscal tear that simultaneously involves one or more ligaments. If untreated, the sprains tend to follow a standard progression best exemplified by the medial collateral ligament. Treatment differs according to the stage reached.

Stage 1

A sprain to a ligament (*Figure 7.29, top*) is accompanied by a secondary traumatic arthritis for 1–2 weeks.

Stage 2

The traumatic arthritis has subsided. But the lesion must not be allowed to heal in immobility, otherwise small adhesions build up at the site of tear, binding ligament to bone (*Figure 7.29, centre*). This sub-acute phase lasts for a further 4–6 weeks.

Stage 3

The tear to the ligament has healed, but unless ruptured the adhesions now preclude full painless mobility indefinitely (*Figure 7.29, bottom*). In this chronic phase there are no symptoms on normal use but attempts at exertion are frustrated by recurrent pain and swelling.

Minor laxity following a sprain seldom causes appreciable disability in those with a sedentary lifestyle. For those who habitually stress the joint, the therapeutic possibilities are surgery (repair or reconstruction) or the provision of a brace. Surgical opinion should be sought.

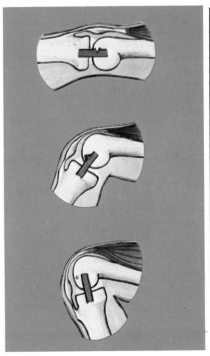

7.29 *After a sprain (top), adhesions may bind the ligament to bone (centre). If untreated, the adhesions will consolidate and must be ruptured (bottom).*

Treatment

Stages 1 and 2 (except the cruciates)

Massage is given, gently moving the ligament over bone to inhibit the formation of adhesions; any fibrils tethering the tissue to bone are disengaged without interfering with the union of normal longitudinal scar tissue.

Forcing the joint towards extension is strongly contraindicated, but after the first week or so the massage is given more strenuously and accompanied by gentle encouragement of movement.

Stage 3

Manipulative rupture of the adhesion is normally only necessary or feasible at the collateral ligaments; during this phase (two months plus after injury) it is the sole remedy.

The medial collateral ligament

Sprain of the medial collateral ligament ranks as the commonest ligamentous disorder in the entire body. The history is of a valgus strain with the pain and an acute traumatic arthritis (often making examination impossible) developing rapidly over some hours. At first the patient can walk, but within half-an-hour he can only hobble with assistance. The pain is localized to the inner side of the knee and although the lesion may lie at one of three sites (*Figure 7.30*), usually it is damaged at the point where it crosses the joint line and is attached to the medial meniscus.

Two weeks after injury the arthritis starts to abate and after three months (if untreated) the symptoms are of an ache following exertion. Except in this chronic stage (see below) the treatment is deep friction. The ligament is never injected with steroid suspension as laxity is apt to ensue.

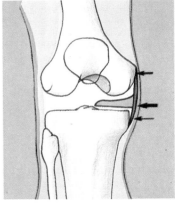

7.30 *The three sites. Unless the lesion is treated, dis-ability is so severe the patient spends some days in bed.*

The medial collateral ligament is first massaged in maximum comfortable flexion (*Figure 7.31*). Then massage is given in maximum comfortable extension (*Figure 7.32*). By the end of the session, increased flexion and extension will be attainable and the joint *must* be taken at least once to its new extremes of flexion and extension, but the latter must never be forced for fear of permanently elongating the ligament. The starting points for subsequent treatments are the new positions of maximum range.

Massage in flexion is administered to the site of the lesion with strong transverse pressure. The ligament lies roughly in line with the longitudinal axis of the tibia and accordingly the sweep of the fingers is diagonal rather than vertical (*Figure 7.33*).

For massage in extension the ligament is horizontal; the massage is thus straight up and down (*Figure 7.34*). The reader is referred to *Figure 7.29* showing the alignment of the medial collateral ligament for varying knee positions.

The treatments – lasting 20–30 minutes each – are given daily for the first few days and thereafter cut back to every other day. In the hyperacute stage the friction must be delivered with a light touch, only penetrating deeply to mobilize the ligament in the last half-minute. Full and painless range should be restored in one to two weeks.

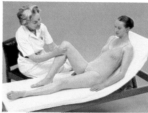
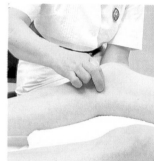

7.31 **7.32**

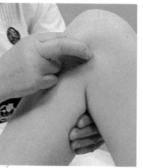
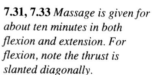

7.33 **7.34**

7.31, 7.33 *Massage is given for about ten minutes in both flexion and extension. For flexion, note the thrust is slanted diagonally.*

7.32, 7.34 *Massage in extension, vertical thrust. With such treatment, most patients get better in two weeks instead of three months.*

In the final stage, adhesions may be found to restrict any of the four passive knee movements, usually lateral rotation and/or flexion. Following deep friction these adhesions must be ruptured by a sharp low amplitude manipulation in the restricted direction. For example, with limitation of lateral rotation the patient half-lies with her knee in flexion (*Figure 7.35*) to eliminate any rotation at the hip. Lateral rotation of the tibia on the femur is forced using the foot as a lever (*Figure 7.36*); the movement is accentuated by an abrupt adduction of the operator's elbow. If medial rotation is also restricted, a thrust is given towards medial rotation (*Figure 7.37*). For the more common restriction of flexion, the thrust is towards flexion.

Further adhesion formation is prevented by instructing the patient to stretch the joint repeatedly into the previously restricted range.

If range of movement diminishes rather than increases despite treatment, Stieda–Pellegrini's disease (in which there is periosteal separation) may be to blame. The bony profileration is normally palpable and the condition shows clearly on the X-ray after a few weeks as a shadow along the whole inner side of the medial femoral condyle. Treatment is useless; recovery takes 6–12 months.

If the patient presents with symptoms of bruising *and* laxity (sometimes in the absence of pain), a complete rupture is suspected and surgical opinion with a view to repair is obligatory.

The lateral collateral ligament is seldom sprained and, although the knee is warm, with fluid, the range of movement is almost full.

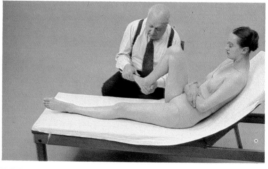

7.35 *Untreated adhesions cause pain after strenuous exertion. They must be ruptured.*

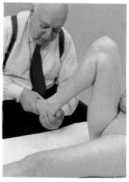
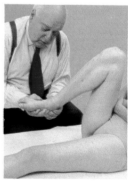

7.36 *The movement is a sharp thrust towards lateral rotation.*

7.37 *Forcing of medial rotation. The grip corsets the heel to avoid spraining the ankle.*

The coronary ligaments

These attach the two menisci to the circumference of the tibial plateau. Accordingly, a rotation strain may overstretch one of the coronaries with or without accompanying tear of the meniscus, depending on the severity of the stress. Unless treated, the sprain resolves slowly over a good 3 months.

The medial ligament *(Figure 7.38)* is more frequently damaged than the lateral. The appropriate passive rotation (i.e. lateral rotation for the medial ligament) will be uncomfortable as is sometimes passive extension; this shifts the meniscus which bulges out against the ligament. The pain and traumatic arthritis are less pronounced (e.g. 2° limitation of extension, 45–60° limitation of flexion) than for the medial collateral ligament. It is a common football injury.

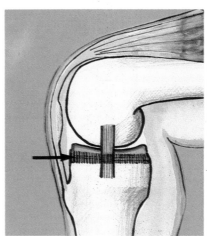

7.38 *The medial coronary ligament. If untreated, the sprain resolves slowly over a good three months.*

The medial coronary ligament

The lesion usually straddles the anteromedial quadrant of the joint line but may on occasion extend behind the medial collateral ligament. The precise location is sought by palpation for tenderness with the knee well bent.

Massage is highly effective and is the treatment whether the strain is acute, sub-acute or chronic. Sessions last 15–20 minutes daily for the first week and are given on alternate days thereafter. The knee is put into flexion *(Figure 7.39)* to open the joint anteriorly and lateral rotation further exposes the ligament.

The temptation is to press straight inwards towards the femur. This is wrong; it massages only bone.

The friction must be directed downwards *(Figure 7.40)* onto the tibial plateau. The tibial condyle is located from above, the superficial tissue indented and the pressure exerted onto the shelf afforded by the tibia. The finger is then pulled to and fro across the site of the sprain, with the index fingernail lying horizontally and uppermost.

However, if the lesion can be localized to the *deep* fibres of the overlying medial collateral ligament (comprising its attachment to cartilage), then 0.5 ml steroid suspension is highly effective.

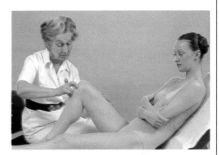
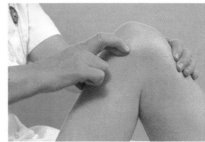

7.39, 7.40 *Massage, group and detail. This is the only treatment for the sprain, which is always traumatic. The fingers press distally on to the ligament, down the axis of the leg.*

The cruciate ligaments

Pain in the absence of laxity on straining the cruciates *(Figures 7.41* and *7.42)* responds to treatment by injection of 2 ml steroid suspension. Sprains here often occur in association with other lesions and may result from any one of a number of different directional stresses. The pain is described as 'right inside the joint'.

The knee is warm and swollen, fluid is present and although full range is possible, all the extremes hurt because the cruciates limit rotation as well as flexion and extension. The collateral and coronary ligaments are palpably normal. Involvement of the anterior cruciate ligament is apt to entail a haemarthrosis.

Spontaneous recovery takes 6–12 months. A single correctly placed injection leads to recovery in one or two weeks, but although it is possible to distinguish which ligament is involved, one cannot always tell at which end.

The tissues are too deep for palpation, so first one end and later, if need be, the other must be infiltrated. If one of the ligaments has become permanently elongated after a strain, the history simulates that of a ruptured meniscus, the knee appearing to 'go out' with a click.

If the finding is of anterior cruciate laxity coupled with weak hamstrings, then in order to enable the patient to regain control of the joint the quadriceps must be rehabilitated, whether by isometric, isokinetic or isotonic exercises, performed both prone and sitting. External support of the knee with a de-rotational brace may also be required. A common error with this syndrome is to work on the hamstrings and neglect the quadriceps.

In the event of rupture of the ligament itself, surgery may be considered, but the results have yet to be fully evaluated.

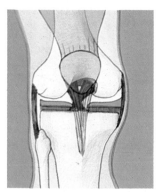

7.41 *The anterior cruciate ligament runs downwards and forwards from the medial surface of the lateral condyle.*

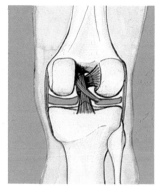

7.42 *The posterior cruciate has two bundles, both running backwards and downwards from the lateral surface of the medial condyle.*

Posterior ligament: posterior end

The posterior ligament is the more commonly injured; the lesion is marked by pain on backwards shearing. Steroid suspension 2 ml is injected (*Figure 7.43*) at the site centred across the exact mid-point of the tibia. With experience the operator can judge the optimum point of entry and aim the needle straight at the tibial attachment.

The crux of the matter is to bypass the popliteal vessels which overlie the lesion. The easiest approach is using one thumb to locate the apex of the lateral condyle (*Figure 7.44*); the 5 cm needle is inserted just there and inclined at about 60° to the horizontal. It thus passes well under the popliteal vessels and heads distally towards the centre of the posterior aspect of the tibia (*Figure 7.45*).

The angle of entry is then progressively modified until the needle eases into the joint. This is just too far and the tip is returned to the previous position (*Figure 7.46*) and the injection given after the point is felt to penetrate the ligament before hitting bone. A series of tiny insertions and withdrawals is made.

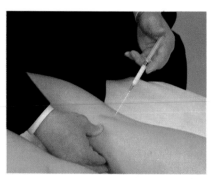

7.43 *Injection, left knee. The posterior end is the more often affected.*

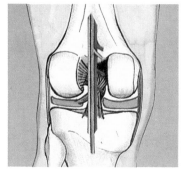

7.44 *The thumb locates the lateral condyle.*

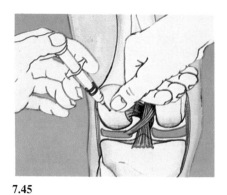

7.45

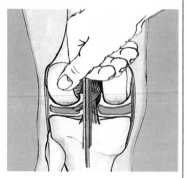

7.46

7.45, 7.46 *This lateral approach avoids the popliteals (shown right) which overlie the lesion.*

Posterior ligament: anterior end

For injection to the anterior end of the posterior cruciate the patient lies supine with her leg extended. The site of the lesion is masked by the patella (*Figure 7.47*).

One hand tilts the patella, lifting it off the femoral condyle. The 6 cm needle is inserted at the patellar margin and enters parallel to the articular surfaces (*Figure 7.48*).

When the needle strikes the lateral aspect of the medial femoral condyle, its position is adjusted until ligamentous resistance is felt. The injection is then made by a series of tiny withdrawals and reinsertions.

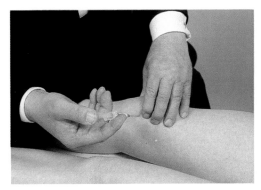

7.47 *Injection, right knee. The free hand raises the patella.*

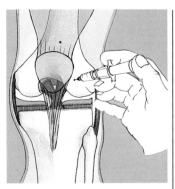

7.48 *The injection obviates months of traumatic arthritis. The site of delivery is marked red.*

Anterior ligament: anterior end

Involvement of the anterior cruciate is marked by pain on forwards shearing. The injection to the anterior end of the anterior cruciate is simplicity itself. The patient flexes her knee to a right-angle and the 5 cm needle pierces the skin immediately below the lower edge of the patella at a slant of about 45° (*Figure 7.49*).

It is aimed for the spine of the tibia; the tip penetrates a resilient tissue – the ligament – before hitting bone (*Figure 7.50*). The infiltration is made as before by a series of tiny withdrawals and reinsertions.

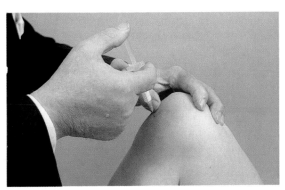

7.49 *Injection, anterior ligament, left knee. Hyperextension can cause the sprain.*

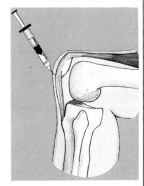

7.50 *Injection is effective whether the sprain has lasted days or years. Delivery site marked red.*

Anterior cruciate: posterior end

The technique mirrors the method for the posterior end of the posterior cruciate, in that the popliteal vessels must be negotiated. But the approach is from the medial side aiming slightly proximally. This time the apex of the medial condyle is identified (*Figure 7.51*) and the needle punctures the skin at an angle about half-way between the horizontal and the vertical. The tip is directed towards the medial surface of the lateral condyle and ligamentous resistance is encountered before reaching bone (*Figure 7.52*). Delivery consists of a series of withdrawals and reinsertions along the line of origin.

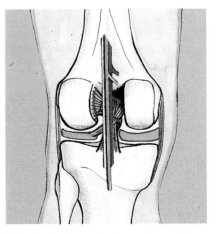

7.51 *Again the popliteal vessels mask the lesion. Left leg shown. Delivery site marked red.*

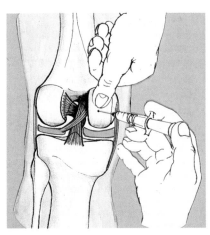

7.52 *The needle passes well posterior to the danger area. The leg is in extension.*

Displacements

The knee has a marked predilection for internal displacements, which fall readily into three categories: menisci, loose bodies and the patella.

Loose bodies can occur either secondary to osteoarthrosis (see page 105) or, in a younger age group, secondary to osteochondrosis dissecans, chondromalacia patellae or a chip fracture.

Their common history is of momentary self-unlocking fixation in extension (as opposed to flexion). The loose bodies possess an osseous nucleus which may or may not be visible radiographically.

The meniscus

The medial meniscus is the less mobile of the two (with a play of only 2mm as against 10mm for the lateral) and consequently more frequently injured. Immediate disabling pain with a click follows a rotation strain during weight-bearing and the joint locks in some 10° of flexion so the patient is incapable of putting her heel to the ground. Secondary effusion occurs.

Recurrent meniscal dislocation nearly always requires excision, particularly since the frequent traumas are prone to set up intractable osteoarthrosis, troublesome by middle age. A strain severe enough to tear the meniscus will most likely have sprained the appropriate coronary ligament as well which will need treatment by deep transverse friction.

A cyst of the lateral meniscus has a history deceptively similar to that of a ruptured meniscus. But then the knee never actually locks and on full extension a small hard bulge is palpable at the joint line. The treatment is to vent the meniscus by puncturing it in a number of different directions with a needle; this liberates the fluid and may result in cure. Surgery is the remaining option.

The short-term treatment for a torn meniscus is manipulative reduction (*Figure 7.53*) followed by consideration of removal if the condition recurs. For the medial meniscus, the medial side of the joint is opened by a valgus strain (*Figure 7.54*), maintained while the knee is being extended (*Figure 7.55*) at the same time as the tibia is repeatedly rotated. The foot is wielded as a lever. At the last moment a further thrust is given towards valgus and extension.

The patient is re-examined after each manipulation and the process repeated until full range is restored; reduction is attended by a click. General anaesthesia is normally desirable.

For the lateral meniscus, varus strain is applied. If internal derangement is not present at the time the patient is seen, the examiner may be able to reproduce the tell-tale click by rotating – or applying a shearing strain to – the knee. The history is also suggestive.

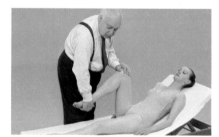

7.53

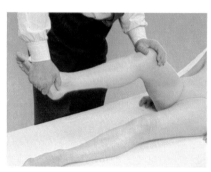

7.54

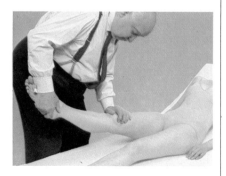

7.55

7.53, 7.54, 7.55 *Manipulative reduction of a subluxated medial meniscus. The fragment must be shifted medially, since it displaces centrally – hence the valgus strain maintained throughout during the extension. The coronary ligament may also require treatment.*

A loose body in the middle-aged or elderly

Initially this condition may resemble rheumatoid arthritis as both warmth and fluid are present.

However, with a loose body the warmth and pain are localized, synovial thickening is absent, the onset is sudden and during attacks the patient complains of twinges and of the knee giving way, especially while walking downstairs. There may be pain-free periods for anything up to years at a time.

Loose body formation is a frequent product of otherwise symptomless osteoarthritic degeneration. This pathology should always be taken into account where a middle-aged patient experiences localized pain in the knee with no history of trauma.

As well as causing twinges and blocking the joint, the loose fragment may momentarily impact under the medial collateral ligament (which is often tender to the touch) from *inside* the joint. Hence valgus strain may prove painful. But no *extrinsic* strain will be reflected in the history – hence its characterization as a 'sprain without a strain' – and a springy end-feel will be felt on either flexion or extension. Limitation of range and degree of discomfort vary with the size and position of the loose fragment, but often full extension is affected and flexion is limited by 5–10°.

Manipulative reduction abolishes the symptoms. There are four techniques. If necessary each is tried several times, the patient being re-examined after each attempt. If one method does not succeed, the operator goes on to the next. Following complete reduction, the patient should be warned that recurrence within a year or two is not unlikely. Avoidance of flexion as far as possible should help forestall relapse but, if it occurs, the patient must attend again.

A large number of small loose bodies formed as a result of attrition of the articular cartilage may produce debris which is best treated by arthroscopic washout.

Manipulation – 1

The operator hooks the patient's foot over his knee and pulls upwards (*Figure 7.56*) while an assistant presses heavily downwards on the thigh to open the joint (*Figure 7.57*). The distracting force is maintained as the operator removes his foot from the couch and then smartly extends and repeatedly rotates the knee using the foot as a lever (*Figures 7.58* and *7.59*). The patient is re-examined and the procedure repeated as necessary, probably several times in a single session.

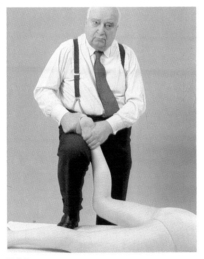

7.56

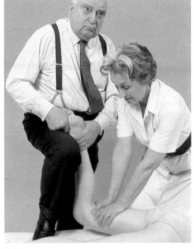

7.57

7.56–7.59 Manipulative reduction, a loose body. The intention is to move the fragment posteriorly from its position between the articulating surfaces. The assistant presses down for some seconds before the manipulation to allow the tibia and femur to come apart. Note how by the final photograph the manipulator has moved right down the couch.

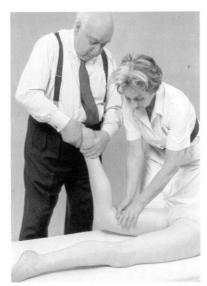

7.58

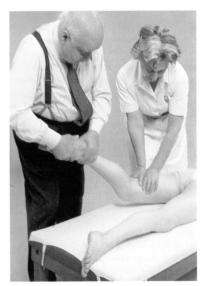

7.59

Manipulation – 2

If flexion remains limited, the next method to try is rocking the tibia on the femur; the movement derives purchase from the fulcrum of an assistant's forearm placed in the popliteal space (*Figure 7.60*).

The anterior movement of the tibia is obtained by jerking the knee strongly towards flexion while simultaneously forcing rotation (*Figure 7.61*); on the beat of the over-pressure the knee is released to let the tibia snap back.

The patient is re-examined and the manipulation repeated as appropriate. For both this and the succeeding variant it is imperative to check that, as flexion eases, the range of extension (the more important movement) does not decrease. If so, these techniques are abandoned immediately and, where necessary, the operator resorts to the first manipulation to re-establish the original range.

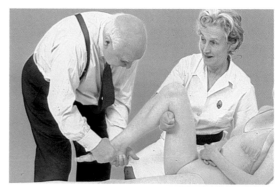
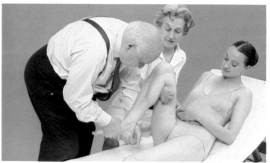

7.60, 7.61 *Flexion during rotation, starting and finishing positions. The foot is repeatedly rotated with a final overthrust towards lateral rotation. A click may be felt, flexion suddenly becoming free.*

Manipulation – 3

The same manipulation is possible when working single-handed; the manoeuvre is as before but omits the rotation – only flexion is forced (*Figures 7.62* and *7.63*).

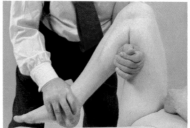
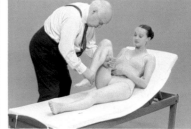

7.62, 7.63 *Rocking the tibia without rotation, starting and finishing positions.*

Manipulation – 4

There is one other method if pain on full extension persists. The patient half-lies, with her leg in slight flexion, and the operator applies varus pressure (*Figure 7.64*).

While this is maintained, the subject co-operates actively by extending her knee. At the last moment a small jerk encourages full extension (*Figure 7.65*). The patient is re-examined and the procedure repeated as necessary.

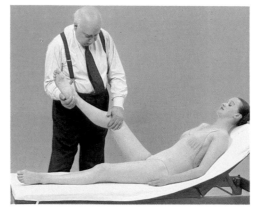
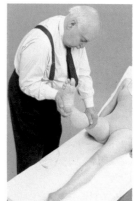

7.64, 7.65 *Full extension can usually be rendered painless provided varus pressure is maintained.*

Contractile structures

The two main groups are the hamstrings posteriorly and the quadriceps anteriorly. Both can be strained at either end.

The extensor mechanism

Painful resisted extension may stem from a lesion of the rectus femoris (at its origin at the anterior inferior spine), the quadriceps belly, the quadriceps expansions, the suprapatellar or the infrapatellar tendon. The last two respond to both massage and injection.

With the exception of the rectus femoris (see page 89) and the quadriceps bellies, they share a history of pain at the front of the knee on walking, climbing the stairs or squatting, with the joint normal. Only resisted extension hurts and palpation reveals the site of the lesion around the patella. In all three cases the massage is angled so that the supinated fingers reach beneath the patella and catch the affected fibres against the edge of the bone.

The patient is frequently an athlete, dancer or one-legged, as amputees put extra strain on the residual leg. Untreated, these conditions may persist for years. Such a history is by no means uncommon and no bar to successful treatment.

An habitual error is to misdiagnose chondromalacia patellae when in fact the trouble is a tendinous lesion around the patella. If resisted extension hurts, the cause is tendinous although, conversely, painless resisted extension does not always exclude a tendinous lesion. Palpation will assist, the more so since chondromalacia patellae should not give rise to localized tenderness.

The quadriceps are most often injured at their insertions; for the site at the anterior inferior spine (see page 89). At the belly, the patient feels something give way at the front of the thigh and afterwards walks slowly with a limp.

Lesions associated with the extensor mechanism

(1) Quadriceps mechanism.
(2) Chondromalacia patellae.
(3) Patellofemoral arthrosis
(4) Osgood–Schlatter's epiphysitis.
(5) Recurrent dislocation.

The suprapatellar tendon

The lesion is found at the insertion of the tendon into the superior border of the patella.

The patient relaxes her quadriceps. For the injection of steroid suspension 2 ml (2 cm needle) one hand presses downwards on the lower pole of the patella (*Figure 7.66*). This tilts the upper border of the patella upwards, tautening the tendon and raising the lesion into prominence. The point of entry is through a spot 1.5 cm proximal to the lesion (*Figure 7.67*). The infiltration is not made until the tip of the needle touches bone whereupon the entire affected area is injected by a series of half-withdrawals and reinsertions. For two days there are painful after-effects and the injection may have to be repeated.

The principles of massage are not dissimilar. The web of one hand presses down on the lower edge of the patella while transverse friction is administered by the other hand in supination.

The pressure is angled distally and anteriorly to catch the fibres against the upper pole of the patella (*Figure 7.68*). The hand must not be held in pronation pressing downwards only; this rubs the wrong part of the tendon (*Figure 7.69*). The massage is very tiring and is given for 20 minutes on alternate days with recovery in under a month.

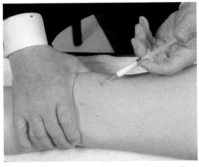 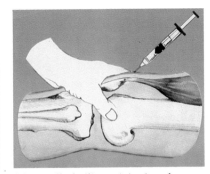

7.66, 7.67 *Pressing down on the distal end of the patella facilitates injection along the tenoperiosteal junction.*

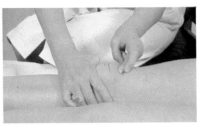 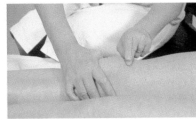

7.68 *Massage, correct. Sprain is usually due to sudden over-contraction of the quadriceps.*

7.69 *Massage, incorrect. The angulation of pressure is wrong, being downwards instead of distally.*

The infrapatellar tendon

Strain of the infrapatellar tendon is commoner than that of the suprapatellar. The clinician palpates the tenoperiosteal junction (*Figure 7.70*) as the tibial extremity of the tendon is rarely at fault (except in Osgood–Schlatter's epiphysitis).

The patient relaxes her quadriceps. Alteration in the angle of the patella is again achieved by downwards pressure of the operator's free hand, but this time it is brought to bear on the upper edge of the patella thus swinging the lower edge upwards. The needle is inserted about 1.5 cm inferior to the mid-point of the tender area (*Figure 7.71*).

When the tip touches bone, a sequence of droplets is distributed fanwise along the tender area – the patient will be sore for two days. Up to three injections may be required, since it is easy to omit some small extent of the lesion.

For massage the free hand tilts the patella while the operative finger, reinforced by its neighbour, presses hard upwards against the tenoperiosteal junction (*Figure 7.72*). The hand is in supination and the whole arm moves to and fro; sessions last about 20 minutes on alternate days and recovery takes anywhere between two and six weeks.

Where there is failure to progress or infrapatellar cysts are suspected, CT scanning or diagnostic ultrasound should be considered.

On occasions an extra-articular fat-pad may become sore from long-distance running or pronounced knee exercise. Capsular and intra-articular signs will be absent; the symptom is tenderness to palpation on both sides of the patella. The condition responds to injection of steroid suspension or ultrasound.

The underlying tibial tubercle bursa may become inflamed (commonly with athletes) and may require steroid injection. MRI scanning will display.

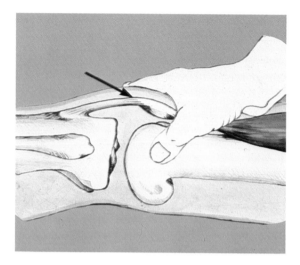

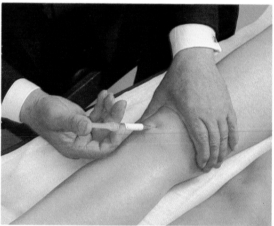

7.70, 7.71 *Injection. The patella is tilted to tauten the tendon, thus facilitating infiltration of the tender extent.*

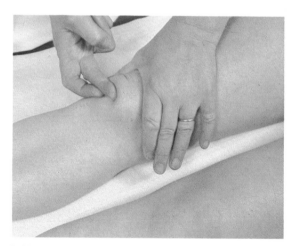

7.72 *Massage. Permanent relief within three weeks is the rule for recent cases.*

The quadriceps expansion

The lesion may lie either side of the patella at the junction between the patella and the expansion (*Figure 7.73*).

The only effective treatment is massage for two to three weeks on alternate days. The first step is for the operator to push the patella towards the affected side using the thumb. This allows the operative finger of the other hand to wedge itself right under the now projecting edge; the hand is held in supination (*Figure 7.74*). The pressure is directed upwards so that the fibres are massaged against the posterior surface of the patella by drawing the finger back and forth.

The quadriceps mechanism also suffers from a number of surgical disorders. Recurrent dislocation of the patella afflicts children aged 8–15; the knee gives way suddenly, painfully and repeatedly.

Patellofemoral arthrosis produces an anterior ache coming on after walking, with pronounced crepitus on weight-bearing.

In young patients the cause – in the absence of trauma – may be chondromalacia patellae, which in turn is often associated with a minor incongruity, for example valgus deformity or dysplasia of the lateral condyle. However, the finding of crepitus should not preclude palpation for tenderness at the attachments of the patellar tendon and retinaculae. Lesions at any of these sites commonly prove to be the cause of pain in crepitating joints – even (perversely) in the absence of pain on resisted extension.

Complete rupture of the belly of the rectus femoris may occur, as can fixation of the muscle at the point of fracture at the lower end of the femur.

The flexor mechanism

The main flexors of the knee consist of the hamstring muscles. These are the semimembranosus and semi-tendinosus (which are also medial rotators), and the biceps femoris which is also a lateral rotator. The popliteus is a very weak knee flexor, its main function being to initiate flexion by unlocking the extended joint with medial rotation.

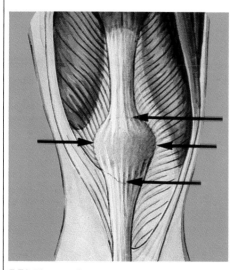

7.73 *The sites lie around the periphery of the patella. Sometimes a direct blow rather than overuse is the cause.*

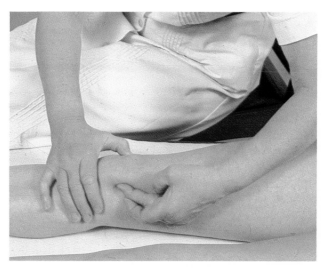

7.74 *Massage. The pressure is straight upwards against the back of the projecting edge of the patella. Recent cases may be better within the week.*

The hamstrings

Pain on resisted flexion points to a lesion of the hamstrings which may be injured at any one of a number of sites (*Figure 7.75*); for the ischial origin and bellies, see page 89. A severe lesion in the latter will also limit straight-leg raise.

Occasionally, painful resisted knee flexion is attributable to a lesion of the popliteus tendon or of the posterior cruciate ligament or even of the upper tibiofibular joint. In these three cases, the pain on resisted flexion is only elicited when the knee is in 90° flexion.

If lateral rotation hurts in addition to flexion, the sensitive area will be discovered in the bicipital tendon near its insertion at the head of the fibula. Painful resisted medial rotation probably indicates a lesion of the semimembranosus tendon as it passes across the head of the tibia; although this condition is rare, it is commonly overlooked. The likely candidate is an athlete running with an externally rotated foot and increased pronation. Massage is the treatment of choice, although the lesion at the semimembranosus site may also respond to injection.

A lesion of the popliteal muscles (rare) can be cleared up either by massage or by infiltration of steroid suspension 1 ml at the tendinous origin. At the belly, only massage works. Both resisted flexion and resisted medial rotation hurt.

Very occasionally a lesion at the upper extent of the gastrocnemius will account for posterior knee pain. But although in this case resisted flexion will be painful, the rotations are painless and rising on tiptoe painful (see page 112).

Lesions at the bellies of the gastrocnemius behind the knee respond to massage. Weakness of the hamstrings coupled with anterior cruciate laxity calls for rehabilitation of the hamstrings.

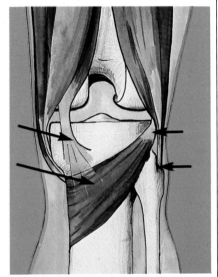

7.75 *The sites. Palpation may be necessary to differentiate between the popliteus (top right and bottom left) and the semimembranosus (top left), since both hurt on resisted medial rotation. The biceps (bottom right) hurts on resisted lateral rotation.*

Frictional inflammation of the iliotibial tract

Over-use may result in inflammation of the iliotibial tract's deep surface where it overlies the lateral epicondyle of the femur. The patient, normally a long-distance runner, complains of a burning or stabbing pain at the lateral aspect of the knee whenever he runs, sufficiently intense to make him desist. As long as running is avoided (in all but the most severe of cases) the knee is asymptomatic, although occasionally inspection reveals a warm swelling over the lateral epicondyle.

Resisted hip abduction proves painful. Alternatively, the standing patient adducts the affected limb behind the other and bends the trunk away from the painful side, thus stretching the affected structure whilst working it eccentrically.

The joint may demonstrate a painful arc between 30° and 50° of flexion as the tract slips posteriorly over the epicondyle, but may equally well prove wholly negative. The history and dearth of findings on examination will lead the clinician to perform an accessory test: active flexion at the knee while digital pressure is maintained over the epicondyle. Reproduction of a painful arc is diagnostic.

Treatment is by friction, hydrocortisone phonophoresis (or occasionally surgery). The knee is fully flexed and laterally rotated to expose the epicondyle and this site treated daily until the condition subsides. More than three weeks' treatment is seldom required and the minor recurrencies which sometimes occur are quickly abolished in the same way, assisted by orthotics if necessary.

Anterior knee-pain syndrome

The normal patella tracks between the femoral condyles. Distortion of this mechanism may cause pain, possibly in association with a disuse fibrillation of the medial patellar facets.

A subluxating patella can also be involved, in which case an apprehension test should prove positive.

Mechanisms that alter tracking
(1) Short leg: (i) anatomical; (b) functional (e.g. camber running).
(2) Over-pronation of foot/short calf muscles.
(3) Tibial torsion.
(4) Genu valgus.
(5) Anteversion of hip.
(6) Female pelvis.
(7) Dysplasia of the lateral condyle.

All the above increase the Q angle – the angle pertaining between the femur and the tibia – by moving the tibia to valgus. The Q angle can be decreased by:

(1) Supination of foot.
(2) Genu varus.

Either way, the treatment is to return the patella's tracking to normal by orthotics, exercises to the vastus medialis obliquus and exercises to the entire extensor mechanism with strapping to hold the patella medially. Over-training should be avoided.

CHAPTER EIGHT

THE LEG

Conditions affecting the leg are simple and diagnosis easy. The lesions most frequently encountered are muscular, routinely tested for by resisted movements, although tight fascial compartments and stress fractures should not be forgotten in athletes.

Referral of pain from local structures is minimal, as they lie superficially and near the distal end of the dermatome.

The usual cause of referred pain in the calf is a fifth lumbar disc lesion compressing the first and/or second sacral nerve. Pain of dural origin below the knee crops up from time to time. Clearly, resisted movements of the leg muscles will not affect pain levels from spinal disorders, but may reveal painless weakness from nerve foot conduction loss.

Examination

Examination begins with inspection for deformity, bruising, a ruptured tendon or loss of muscle mass.

Resisted movements

The patient stands on tiptoe, first on one leg and then the other (*Figure 8.1*). This tests both the ankle plantiflexors: the gastrocnemius and the soleus. The finding may be of painless weakness (L5 conduction loss), pain and weakness (a ruptured muscle or tendon) or pain alone (a muscular lesion).

The four resisted movements then assess the contractile structures. Resisted dorsiflexion (*Figure 8.2*) puts strain on the tibialis anterior.

Resisted plantiflexion (*Figure 8.3*) again tests both the soleus and the gastrocnemius.

Resisted inversion (*Figure 8.4*) puts strain on the tibialis posterior.

Resisted eversion (*Figure 8.5*) tests the peronei.

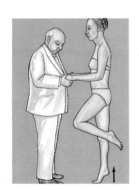

8.1 Repeatedly rising on tiptoe, the most potent test for plantiflexion.

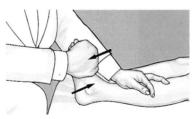

8.2 Resisted dorsiflexion.

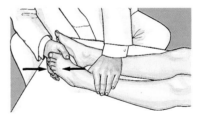

8.3 Resisted plantiflexion.

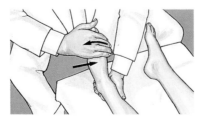

8.4 Resisted inversion.

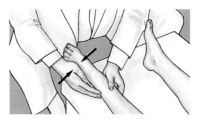

8.5 Resisted eversion.

Findings

The plantiflexors
'Tennis leg'

Sprain of the gastrocnemius ('tennis leg') is the commonest muscle lesion in the leg. Pain on resisted plantiflexion puts strain on both the gastrocnemius and the soleus. But they can be distinguished by resisted plantiflexion with the knee flexed. This excludes the gastrocnemius, so pain on resisted plantiflexion which disappears on knee flexion is a sure sign.

The patient reports a sudden severe twinge at mid-calf with pain on walking ever since. It emerges that although dorsiflexion with the knee extended is limited by muscular spasm, full range is attainable merely by flexing the knee to a right angle. The lesion is substantial and normally lies in the muscle about 5 cm above the musculotendinous junction; the exact spot is tricky to find, but in severe cases a gap as much as 1 cm wide is palpable. Treatment consists of three co-ordinated measures: local anaesthesia, massage and a raised heel.

Whether the patient is seen on the day of injury or some days later, local anaesthesia is immediately induced at the site of rupture (*Figure 8.6*) with a solution of 0.5% procaine 20 ml. Following injection the patient actively mobilizes the muscle for a quarter of an hour or so. These active exercises continue daily until recovery.

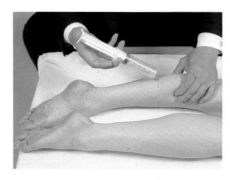

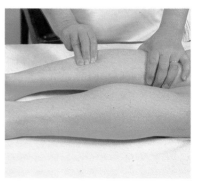

8.6 *Often the site can only be located approximately; thus 50 ml local anaesthetic is advisable.*

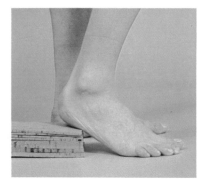

8.7, 8.8 *The muscle is shortened by spasm: a cork support inside the shoe is needed temporarily. The next day, massage is given; in recent cases, recovery should take about 10 days.*

Bruising and bleeding in the first 48 hours should be controlled by compressive support and elevation. Rates of healing can be improved initially by ultrasound and laser, but the control of scar tissue adhesion is best maintained by frictional massage commencing the day after the injection and continuing daily for three days, thereafter reduced to alternate days. Sessions last 20 minutes.

The fingers are placed on the affected area and the friction imparted by drawing the hand to and fro horizontally (*Figure 8.7*). In chronic cases, relief may take up to a month.

Meanwhile, a heel-raise is fitted to the inside of the shoe to compensate for the limitation of dorsiflexion (*Figure 8.8*). The support enables the patient to use the unaffected part of the muscle without straining the healing breach, and is lowered daily as range returns. It may be discarded at the end of a week or 10 days.

Short plantiflexor muscles

Plantiflexor muscles of inadequate length are indicated by painless limitation of dorsiflexion to about 90°. A number of conditions may result:

(1) Excessive range of movement at the mid-tarsal joint (see page 133). Since the ankle itself cannot be fully dorsiflexed, the patient transfers this movement to the adjacent joint. Normally, pain results only in middle age and the patient may not present until then. But if the patient is five or under, the calf muscles can be stretched.

(2) Eversion of the tibia. This deformity allows the patient to put her heel to the ground, but the eversion means with each forward step less distance is covered since disproportionate width, not the length, of the foot is employed for forward motion and the normal toe 'push off' is lost.

Accordingly, the patient is often a very poor runner at school and has an awkward gait.

There is no pain. If circumstances warrant, particularly in the young, osteoclasis of the tibia is carried out and the bone reset with the foot straight. A raised heel may be provided if necessary.

(3) Metatarsalgia. In this condition the patient cannot rest her heel on the ground, so the whole body weight is transferred to the forefoot. Pain on weight-bearing results and the patient commonly complains of pain/fatigue on standing, even for short periods. Symptoms generally do not appear until the patient is over 20 and often follow a period of rest in bed sufficiently long for the short flexor muscles to weaken. A raised heel is required.

(4) Plantar fasciitis (see page 132).

The tendo Achillis

The pain is at the back of the heel. Standing on tiptoe hurts. Resisted plantiflexion is normally the only other painful movement, but passive dorsiflexion may be uncomfortable. There is no limitation and the condition is often correctly diagnosed by the patient.

Although the lesion is usually at the narrowest part of the structure, it must be ascertained which aspects are affected. Often both sides as well as the anterior surface are involved. If so, all three must be treated. The posterior surface is never at fault (*Figure 8.9*). As a rule, acute strains respond well to therapy.

The injury can affect just the paratenon or, in more severe cases, go on to involve the tendon itself. The former has a history of stiffness and pain in the morning and after rest, improved by exercise; the condition is primarily an inflammatory response with fibrosis and thus responds well to either massage or injection.

The latter – the tendinopathy – has a history of pain with exercise and shows histological degenerative changes. Neither steroids nor physiotherapy are of much assistance.

However, as most lesions are combined, the treatment is directed towards controlling the paratenon and rehabilitation of the tendon through increased graduated exercises. It may be that magnetic resonance imaging has a role to play in accurate diagnosis of the affected tissues.

Massage is the treatment of choice. Sessions last 20 minutes on alternate days, with a three-week recovery in appropriate cases. For the lateral and medial aspects of the tendon the patient's foot projects over the edge of the couch and dorsiflexion is maintained by the operator's knee (*Figure 8.10*); this keeps the tendon on the stretch. The tendo Achillis is then squeezed firmly between finger and thumb, and friction imparted simultaneously to both sides by drawing the hand up and down (*Figure 8.11*). It is

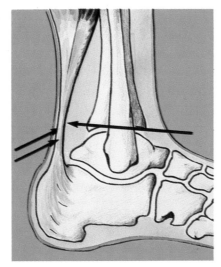
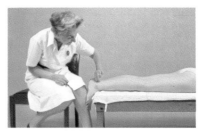
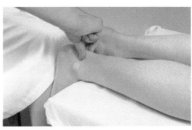

8.9 *Any aspect apart from the posterior surface may be involved; treatment must reach every affected portion. After-care includes close attention to footwear and gait.*

8.10, 8.11 *Massage to the lateral and medial aspects. Note the foot is clamped in dorsiflexion. Recovery after friction is nearly always permanent, but the patient should walk as little as possible until well.*

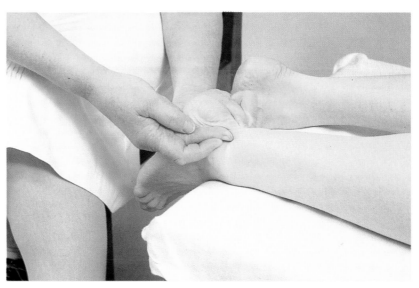

8.12 *Massage to the anterior aspect is only practicable if the tendon is pushed sideways with the free hand. The massage is rotary with upwards pressure.*

hard work and the operator may wish to change hands mid-session.

For the anterior aspect, the foot is fully plantiflexed to relax the tendon so it can be pushed sideways by the free hand. This brings the anterior surface within reach of the operator's supinated fingers.

Friction is delivered by supination and pronation of the forearm with upwards pressure maintained by elbow flexion (*Figure 8.12*). The finger, hand and forearm are held in line with the patient's lower leg.

Injection of steroid suspension 2 ml is effective but relapse often occurs. Massage is to be preferred, particularly for athletes or if the lesion is extensive. Infiltrating the anterior aspect of the tendon is difficult if not impossible.

The patient lies prone with her foot dorsiflexed. The needle (5 cm) is inserted almost horizontally some 3 cm distal to the lesion and the tip is pushed forwards to the proximal edge of the lesion. The needle runs parallel to the tendon along its surface (*Figure 8.13*). The *substance* of the tendon must never be injected since the steroid has no therapeutic effect on the pathology and may cause weakening for approximately three weeks. Steroid suspension 0.5 ml is delivered to the paratenon along the surface of the tendon as the needle is drawn back to the near edge of the lesion. Three or four more lines of fluid are injected in the same way until the entire solution is exhausted (*Figure 8.14*). Sero-negative peritendinitis also benefits from this treatment.

Although small strains normally respond permanently, the less localized lesions arising from over-use, often associated with diffuse swelling and crepitus, have a strong tendency to recurrence since the underlying tendon is damaged. An alternative to injection, particularly with the larger diffuse lesions, is hydrocortisone phono-phoresis. Clinical experience suggests that steroid administered by this means cannot penetrate structures as dense as

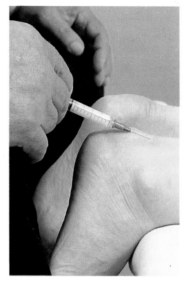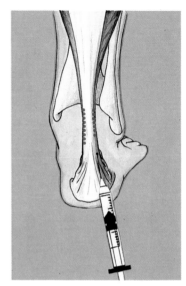

8.13, 8.14 *Relapse may follow even successful injection. Steroid is introduced in lines along the tendon's lateral surfaces.*

the Achillis itself and accordingly is deposited on the paratenon.

A heel-raise in the initial stages of inflammation reduces the stretch on the healing tendon, thus allowing firm union which must later be stretched up to its full functional length. The support should also lift the affected part away from the rear shoe-rim against which it would otherwise impinge during plantiflexion.

Other aggravating factors must be

minimized. Inappropriate footwear (e.g. heel-tags, hard heels) dig into the tendon. Collapsed or weakened heel-cups and longitudinal arch supports allow excessive pronation and detrimentally increase lateral 'bowing' of the tendon.

Training into fatigue – e.g. too many repetition sprints – causes dislocation between the quadriceps and the calf muscles and hence strains of the tendo Achillis.

Plantiflexors: other findings

Rupture of the tendo Achillis results in gross weakness on resisted plantiflexion coupled with excessive range or dorsiflexion. Active plantiflexion is just possible but, on prone-lying, the injured foot hangs vertically while the normal foot has a plantiflexed attitude. This relationship

may be better displayed with the prone knees bent to a right angle, when the damaged foot again lies horizontally while the normal one is in slight plantiflexion.

If rupture is complete, there will be no plantiflexion when the calf muscle is squeezed ('the calf-squeeze test').

Treatment consists of operative suture and is only beneficial during the first 10 days; thereafter spontaneous healing occurs, but only gradually, leaving permanent discomfort which should be controlled with plantiflexed plaster of Paris.

Intermittent claudication

Owing to the exceptional arrangement of its nutrient arteries, the gastrocnemius muscle is particularly susceptible to ischaemia as the result of arteriosclerosis. The history is characteristic. An elderly patient relates that pain in one calf is brought

on by walking a short distance and relieved by rest; repeated and rapid dorsiflexion and plantiflexion evoke the pain. The condition must not be confused with spinal claudication or the 'mushroom phenomenon' (see page 206) and may also be mimicked

by the compartment syndrome (see page 117).

Provided the lesion does not lie at or distal to the popliteal bifurcation, the treatment of choice is the restoration of a patent artery by surgery.

The evertor muscles

The peronei

Painful resisted eversion of the foot indicates that the peroneal muscles are at fault. The site of tenderness defines the position of the lesion which is seldom localized enough for steroid infiltration. The cause is either over-use or a single strain often occurring concurrently with a sprained ankle (see page 122) and persisting after the ankle has healed. There are four sites, one at the musculotendinous junction and three on the tendon – above, at and below the malleolus (*Figure 8.15*). As the lesion is seldom sufficiently localized for injection, the treatment of choice is massage, with the foot held in inversion to stretch the tendons.

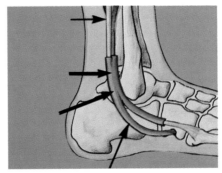

8.15 *The four sites. The thick arrows point to the commonest locations. The lesion is seldom localized enough for an injection of steroid.*

The technique varies with the site of the lesion. At the upper site only one finger is used, reinforced if need be (*Figure 8.16*). Above the malleolus three fingers are required (*Figure 8.17*) and below it two suffice (*Figure 8.18*). The fingers are drawn briskly to and fro across the lesion; recovery in two to three weeks is the norm.

Behind the malleolus the friction must be imparted by rotation because the tendon is shielded from direct pressure (*Figure 8.19*).

Spasm of the peroneal muscles results in fixation of the talocalcanean and mid-tarsal joints, produced by arthritis. 'Spasmodic pes planus' (see page 133) is the old-fashioned term.

Weak peronei may be due to S1 root conduction loss (most likely a fifth lumbar disc protrusion), an upper motor neuron lesion or peroneal atrophy. But more often it is failure to rehabilitate strength into this muscle group after injury that leads to persistent problems. Conversely peroneal hypertrophy can occur following ankle instability and give rise to compartment pressure.

Occasionally a clicking, unstable ankle may be caused by subluxation of the peroneus longus from its groove behind the lateral malleolus ('the

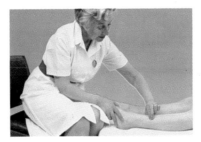

8.16 *Massage, upper site. Tenderness is sought from the musculotendinous junction downwards. Walking is avoided pending recovery.*

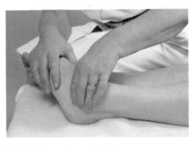

8.18 *Below the malleolus.*

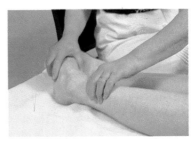

8.17 *Above the malleolus.*

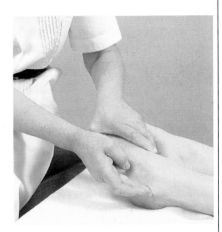

8.19 *At the malleolus. Massage by rotation.*

snapping ankle'). Generally treatment consists of the avoidance of excessive strain, and strapping with padding to the posterior element of the fibula to prevent anterolateral subluxation. But surgery may be required.

The invertor muscles

There are two invertors – the tibialis anterior and the tibialis posterior. However, the anterior tibialis also controls dorsiflexion and will evoke pain on both resisted inversion and resisted dorsiflexion.

The tibialis posterior

If resisted inversion hurts but dorsiflexion does not, the pain originates in the tibialis posterior. The unwary may confuse the condition with the tendo Achillis, as resisted plantiflexion may hurt.

The underlying cause can be a congenital deformity maintaining the heel in valgus, the outcome of which is lateral rotation of the forefoot ('pes planus'). This posture imposes constant strain on the posterior tibial tendon and calls for a permanent support. An orthotic with a medial heel-wedge and longitudinal arch support (accompanied occasionally by a medial post over the first metacarpal head) realigns the foot. The support, permanently required, tips the heel into varus and encourages the forefoot towards medial rotation. A full podiatric assessment may be necessary. In the absence of treatment the pain goes on indefinitely, although often only starting in middle age. Both massage and support are needed (except in cases of non-postural strain, where treatment is confined to deep

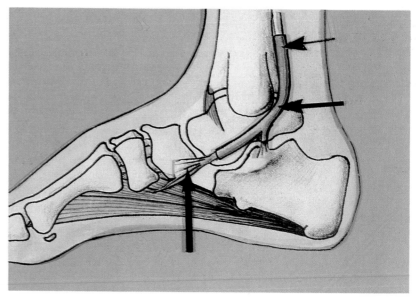

8.20 *Possible sites of a lesion to the tibialis posterior. Athletes call the condition at the upper end 'shin-soreness'.*

friction). Steroids injected into the posterior tibial sheath can also be effective.

There are three sites (*Figure 8.20*) separated in all by several inches. For massage, the tendon is put on the stretch; sessions last 20 minutes twice a week for a month or less.

Above the maleolus, massage is angled directly across the tendon (*Figure 8.21*). For the calcanean extent the fingers massage across the tendon using the thumb as a fulcrum (*Figure 8.22*). At the malleolus, the tibialis posterior is recessed in a groove and is inaccessible to transverse pressure; here the transverse element is achieved by laying the finger flat on and in line with the affected sector and rotating the forearm (*Figures 8.23* and *8.24*).

Acute injuries of the tibialis posterior may also be supported by strapping the foot and heel into varus.

Healing may take longer if an accessory navicular is present.

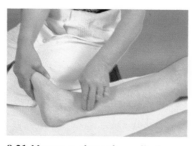

8.21 *Massage; above the malleolus.*

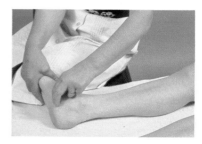

8.22 *The calcanean extent.*

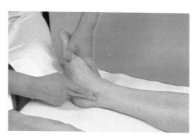

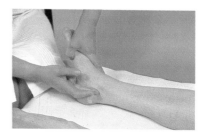

8.23, 8.24 *At the malleolus. The fingers rotate in the sulcus between tendo Achillis and tibia.*

The dorsiflexor muscles

The tibialis anterior

Painful resisted dorsiflexion may hurt just above the ankle; resisted inversion should also be painful. These symptoms suggest the tibialis anterior which boasts a tendon of great length. The lesion is not at the ankle but a good six inches higher, at the musculotendinous junction next to the anterior border of the tibia. Crepitus is felt on movement.

The treatment is massage. The thumb is placed on the lesion and the forearm pronated and supinated (*Figure 8.25*). Recovery usually takes 2–3 weeks.

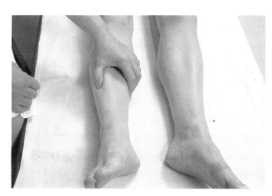

8.25 *Massage, tibialis anterior.*

Other findings

Weakness

Weakness on dorsiflexion is a common finding with lumbar displacements at the fourth level, upper motor neuron lesions and anterior poliomyelitis.

Tight fascial compartment

A tight fascial compartment may cause compression of the anterior tibial muscles, the tibialis posterior, the gastrocnemius or the peronei (very rare). There is a superficial resemblance to intermittent claudication.

Severe cases usually accompany major trauma and/or fracture. Minor forms often occur among athletes. In the most minor cases an ache is produced by exertion and persists for some time. In the severest, intra-compartmental pressure may become sufficiently high to produce paralysis of the muscles after use and, eventually, irreversible ischaemic changes.

Diagnosis in severe cases is thus easy, in minor cases less so. The muscle is found to be hard – maybe rock hard – at rest, and although resisted movements are painless, rapidly repeated contractions provoke the symptoms. Passive stretching may well be resented by the affected muscle. Pressure studies may be needed for assessment and/or to decide if surgical fasciotomy is necessary.

Conservative treatment in the form of rest, elevation, ice, effleurage and a cautiously gradated return to full activity is slow and uncertain. Surgical division of the fascia is the treatment of choice, and should be performed urgently if necrosis is impending.

Peroneal compartment compression may occur due to muscle hypertrophy secondary to lateral ankle instability.

Proximal tibiofibular joint

The proximal tibiofibular joint may be stressed, causing local discomfort and referred pain similar to compartment or stress fracture symptoms in the anterior and lateral compartments of the leg.

The pain is produced by irritation of the common peroneal nerve as it swings round the neck of the fibula and often occurs in polo players through 'riding off'. Adequate protection is required.

Although difficult to treat, desensitization of the nerve with procaine and steroids may help. Surgery to relieve the constriction may be necessary.

Ligamentous strains of the proximal tibiofibular joint respond to local steroid and classical ligamentous treatment. However, prolonged rest from running is advisable.

Stress fracture

Stress fractures occur fairly commonly, particularly with athletes, at the tibia and fibula, normally at the junctions of the upper and middle or middle and lower thirds of the tibia. If half-way along the tibia, the stress fracture is horizontal. In this case a bilateral lesion must be suspected which may proceed to total fracture and may be multiple.

The commonest site of the fibular stress fracture is 5–6 cm proximal to the tip of the fibula and pain in this area should be regarded as a stress fracture until excluded.

Activity is painful, particularly in the early stages, and cannot be worked off. As in all fractures, angulation stresses of the bone produce pain as may distant pressure on the fibula.

The patient may present with apparently bizarre signs. For example, all resisted movements may hurt, or some passive and some resisted movements may be painful in an incongruous pattern. In particular, if resisted inversion causes pain at the lower lateral part of the leg, this almost always denotes a fracture of the lower fibula. Such a sign could easily lead to a mistaken diagnosis of hysteria.

Sometimes palpation reveals warmth and swelling, but there is nearly always a marked local bony tenderness which can occasionally be traced linearly around the shaft of the bone.

Stress fractures may be differentiated from shin splints – a fascial pull on the periosteum – by:

(1) the area of tenderness, the stress fracture being limited to 1–2 cm, while the shin splint extends over several centimetres;
(2) bone scan, when the stress fracture shows as a horizontal line and the shin splint as a vertical line.

The shin splint may often appear in the early blood phase on the bone scan.

The conditions may often occur as combined lesions, and both may have low compartment pressures.

Lowdon's ultrasound test, while prone to false-positive findings, is useful nevertheless. Radiography is often inconclusive but at least excludes tumours and infections.

Stress fracture management hinges upon the avoidance of all painful activities – usually running (although cycling, swimming, etc., can be continued). As the symptoms abate the patient becomes increasingly able to use the limb.

Angulation and rotational stresses (e.g. pronation, supination, camber running) may be helped both by corrective orthoses and an awareness of the causative mechanism, leading to – say – running on opposite sides of the camber, thus correcting apparent leg-length inequalities. True leg-length inequalities will also require correction.

Restoration of full function may take as little as 6–8 weeks or several months. Following resolution, care must be taken to minimize untoward stresses through the bone by, for example, the use of shock-absorbent insoles, running on grass rather than roads and firmly discouraging such practices as running with weights.

CHAPTER NINE

THE ANKLE AND FOOT

The ankle joint itself is simple as it permits only two movements in one plane. But a sprained ankle can involve any one of a number of ligaments and tendons at different sites, readily distinguished; a lesion of the anterior talofibular ligament is much the most frequent.

The foot consists of a highly intricate series of joints which give rise to a multiplicity of possible conditions. Accurate diagnosis is nevertheless practicable and the conditions respond well to treatment. The patient can usually point to the site of the lesion, which is usually palpable.

In cases of trauma to the foot, a detailed history will establish the mechanism of injury and thus help define the exact strains imposed on the joint.

Dural pain does not extend below the ankles. But root pain (which will not be confined to the foot) and/or paraesthesia from a lumbar disc lesion is common (see page 237).

Examination

After a careful history, the foot is inspected, once with the patient standing and walking, and again with her supine. This is because the physical examination conducted when the patient is not weight-bearing may reveal nothing, since the momentary stress imposed by manual testing is sometimes insufficient to evoke the pain caused by sustained weight-bearing.

Changes in the contours of the foot may be apparent when the patient stands. Any minor deformities or alteration in shape show where undue strain falls and, by corollary, where it should be diminished. Inspection is made for over-pronation or supination. Many conditions can be treated simply by providing a carefully structured orthotic cast in the neutral position to support the foot and alleviate strain.

Hallux valgus may indicate functional eversion and over-pronation in an otherwise apparently normal foot.

Short plantiflexor muscles may account for a number of disorders in the foot (see page 112). Minor misalignments of the tibia can also cause abnormal stresses in the foot.

The ankle

The capsule at the ankle joint is evaluated by two passive movements – dorsiflexion (*Figure 9.1*) and plantiflexion (*Figure 9.2*). The ligaments stabilizing the ankle cross the talocalcanean and mid-tarsal joints which are thus included in the ankle examination.

The talofibular, calcaneofibular and the lateral mid-tarsal ligaments are tested by passive inversion during plantiflexion (*Figure 9.3*).

The middle and anterior fasciculi of the deltoid ligament – less frequently strained than the ligaments at the lateral side – are assessed by passive eversion, again during plantiflexion (*Figure 9.4*).

Strong varus is applied (*Figure 9.5*). This tests both the tibiofibular ligament and the talocalcanean joint. If the ligament is at fault, a click is felt as the talus over-tilts in the enlarged and unstable mortice; there is thus pain and excessive range. Stress X-rays may confirm the diagnosis. Conversely, if the talocalcanean joint is involved there will be pain and limitation, the limitation increasing as the condition advances. In both cases, valgus strain (*Figure 9.6*) proves full and painless.

Anterior gliding of the talus in the tibiofibular mortice may either be painful or be increased by anterior tibiofibular or anterior talofibular ligament instability.

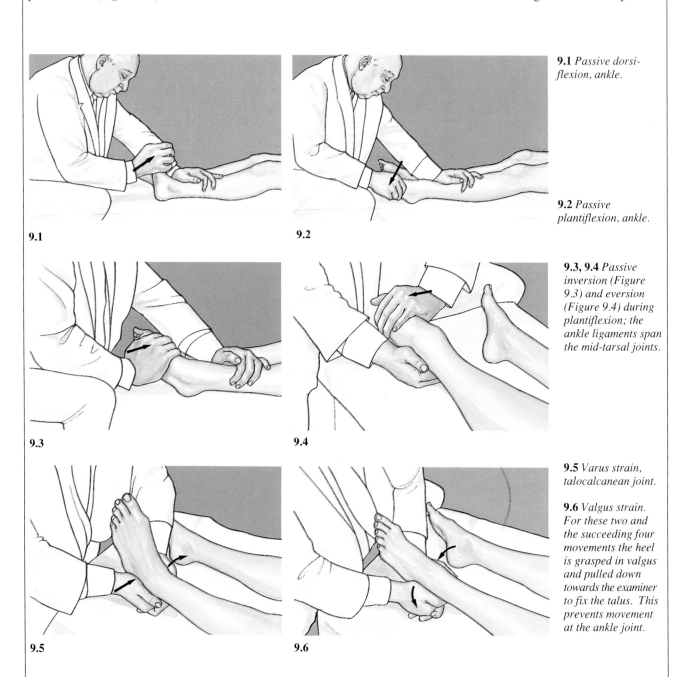

9.1 *Passive dorsiflexion, ankle.*

9.2 *Passive plantiflexion, ankle.*

9.1

9.2

9.3, 9.4 *Passive inversion (Figure 9.3) and eversion (Figure 9.4) during plantiflexion; the ankle ligaments span the mid-tarsal joints.*

9.3

9.4

9.5 *Varus strain, talocalcanean joint.*

9.6 *Valgus strain. For these two and the succeeding four movements the heel is grasped in valgus and pulled down towards the examiner to fix the talus. This prevents movement at the ankle joint.*

9.5

9.6

The mid-tarsal joint

This is now examined by six movements:

(1) Passive dorsiflexion (*Figure 9.7*).
(2) Passive plantiflexion (*Figure 9.8*).
(3) Passive adduction (*Figure 9.9*).
(4) Passive abduction (*Figure 9.10*).
(5) Passive inversion (*Figure 9.11*).
(6) Passive eversion (*Figure 9.12*).

The capsular pattern is determined by peroneal spasm and consists of limitation of adduction and medial rotation.

If necessary, the examination takes in the toes. Resisted movements for the leg may also have to be tested (see page 111).

Finally, the examiner feels for pulsation both of the posterior tibial artery just behind the medial malleolus (*Figure 9.13*) and of the dorsalis pedis on the front of the mid-tarsal joint. If pulsation is absent, the artery is blocked and requires further evaluation.

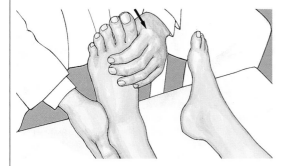

9.7 *Passive dorsiflexion.*

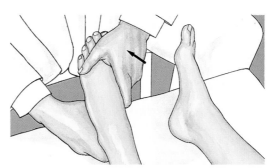

9.8 *Passive plantiflexion.*

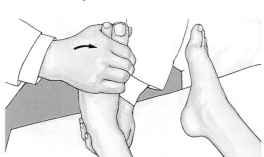

9.9 *Passive adduction.*

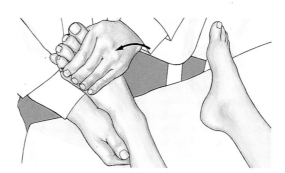

9.10 *Passive abduction.*

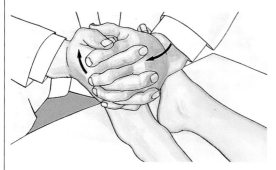

9.11 *Passive medial rotation.*

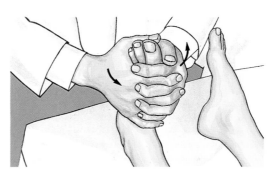

9.12 *Passive lateral rotation.*

The ankle joint

Capsular lesions

Capsular lesions at the ankle are unusual. Rheumatoid arthritis does not occur and the only common conditions are osteoarthrosis and reactive arthritis. Conservative treatment of osteoarthrosis is seldom satisfactory but if the symptoms warrant, arthrodesis is highly effective.

Inflammatory arthritis responds to steroid injection, either intra-articular or pulsed.

The capsular pattern is some limitation of dorsiflexion and more limitation of plantiflexion, coupled with a hard end-feel. But if short calf muscles restrict dorsiflexion in the normal joint, only these last two findings will be apparent.

Ligamentous sprains

These are very common and need careful differentiation for treatment to be effective. Following examination by selective tension, the clinician palpates for tenderness of the affected structure. If gross oedema renders this impossible, the swelling is first reduced by effleurage.

Valgus sprains are uncommon and considered at page 127. Varus sprains are routinely encountered and the sites (*Figure 9.13*) are listed in order of descending frequency:

(1) The anterior talofibular ligament at the fibular origin.
(2) The calcaneofibular ligament at the fibular origin.
(3) The anterior talofibular ligament at the talar insertion.
(4) The calcaneocuboid ligament.
(5) The peroneal tendons (see page 115).
(6) The extensor longus digitorum (very rare).
(7) The anterior talotibial ligament (rarer still).

A double lesion is the commonest of all – the combined sprain of the talofibular and calcaneocuboid ligaments.

Most sprained ankles clear up of themselves in due course, but provided there is no actual rupture with consequent instability, full painless mobility can be greatly expedited by proper treatment. This varies according to the period elapsed since tissue damage.

Acute stage
During the first 24 hours, steroid suspension 2 ml is injected into the ligament – the sooner the better. Deep effleurage may be needed first to

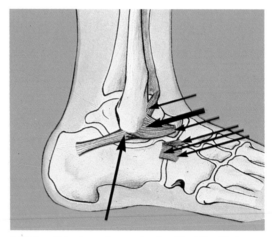

9.13 *Possible sites of a sprained ankle. The fibular origins of the two main ligaments (the two large arrows) are by far the commonest sites of tear. Note the lesion may lie at various locations within individual ligaments. The peronei and the extensor digitorum can also suffer.*

diminish oedema and facilitate localization. Transverse friction follows the next day and continues daily until recovery.

Sub-acute stage
Deep massage moves the ligament in imitation of its normal behaviour, preventing the formation of adhesions both in the ligament and between it and bone. After effleurage, massage is given to the site of the tear, at first for a few minutes but for longer at later treatments. After each session the joint is encouraged towards its new extreme of range by gentle passive movements, a process continued by the patient at home by active movements within the painless range.

Ultrasound and laser in the early stages may improve the rate of healing, but frictional massage is essential to prevent adhesions which may otherwise give rise to chronicity.

Chronic stage
Pain on prolonged exertion persisting some months later is treated by manipulative rupture of the adhesions. Peroneal tendinitis following a sprained ankle is often mistaken for adhesions and manipulated in vain; resisted eversion must be tested to avoid this error.

None of the foregoing procedures has any bearing on the interosseous talofibular ligament. Sprain here results in elongation and attendant instability of the mortice joint and frequent recurrent episodes as well as twinges suggestive of a loose body (see page 128).

If an inversion and plantiflexion injury is accompanied by both lateral and medial bruising, this suggests deeper and more widespread ligamentous disruption. Like the rare valgus injuries, this will not recover spontaneously (see page 130).

Varus sprain

The anterior talofibular ligament

This may be sprained at either end of the fibular origin or talar insertion (see *Figure 9.13*). Passive inversion during plantiflexion is the most painful movement and treatment is identical irrespective of the site. Swelling should first be dispersed with effleurage.

Where the injury occurred within the previous 24 hours and there is no evidence of instability, steroid suspension 2 ml (3 cm needle) is injected.

The foot is held in maximum possible plantiflexion and inversion and the insertion made about 2 cm distal to the lesion – most often at the fibular origin. The needle is thrust in almost horizontally (*Figure 9.14*) until it meets bone and a series of droplets distributed fanwise. The pain is quite considerable for 48 hours, but then the symptoms resolve rapidly until the patient is well in a couple of days. Usually massage will not be necessary.

Though ultrasound and laser improve the initial rate of healing, massage is essential to prevent adhesions and – accompanied by proprioceptive work and isometrics to the strap muscles – is the only treatment if the injection is too painful for the patient or too late for the condition.

For massage, the foot is again put in maximum plantiflexion and inversion with the finger lodged against the lower anterior part of the malleolus. The hand is in pronation and the fingers press medially and proximally to rub the ligamentous fibres against their origin from the bone (*Figure 9.15*).

The principles of treatment are the same at the talar site. For injection the needle is thrust directly into the lesion (*Figure 9.16*). With massage, the pressure is directed medially only, while the fingers travel in a straight line across the fibres (*Figure 9.17*).

At either site the massage is gentle in the acute stage; less than two weeks' treatment is the rule.

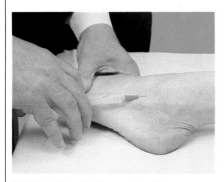

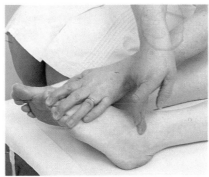

9.15 *Massage, fibular origin. In recent cases, deep friction is only necessary or tolerable for a few minutes. Treatment may have to be preceded by effleurage.*

9.14 *Injection, fibular origin. The sooner the infiltration the better.*

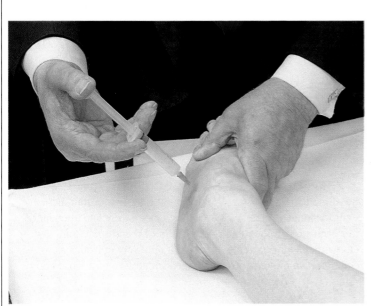

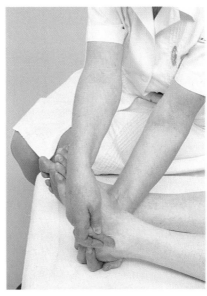

9.16 *Injection, talar insertion. The two sites are hardly more than 1 cm apart.*

9.17 *Massage, talar insertion. Whatever the site, the treatment must include instruction on normal heel-and-toe gait to ensure mobility of the ligament.*

The calcaneofibular ligament

As the ligament spans the talocalcaneal but not the mid-tarsal joint, the only painful movement is varus and the tenderness is found just below the lower edge of the fibula (see *Figure 9.13*). Treatment is by infiltration (*Figure 9.18*) with steroid suspension 1–2 ml during the first few days and massage thereafter (*Figure 9.19*).

Sometimes the ligament is totally or partially ruptured, producing instability and pain on movement. The foot must be maintained in full valgus by fixing an adhesive strapping to the inner aspect of the heel and tightly drawing it up the outer aspect of the leg (*Figure 9.20*). For athletic performance, an air cast or hinged brace splinting may be vital. After three weeks the ligament should have healed.

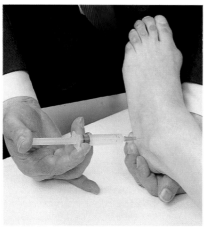

9.18 *Injection is the treatment immediately following injury.*

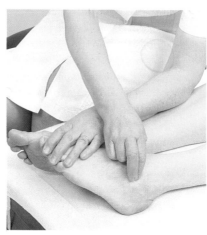

9.19 *Massage may be needed a few days after the injection, or by itself as the treatment of choice.*

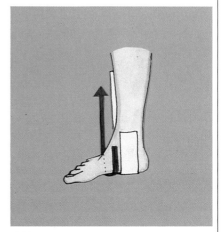

9.20 *If the ligament is ruptured, firm strapping prevents varus movement.*

The calcaneocuboid ligament

Often this is injured at the same time as the anterior talofibular ligament during a varus ankle sprain. But the calcaneocuboid can be tested in isolation by holding the foot in both dorsiflexion and valgus via the heel, which is maintained stationary while medially rotating the forefoot. Pain arising from the calcaneocuboid joint is felt at the outer side of the mid-foot.

In a recent sprain, after effleurage the joint is injected with steroid suspension 2 ml (2 cm needle). The needle punctures the skin just above the lowest palpable extent of the joint line and a series of droplets is injected into the ligaments and a small amount into the joint (*Figures 9.21* and *9.22*).

The resultant pain is severe enough to make walking difficult for a day or so. Then the symptoms rapidly abate.

Massage is given the next day or as the only treatment (*Figure 9.23*). The foot is held in adduction, bringing the

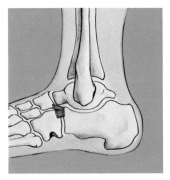

9.21 *The ligament binds the calcaneus, cuboid and navicular bones. Injection sites shown red.*

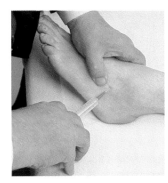

9.22 *Injection is painful but the results uniformly good.*

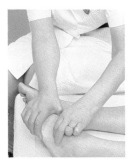

joint into prominence, and the finger is placed on the joint line. Friction is imparted by a movement of the whole forearm. Treatment on alternate days for a week should result in recovery.

9.23 *Massage is given by vertical movements.*

Rupture of adhesions

Adhesions may develop following an untreated sprain of the talofibular or calcaneocuboid ligaments, causing pain and slight swelling persisting for some days after extended exertion. The treatment is manipulative rupture. One sharp twist generally suffices; there is a tiny crack, and the patient is cured.

No anaesthesia is required apart from accurately delivered transverse friction.

For the manipulation, one hand grasps the heel forcing it into full varus and keeping it there throughout (*Figure 9.24*).

The other hand puts the patient's foot into the starting position, consisting of the fullest possible plantiflexion, adduction and medial rotation (*Figure 9.25*). The operator then gives a sharp thrust to accentuate this position by crisply bringing his elbow in towards his side (*Figure 9.26*).

The patient is manipulated only once per session and if re-examination shows no – or incomplete – improvement, the patient attends again the next day.

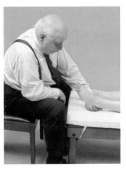

9.24 *Manipulative rupture: starting position, anchoring hand. Despite the adhesions, the foot is adequate for ordinary purposes and only aches after vigorous use.*

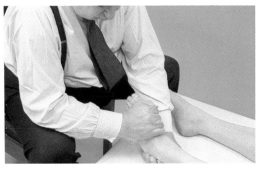

9.25

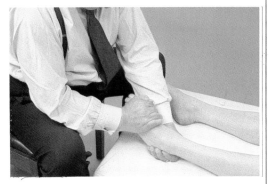

9.25, 9.26 *The manipulative movement is into plantiflexion, adduction and medial rotation.*

The anterior tibiofibular ligament

A strain here (*Figure 9.27*) is almost invariably part of a composite varus sprain. The treatment is massage, with foot held in full plantiflexion to render the ligament accessible (*Figure 9.28*).

Air cast bracing may also help. If the interosseous tibiofibular ligament is sprained, un unstable mortice joint may result, provoking momentary pain within the ankle which turns over easily with a click. The two malleoli can be felt to move apart, and a history of tibiofibular sprain some years previously is suggestive.

In a recent case, strapping is applied to restrict movement at the mortice. Crutches and a heel-raise are provided and surgical opinion sought. In chronic cases, a floated heel (*Figure 9.29*) or injection of sclerosants may make surgery unnecessary.

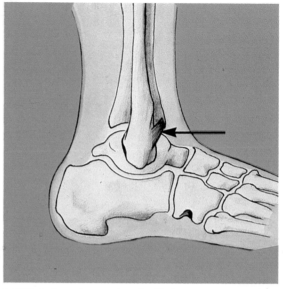

9.27 *Pain from the anterior tibiofibular ligament (arrowed) is never severe but may last for years.*

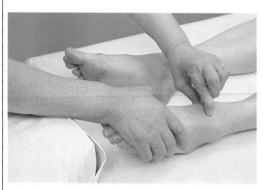

9.28 *Massage is extremely effective.*

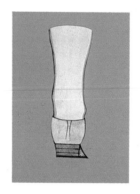

9.29 *Unstable mortice joint. A false heel can be floated on the outer side of the shoe to prevent recurrent strain.*

Recurrent sprain

The occasional individual complains of recurrent minor sprain during ordinary usage. There are two main explanations.

The first is a chronic interosseous tibiofibular sprain (see above) giving attacks lasting a day or two. Alternatively, a sluggish reflex arc between the lateral ligaments and the peroneal muscles leads to delayed contraction of the peronei. The muscles therefore fail to prevent varus strain during walking.

This latter condition is managed by proprioceptive training of the peronei on a wobble board or balancing exercises at home to speed up the reflex arc, accompanied by isometric exercises to the muscle. A floated heel at the outer side of the foot is seldom necessary.

Valgus strain

The deltoid ligament

It is unusual for a valgus strain to end in a sprain of the deltoid (*Figure 9.30*). Chronic strain is usually secondary to a valgus foot and the pain may continue even for years, as the ligament is re-strained at every step. Massage is useless; manipulation and stretching positively harmful. Full passive eversion during plantiflexion is the painful movement.

As soon as the patient is seen, an anti-pronation orthotic controlling calcanovalgus and pronation is fitted to avoid the repeated stretch at every step. It is worn for months.

In addition and provided that there is no instability, steroid suspension 2 ml is injected to settle the persistent traumatic inflammation at the tibial origin. The foot is held in eversion and the 3 cm needle enters 2 cm below and distal to the ligament (*Figure 9.31*). The tip heads towards the inferior aspect of the tibia and a series of droplets is deposited fanwise along the affected extent of the ligamento-osseous junction. A painful reaction can be expected for 24 hours.

The posterior tibialis is invariably weak and requires isometric and proprioceptive rehabilitation with the orthotic *in situ*. Additional supporting strapping may be required for physical activities.

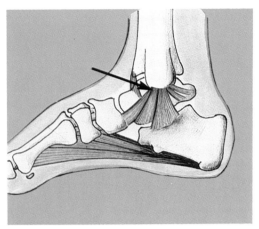

9.30 *Tenderness is found along the tibial origin (arrowed).*

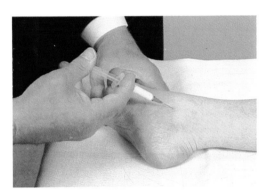

9.31 *Injection. Beads of fluid are delivered all along the affected extent.*

The anterior tibiotalar ligament

Sprain here is an uncommon result of a pure plantiflexion stress. The pain may persist for years but is never severe; symptoms are felt at the front of the ankle on full plantiflexion. To palpate, the extensor tendons must first be pushed aside.

Massage is the treatment of choice (*Figure 9.32*).

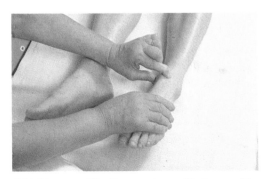

9.32 *Massage. The ligament is too thin for steroid infiltration; it is just visible to the left of the head of the arrow in Figure 9.30.*

A loose body and other conditions

After a sprain, a small fragment of cartilage may become detached within the ankle joint. The patient complains of sudden erratic twinges on plantiflexion, often when walking downstairs.

A loose body may also be caused by osteochondritis dissecans of the talus. This lesion may be symptomatic or asymptomatic and displays on X-ray or magnetic resonance imaging, but as the subluxation itself is momentary it will not be revealed by radiography.

The pain is momentary and the displacement self-reducing. Thus the patient is well at the time of attendance and treatment must be conducted without the framework of symptoms and signs that normally guide the manipulator, since the patient cannot immediately report whether the loose body has been shifted to a more favourable position.

The patient therefore returns a week after treatment, stating whether attacks are now spaced at wider intervals. In the absence of improvement, the manipulation for the talocalcanean joint can be tried instead. An alternative is to fix an anterior wedge to the heel of the shoe.

For the manipulation the patient lies on a high couch, her heel level with the edge (*Figure 9.33*). An assistant at the other end supplies traction.

The operator's lower hand does not move. Instead it acts as a fulcrum, protected from the hard edge of the couch by a foam rubber pad.

The upper hand grasps the dorsum and the operator leans back, pulling hard to distract the talus from its mortice. A strong circumduction movement is then carried out several times while traction is maintained (*Figure 9.34*).

Footballers can show signs of repeated trauma around the ankle joint where bony and calcium flakes may be seen in the capsular ligaments. These can be treated symptomatically, unless they move in between the articular surfaces to present as episodic acute pain.

Compression, not distraction, of the talus on the fibula is a rare cause of pain in high-jumpers.

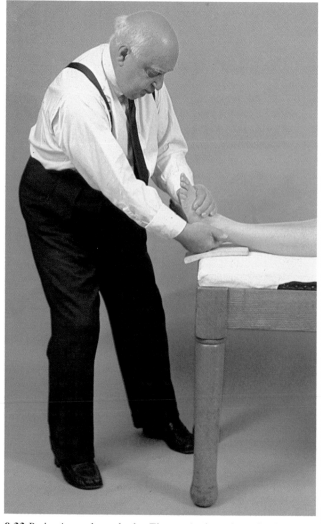

9.33 *Reduction, a loose body. The manipulator leans back and distracts the joint; an assistant at the other end supplies counter-traction.*

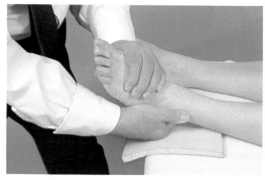

9.34 *The foot is used as a lever to distract talus from mortice during a circular movement in plantiflexion. About half the cases are relieved.*

The talocalcanean/sub-taloid joint and heel

Capsular lesions

Most cases are due to either an inflammatory arthritis or osteoarthrosis. Recovery after a sprained ankle may be retarded by a sub-acute traumatic arthritis, a condition readily distinguishable from ligamentous adhesions following strain by the limitation of movement at the talocalcanean joint.

Rheumatoid arthritis is often bilateral and is characterized by palpable warmth and synovial thickening. There is no history of sprain. Osteoarthrosis follows fractures involving the articular surface of the calcaneus. Persistent pain, which can only be helped by arthrodesis, is apt to result.

As the capsular pattern encroaches, the full range of varus of the normal joint becomes increasingly limited and in due course fixation in full valgus results (*Figure 9.35*).

Rheumatoid arthritis and sub–acute traumatic arthritis respond well to one or two injections of steroid suspension 2 ml. Since the heel is fixed in valgus, the simpler approach is from the medial side.

The sustentaculum tali is identified and the 2 cm needle thrust in above it, parallel to the joint surfaces (*Figures 9.36* and *9.37*), and usually strikes bone at 1 cm. The tip is manoeuvred until it slips in further without resistance and steroid suspension 1 ml is injected into the anterior joint, the needle partly withdrawn, reinserted at 45° posteriorly and a further 1 ml discharged into the posterior compartment. Failure after two injections is the exception and indicates several months' immobilization in plaster.

An alternative approach is via the sinus tarsi where the ligament to the neck of the talus is infiltrated. This often requires short-lasting general anaesthesia.

Post-traumatic osteoporosis ('Sudeck's atrophy') can involve the

talocalcanean joint, in which case the capsular pattern amounts to fixation in the mid-position rather than full valgus. The condition is visible radiographically, the whole foot hurts, the nails stop growing and when the leg is dependent the foot turns all but black. No treatment avails but the condition improves within two years.

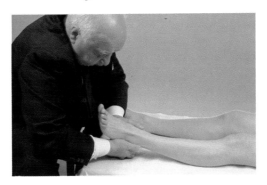

9.35 *Arthritis. The foot cannot be persuaded into varus.*

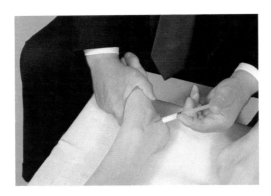

9.36 *In advanced rheumatoid cases the injection cannot restore range but still abolishes pain.*

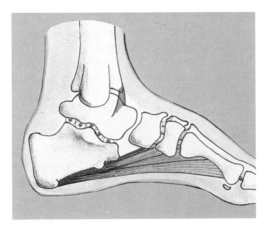

9.37 *The suspension (marked red) is delivered into the entire length of the joint.*

Non-capsular lesions

Dancer's heel

Despite its name, this condition is also seen *inter alia* in the footballer whose kick has been blocked, a javelin thrower's lead leg, a field hockey player braking on imitation turf (e.g. Astroturf), squash players and so on. Furthermore, the chronic ankle with widespread ligamentous disruption may show this condition, caused by trauma to tissues around the posterior articular margin of the tibia (*Figure 9.38*) precipitated by the impingement of the upper surface of the calcaneus.

Full passive plantiflexion of the foot is painful, especially when the patient lies prone and the examiner abruptly jerks the calcaneum into contact with the posterior surface of the tibia, setting up pain at the back of the heel. Because rising on tiptoe may hurt, it is often erroneously diagnosed as an Achillis tendinitis which would not, however, be affected by full passive plantiflexion.

In dancers the cause is over-pointing (i.e. plantiflexion beyond 180° when the dancer is *sur les pointes*). The other activities listed above achieve the identical position by almost the reverse posture, driving the heel into the ground with the foot plantiflexed.

The length of the articular margin is palpated for tenderness. For injection of steroid suspension 2 ml (4 cm needle) the patient lies prone. The posterior articular margin of the tibia is identified about 2 cm superior to a line joining the tips of the malleoli; the needle enters to one side of the tendo Achillis (*Figure 9.39*).

The tip is adjusted until it rests on the tibial edge (*Figure 9.40*). This is about 1 mm above the point at which the bone gives way to articular cartilage, and when the tip contacts the periosteum a number of droplets are delivered along this horizontal line (*Figure 9.41*). The chronic ankle may respond very well to this treatment.

Dancers must not rise *sur les pointes* for a week and should take care not to over-point.

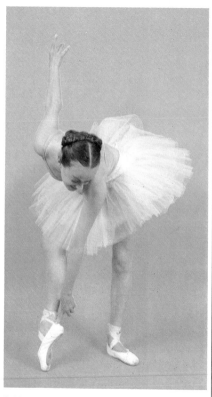

9.38 *Site of dancer's heel. Sometimes the pain is mistakenly ascribed to the tendo Achillis.*

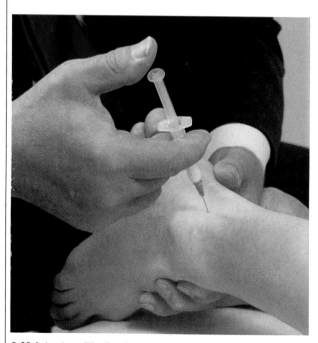

9.39 *Injection. The foot is plantiflexed so that the tendo Achillis can be pushed aside with the thumb.*

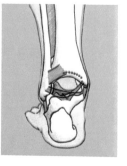

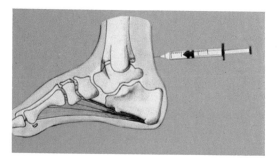

9.40, 9.41 *The injection (shown red) is made all along the bruised edge.*

Immobilization limitation

Immobilization in plaster for several months following a tibiofibular fracture may result in permanent limitation as the sub-talar joint becomes fixed in the mid-position (cf. arthritis). The capsule must be stretched out, but the treatment is heavy going because of the difficulty in getting much leverage. But if only half the normal range can be restored, the lesion ceases to trouble the patient.

The heel is clasped as strongly as possible between the two palms. By alternately swinging one elbow away from, and the other towards, herself the operator imparts a varus and valgus movement (*Figures 9.42* and *9.43*). This forcing is repeated with the utmost vigour a great number of times. Sessions take place twice a week for anything up to several months, and after some range of movement is regained the symptoms may well abate of themselves.

Sometimes mobilization may be facilitated by injections around the ankle joint as for the dancer's heel, together with manipulation under anaesthetic.

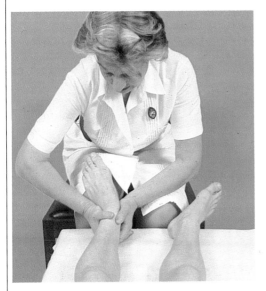 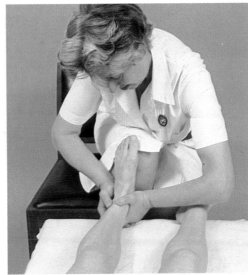

9.42, 9.43 *Capsular stretching. The operator grips the heel firmly below the malleoli and swings her trunk and arms from side to side. Note the patient's foot is maintained in comfortable dorsiflexion against her knee.*

Subcutaneous nodules

A nodule about the size of a small pea may form spontaneously in the subcutaneous fascia. It engenders severe momentary pain but only when pinched at the back of the shoe. Division by subcutaneous tenotomy (*Figure 9.44*) under local anaesthesia achieves good results. Shoes with a gap posteriorly are an excellent alternative.

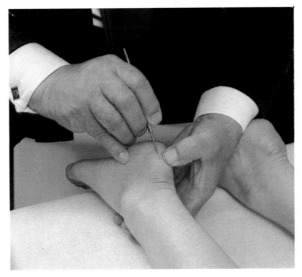

9.44 *Tenotomy gives results as good as excision.*

Plantar fasciitis

Chronic strain is a common cause of pain arising from the plantar fascia. It normally stems from prolonged strain during standing by patients with an over-arched foot ('pes plantaris') or short calf muscles. The most distinctive symptom is severe pain at the heel on first getting up to walk after sitting, symptoms rapidly relieved by avoidance of weight-bearing. Occasionally, the patient may be woken at night because of irritation from the medial calcanean nerve under pressure from a calcanovalgus heel.

Alternative pathologies are:

(1) Degeneration of the fat/stroma pressure mechanism, allowing the shock-absorbing nature of the subcutaneous tissue to be dissipated sideways, thus diminishing its effectiveness.
(2) Sero-negative reactive arthritis, particularly in Reiter's syndrome.

Continued over-strain may pull the periosteum away at its origin from the calcaneus. A bony spur results which is symptomless of itself and has no bearing on treatment.

On examination, foot movements are normal and painless: all findings are negative. The tender spot is palpable and always at the inner aspect, just distal to the origin from the calcaneus (*Figure 9.45*). For confirmation, the discomfort produced by pressure there will be diminished by simultaneously squeezing the lateral and medial borders of the subcutaneous tissue together between thumb and fingers.

The fascia must be relaxed by dropping the forefoot, accomplished by raising the heel of the shoe while keeping horizontal the platform on which the patient's heel rests (*Figure 9.46*). More permanent support is achieved by a wedge applied to the heel, the thick end lying anteriorly (*Figure 9.47*). These measures should afford immediate relief.

An alternative is to prevent flattening of the fat-pad by a cupped orthotic and arch support, heel-cups and strapping during sports.

However in obdurate cases the patient is injected with steroid suspension 2 ml. The foot is dorsiflexed to tauten the plantar fascia. The skin must be sterilized and the point of entry is some 3–4 cm anterior to the lesion. The approach is oblique (*Figure 9.48*).

As the needle advances it traverses fascia before touching bone and the affected area is infiltrated all over by a series of minor withdrawals and reinsertions (*Figures 9.49* and *9.50*). Severe discomfort is provoked lasting two days, making walking painful, and a strong analgesic is prescribed.

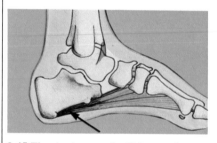

9.45 *The site (arrowed). If the muscles are inadequate to support prolonged standing, the strain falls on the plantar fascia.*

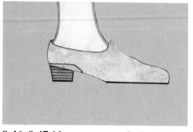 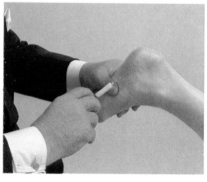

9.46, 9.47 *Most cases are dealt with by a modified heel. An internal or external wedge raises the front edge of the heel so the platform is horizontal.*

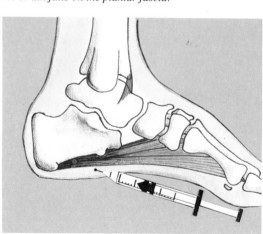

9.48 *Injection (marked red).*

9.49, 9.50 *The patient lies prone with her knee flexed. The point of entry is some distance from the lesion, as the plantar skin overlying the site is too thick for sterilization.*

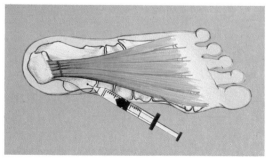

The mid-tarsal joint

The mid-tarsal joint is made up of the talonavicular and calcaneocuboid joints. They extend the full width of the foot and permit movement in six directions, each of which are tested during the examination.

Capsular lesions

Osteoarthrosis – unless gross – causes no symptoms of itself and this radiographic finding should not preclude consideration of alternative causes of pain from, e.g., mid-tarsal strain, but the mid-tarsal and other tarsal joints are prey to several types of inflammatory arthritis.

Rheumatoid mono-arthritis may present with oedema and synovial swelling at the dorsum of the foot. Joint aspirate should be tested for rheumatoid factor to confirm the diagnosis. Treatment is by local injection of steroids or by systemic anti-rheumatic agents if other joints are involved.

Sub-acute arthritis in middle age and adolescence is dealt with below.

The capsular pattern, determined by peroneal spasm, is limitation of adduction and inversion with the other movements full.

Sub-acute arthritis in middle age

Over-use far outweighs an isolated strain as the cause; usually the patients are stout women. An inversion movement at the talocalcanean and mid–tarsal is partially restricted by muscular spasm. Without treatment, the condition appears to continue indefinitely.

If, as sometimes happens, only one joint is affected, it can be injected with steroid suspension 2ml delivered in droplets over the entire extent of the tender area (*Figures 9.51* and *9.52*). One injection should suffice.

But where the lesion is diffuse, treatment is by rest. This entails maintaining the heel in varus by application of a figure-of-eight adhesive strapping (*Figure 9.53*) to hold the forefoot in maximum inversion. At least two layers of strapping are required. The patient is seen every few days to renew tension on the bandage, which is worn for some months.

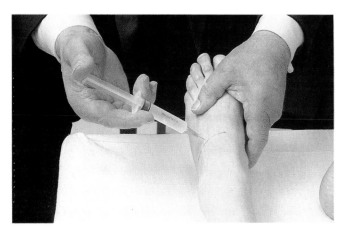

9.51 *Injection, calcaneocuboid joint (marked in blue); the likelies site.*

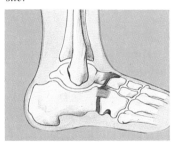

9.52 *The lesion can lie anywhere on the joint line, marked in blue.*

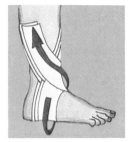

9.53 *Strapping is the alternative.*

Sub-acute arthritis in adolescence

This condition presents as a painless deformity: the foot is fixed in valgus at the heel and in eversion and abduction of the forefoot. The most obvious symptom is a clumsy gait. It is often called spasmodic pes planus because of the secondary spasm of the peroneal muscles which accompanies the arthritis. The condition is brought on by prolonged standing and is rarer than formerly. The basis of treatment is support for the joint and relief from weight-bearing. The patient needs a sedentary job, a bicycle to shorten long walks, a medial wedge on the heel of her shoes and strapping (see above). Full range of movement is normally restored in 6–12 months.

The mid-tarsal ligaments

These (see *Figure 9.56*) are susceptible to two contrasting disorders. Strain may lead to pain with excessive range, and contracture to pain and limitation.

Mid-tarsal strain

This condition, like non-inflammatory plantar fasciitis, can be anticipated in patients with an over-arched foot or an equinus deformity caused by short calf muscles. In such cases, weight-bearing dorsiflexes and therefore abducts the foot at the mid-tarsal joint. First the foot becomes wobbly. Later, an ache appears at the extremes of passive range, especially rotation, and finally increasing abduction of the forefoot puts undue strain on the calcaneonavicular ligament.

Treatment consists of a combination of four measures.

First, the heel of the shoe is raised to allow the forefoot to adopt a more plantigrade position.

Second, the short flexor muscles are given resisted exercises so they become strong enough to take the strain of weight-bearing.

Third, the joint is mobilized (see below); this is the only example of manipulation at a joint already possessing excessive range.

Fourth, the sprained calcaneonavicular ligament is infiltrated with steroid suspension.

The aim of mobilization is to attain full painless range of eversion. Repeated strains during healing of minor ligamentous ruptures will have led to the formation of adhesions (giving discomfort at the extremes of range) which must now themselves be ruptured. The operator clasps his hands about the outer aspect of the forefoot; great strength is required. The heel of the dorsally placed hand presses chiefly on the first metatarsal bone, the heel of the other hand acts in the main against the plantar surfaces of the fifth metatarsal bone, and the rotation is imparted by the operator forcibly swinging his elbows, one towards and the other away from himself (*Figures 9.54* and *9.55*). This movement is repeated scores of times each session for three or four treatments.

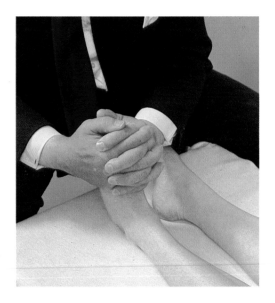

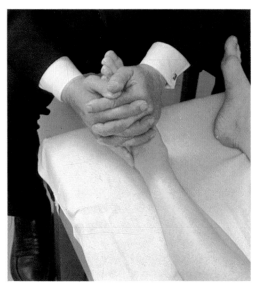

9.54, 9.55 *Forcing lateral rotation. Surprising vigour is necessary; the operator's widely spread legs give him a stable platform.*

Mid-tarsal ligamentous contracture

Limitation of movement at the mid-tarsal joint may arise from ligamentous contracture following some months in a plaster cast for, for example, fractures of the lower leg. The shortened ligaments on the dorsum of the foot are tender and although walking is painless, more pronounced exertion provokes immediate symptoms.

Mobilization does not work. Instead, the affected ligaments are infiltrated with steroid suspension 2–5 ml. The solution is injected along their length wherever they are tender (*Figure 9.56*). There is no increase in range, but the pain is much diminished.

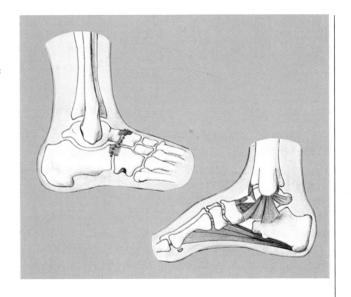

9.56 *The tender area lies anywhere (marked red) on the joint line across the dorsum.*

Other conditions

Stress fractures occur, particularly in the calcaneus and navicular where a history of pain on activity should alert the clinician. X-rays are invariably negative and a bone scan is required to confirm the diagnosis. It requires about eight weeks non-weight-bearing and takes some 14–16 weeks to heal. An accessory navicular may sometimes be mistakenly interpreted as an avulsion fracture of the posterior tibialis.

The cuneo-first-metatarsal joint

Only one condition affects the joint – osteoarthrosis of insidious onset, usually bilateral, probably the legacy of a previous adolescent osteochondrosis. Pain for some months may result from osteophytes pinching the skin when cramped by the uppers of a tight shoe. The osteophyte is palpable as a small projection at the dorsum of the foot.

The pain is localized and the problem can normally be resolved by wearing footwear no part of which touches the joint. At worst the osteophyte may have to be chiselled away, but in any case recovery from the pain is a certainty.

The metatarsal shafts

A marching fracture

This, the common cause of pain in the forefoot, is typified by unilateral localized warmth and oedema lying in a circular patch over the metatarsus. The history may be devoid of injury or even over-use. The condition is a stress fracture, most often at the neck of the second or fourth metatarsal bone. X-ray changes may only become apparent after two weeks but can be displayed earlier by bone scan.

Spontaneous recovery within six to eight weeks is facilitated by strapping the foot so the intact bones splint the fracture, and if necessary, fitness in athletes may be maintained by non-running regimens such as cycling, rowing, swimming, etc.

A short metatarsal bone visible radiographically is compatible with full painless function.

Differential diagnosis

Localized warmth, swelling and tenderness at the dorsum of the distal part of the foot are also features of a number of other conditions, all relatively rare, listed below:

(1) Strained interosseous muscles secondary to a marching fracture – massage.
(2) Gout – indomethacin.
(3) Gonorrhoea – penicillin.
(4) Rheumatoid arthritis of the metatarsophalangeal joint – steroid suspension
(5) Freiburg's arthritis.
(6) Sarcoidosis and Reiter's disease – systemic treatment.
(7) Ringworm.
(8) Morton's metatarsalgia – see page 138:

The toe joints

Capsular lesions

The first metatarsophalangeal joint

Gout, adolescent arthritis or osteoarthrosis may attack the first metatarsophalangeal joint which, when normal, is capable of 30° of flexion and 90° of extension – the latter is the one that matters. The capsular pattern is gross limitation of extension and some limitation of flexion. Fixation in the neutral position (hallux rigidus) eventually results.

Arthritis in adolescence may follow osteochondrosis dissecans. Onset is slow and unprovoked and the patient is normally male, aged 15–20. Conservative treatment consists of the prescription of a rocker to the sole of the shoe, thus relieving the big toe from the necessity of extension during walking.

Osteoarthrosis in middle age produces no symptoms until extension is limited by about 45°. After that, each step results in a forced extension of the toe joint producing a superimposed traumatic arthritis.

Rheumatoid arthritis is frequently encountered and treated by an injection of steroid. The so-called 'Astro toe' is caused by fast checking or stopping on an artificial surface, driving the big toe into the shoe. This may produce a sub–ungual haematoma which can be relieved by trephining the nail with a needle or hot cautery. It is accompanied by traumatic arthritis of the big toe joint and sometimes even partial rupture of the capsular ligaments.

Whatever the cause, the pain is accurately localized and the joint tender. Resisted flexion proves painless, thereby excluding sesamoiditis. Steroid suspension 1 ml is injected into the joint. The patient lies on the couch while the assistant grasps the big toe and pulls hard to distract the joint surfaces (*Figure 9.57*).

Rotation of the toe facilitates identification of the proximal phalanx. The needle passes into the space between the two bones and the injection is given there (*Figure 9.58*), provoking considerable pain for some 12 hours. This procedure is also appropriate for the same lesions at the interphalangeal joint. But both rheumatoid arthritis and osteoarthrosis are normally relieved for a year or longer.

Typically gout affects the big toe in elderly men. The attacks are mechanically unprovoked, recurrent, excruciating, accompanied by swelling and skin reddening, and frequently switch from one foot to the other. Often the joint is normal for some years at a stretch. Indomethacin resolves the symptoms within a day or two. In periods of respite, the excretion of urates is increased by aspirin, probenecid or allopurinol.

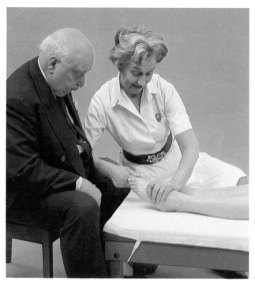

9.57

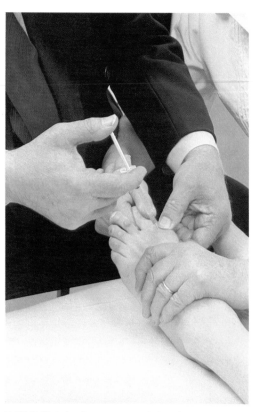

9.57, 9.58 *Injection, group and detail. The assistant opens the joint space to facilitate entry of the needle.*

Sesamoiditis

Over-use may set up a traumatic arthritis at the sesamo-first-metatarsal joint. Patients with short calf muscles fixing the foot in plantiflexion are particularly susceptible. They come down too hard on the forefoot. Resisted flexion of the hallux is painful and, contrary to expectation, the position of the tender spot is unaltered by flexion and extension of the big toe.

The treatment is injection of steroid suspension 1ml. Recurrence is prevented both by fitting a metatarsal support and by raising the heel of the shoe while maintaining its upper surface horizontal.

Fractures can occur but they are difficult to diagnose as the sesamoids may be bi–, tri– or even quadripartite.

The other toe joints

Traumatic and inflammatory arthritis

The capsular pattern is restricted flexion with little limitation of extension (cf. the first metatarsophalangeal joint). An injection of steroid suspension 1ml is curative, although the infiltration provokes a severe reaction lasting some 12 hours. In advanced rheumatoid cases, the toes become fixed in the clawed position; it is then too late to inject. The only effective measure is a support relieving the metatarsal heads from weight-bearing.

Freiburg's arthritis

This condition is normally confined to the second metatarsophalangeal joint. It is a late result of osteochondrosis dissecans starting in adolescence and continuing indefinitely. A support can be fitted to stop the joint touching the ground while walking. Alternatively, the head of the bone is removed.

Hallux valgus

This condition often accompanies an over-pronated forefoot, frequently aggravated by narrow pointed shoes with high heels (for females).

An orthotic to limit pronation together with medial forefoot posting may elevate the first ray of the foot, so the toe to drop into the correct position. With females, an internal horizontal platform to the heel prevents the foot slipping downwards into the constricted toe-cap. Wider toed low-heeled shoes prevent the deterioration which may lead to operation.

Metatarsalgia

Pain at the plantar aspect of the forefoot is called metatarsalgia. In the acute form (rare) it is due to a bursitis pressing on the digital nerve, or occasionally a neuroma, and is known as Morton's metatarsalgia. The standard history is of agonizing pain at the outer border of the forefoot on walking.

Attacks are brief, lasting for a minute or so during which the patient stands still on the other foot. After a couple of minutes the twinges cease but the foot becomes warm and remains so for several hours. Incidents are normally separated by intervals of some months.

The aetiology is either a bursitis at or a neuroma of the fourth digital nerve proximal to its point of diversion. This is nipped between the heads of the fourth and fifth metatarsal bones.

Examination between attacks is wholly negative. Conservative treatment consists merely of a small support under the toe to alter the alignment of the metatarsal heads (*Figure 9.59*), but if this fails, the nerve with its neuroma should be excised.

Chronic metatarsalgia affects the middle three toes; it arises in conditions where an excessive proportion of the body-weight falls on the forefoot. Pain is brought on by standing or walking and relieved by rest. The causes are:

(1) Short calf muscles commonly following a tibial/fibular fracture (Volkmann's ischaemic contracture can occur in as much as 10% of these fractures, resulting in long toe flexor contracture).
(2) Pes plantaris.
(3) Weak flexor and intrinsic muscles.
(4) Local lesions of the metatarsal joints.
(5) Splay forefoot with a dropped transverse arch.
(6) Shoes that are too short,

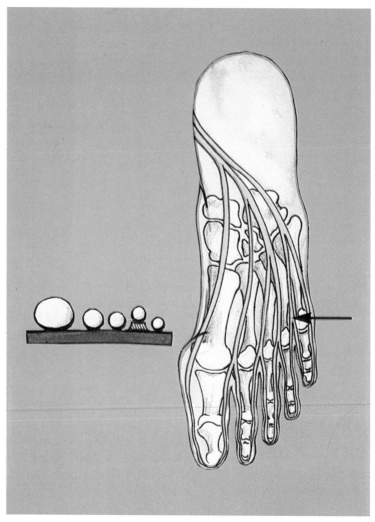

9.59 *Morton's metarsalgia. A small fibrous tumour on the digital nerve causes severe twinges at the outer toes. A support (shown left) under the head of the fourth toe keeps the bones slightly out of line and prevents the nerve from being squeezed.*

provoking functional clawing of the toes and thus a prominent metatarsal head.
(7) Shoes that are too narrow and compress the transverse arch.

Treatment is a combination of two measures – a support and exercises. For the former, a metatarsal pad or bar (proximal to the metatarsal heads under the neck of the second, third and fourth metatarsal bones) transfers the weight from the head to the shaft. The support can be modified to address any underlying problem. In the case of short calf muscles, for example, it would incorporate a heel-raise component. Exercises are directed at strengthening the flexors and the intrinsic muscles. This ensures the toes flex properly at every step and carry weight on their tips, thus taking load off the joint capsules.

Dancer's metatarsalgia is confined to those who do much tiptoe work (not *sur les pointes*). A bruised pad of fibrous tissue is found in the sole lying anterior to the second, third and fourth meta-tarsophalangeal joints. The ballet shoes are fitted with a semi-lunar pad so the proximal phalanges bear more weight.

Arteriosclerosis
In advanced cases the circulatory defect may show itself at the sole rather than in the calf muscles; it is provoked by walking. The dorsalis pedis and posterior tibial pulses are both absent, and the X-ray may show the arteries to be calcified.

The tarsal tunnel syndrome
This is caused by pressure on the tibial nerve as it passes around the medial malleolus. It is precipitated by over-pronation and calcanovalgus and will produce pain coupled with pins and needles over the medial forefoot, sometimes rising up the leg.

Occasionally pressure over the deep peroneal nerve as it passes anterior to the talar joint will produce pain and pins and needles in the big toe.

Paraesthesia
The cause of pins and needles in the feet normally lies in the spine (see Appendix II):

Cervical disc lesion – cord sign.
Thoracic disc lesion – cord sign.
Lumbar disc lesion – root pressure.
Spondylolisthesis – root pressure.
Spinal claudication – lack of arterial blood supply.

Other conditions of the foot

(1) Sever's disease is an epiphysitis of the calcanean epiphysis occurring in adolescents and caused either by traction from the tendo Achillis or compression from heel strike. It is associated with too much athletic stress, and can be treated circumspectly, managing the child's activities within his pain threshold.

(2) Impingement periostitis may occur on the navicular, talus and tibia in sports such as gymnastics, when forced dorsiflexion from, e.g. a vault, occurs on landing.

(3) An os trigonum in professional dancers and athletes may have to be removed surgically.

(4) Inflammation may arise in the retro-calcaneal bursa (or sub-Achilles) which lies between the tendo Achillis near its insertion and the calcaneus. The signs resemble those of a dancer's heel. Pinching the bursa between thumb and forefinger sets up the pain. One or two injections of steroid are normally curative. Alternatively, steroid phonophoresis may be used.

(5) An adventitious Achilles bursitis, or so-called 'pump bumps', requires adjustment of the shoes to prevent rubbing. Calcanovalgus may be present.

The condition responds well to ultrasound and steroid injections.

(6) Children may have a number of locally tender superficial bursae around the calcaneum which settle with rest.

PART THREE

THE SPINE

CHAPTER TEN

PRINCIPLES OF EXAMINATION

As at other joints, diagnosis at the spine is dependent on assessment of function. At all spinal levels – cervical, thoracic and lumbar – a number of general anatomical considerations hold sway which together dictate the examination's format. In order to cover the basic theory this chapter treats the spine in its entirety. But in practice the clinician will consider one region at a time and the three subsequent chapters deal with each level in turn.

Because disc lesions are common and generally responsive to treatment, the examination sets out to differentiate between disc lesions and other sources of pain as well as establishing the particular treatment that will benefit any given displacement.

As elsewhere in the body, displacements give rise to certain characteristic signs and symptoms.

First, the history is suggestive.

Second, any loose fragment in the joint restricts spinal movement in some but not all directions, producing the non-capsular pattern characteristic of internal derangement.

Third, a displacement protruding posteriorly interferes with the dura mater. Apart from pain – referred extra-segmentally – this adversely affects the dura's normal mobility.

Fourth, a displacement protruding posterolaterally impinges on the appropriate nerve root. Where the pressure is mild, only the nerve root's dural sleeve suffers resulting in pain in the dermatome and restriction of the nerve root's mobility. But if pressure is severe, conduction loss results together with weakness in the relevant muscle groups and sensory and reflex changes.

Examination for a disc lesion is thus conducted for each of the above. However, in many cases the dural signs, nerve root symptoms and nerve root signs are absent, leaving the diagnosis to be made on history and joint signs alone.

Finally, compression of the spinal cord is an absolute bar to manipulation, which is the primary treatment for cartilaginous displacements. Accordingly, the examiner always checks for cord signs.

The basic clinical principles do not differ greatly from one spinal level to another and repay close study; lesions of the spine account for about half of all orthopaedic medical cases. Moreover, symptoms of spinal origin often affect the upper or lower limb and thus a sound grasp of peripheral pain is founded on an understanding of the spine.

In the following pages, the various structures involved are discussed in detail and the inferences drawn are progressively tabulated under the appropriate headings. Discussion commences with the dura mater, as its role is paramount. It provides the main source of spinal pain.

EXAMINATION FOR A SPINAL DISPLACEMENT: SUMMARY I

History	Joint Signs	Dural Signs	Nerve Root Signs		Cord Signs
			Mobility	Weakness	
Always characteristic	Always characteristic	Sometimes present	Sometimes present	Sometimes present	Rare

The dura mater

This tough membranous tube extends from the foramen magnum of the skull down to the caudal edge of the first or second sacral vertebra (*Figures 10.1* and *10.2*). It houses the spinal cord surrounded by cerebrospinal fluid and provides a dural sleeve for the emergent nerve roots.

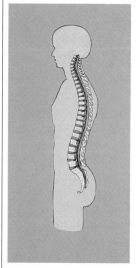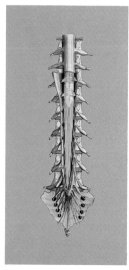

10.1, 10.2 *The dura mater. This membrane runs the length of the spine and is sensitive anteriorly, where it is vulnerable to pressure from intervertebral displacements. Likewise, the nerve root sheaths carry a dural investment.*

Two important characteristics of the dura mater are not always appreciated:

(1) It is sensitive, being innervated from the sinuvertebral nerve by three separate routes[1]. However, these fibres all run to the ventral aspect of the dura and no nerves have been traced to or discovered at the dorsal surface of the membrane. This partial innervation, confined to the anterior aspect of the dura, explains why no pain is felt at lumbar puncture. At its anterior aspect the dura is sensitive to two stimuli: stretching and compression. In addition, pain may be provoked by a vascular jolt (e.g. coughing) which momentarily enlarges the intradural veins and starts an impulse transmitted through the cerebrospinal fluid.

   At any spinal level, the dura may cause not only referred pain, but also referred tenderness, which can be exacerbated locally by deep palpation since this increases afferent input to the sensory cortex.

(2) It moves slightly in relation to the vertebrae it traverses. Thus neck flexion lifts the dural tube cranially by an average of 3 cm and draws the thoracic extent with it. The dura can, of course, be stretched from below (e.g. by straight-leg raising via the sciatic nerve).

The dura mater is thus an inert, mobile and sensitive structure. Accordingly, its function can be examined by stretching, and any compression limiting mobility will result in pain and limitation on passive movements.

As noted previously, dural pain is not subject to the rules of segmental reference.

At the cervical level (*Figure 10.3*) pain of dural origin may be felt running up the neck and over to the forehead – C2 and C3 dermatomes – or down towards the mid-scapular area – T3, T4, T5 and T6 (but never down the arms). The commonest symptom of a cervical disc lesion is scapular and shoulder pain.

Thus in the stages of central and posterolateral dural pressure, pain is usually felt in areas derived from a segment quite other than that which in due course is found to contain the lesion. The small area of tenderness within the painful area identified by the patient as the source of his troubles is, like the pain, a referred phenomenon.

Interference with the dura mater at thoracic levels may give rise to posterior pain spreading to the base of the neck or down to the mid-lumbar region (*Figure 10.4*) and, in particularly misleading guise, round to the front of the thorax.

Extrasegmental reference is also common at the lumbar region (*Figure 10.5*). The pain often radiates to the abdomen or up to the back of the lower chest. In acute lumbago, the symptoms are frequently referred to one or both groins or iliac fossae, thus encroaching on the lower thoracic segments. Dural reference to the buttock or one or both legs is common, but it never extends beyond the ankles.

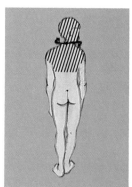

10.3, 10.4, 10.5 *Dural pain and extrasegmental reference. The figures show the extensive areas to which pain can be referred from cervical, thoracic and lumbar displacements respectively.*

10.3

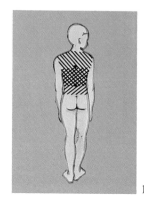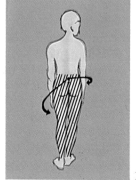

10.4   **10.5**

EXAMINATION FOR A SPINAL DISPLACEMENT: SUMMARY II

Spinal level	CERVICAL	THORACIC	LUMBAR
History *Always characteristic*	Usually unilateral scapular pain almost always referred extrasegmentally	Posterior trunk pain, often referred extrasegmentally	Pain in lumbar region, buttocks, legs, often referred extrasegmentally
Joint Signs			

Dural Signs
 Sometimes present
	Painful neck flexion (ambiguous; stretches thoracic extent of dura)	Painful neck flexion (ambiguous, see left)
		   Check for pain on moving shoulder girdle backwards, forwards and upwards
		   Ask if deep breath or coughing painful
			Test for bilateral limitation on SLR
			   Ask if deep breath or coughing painful

Nerve Root Signs			
Cord Signs			

Dural signs

Dural involvement may give rise to any of the following signs:

At cervical level

Painful neck flexion. This tugs the dura mater upwards. If mobility is restricted pain results, but it is an ambiguous finding as dural mobility could also be impaired at the thoracic level.

At thoracic levels

(1) Painful neck flexion (see above).
(2) Scapular approximation pulls on the first and second nerve roots, thereby raising the dura's thoracic extent. Bringing the shoulder girdle forwards or upwards may also (although less often) have the same effect. If mobility is impeded, pain will result.
(3) Pain on a deep breath or (less often) coughing.

At lumbar levels

(1) Painful straight-leg raise and its variant, the 'slump test'. This stretches the dura mater via the sciatic nerve. A central protrusion limiting dural mobility would thus produce pain on bilateral straight-leg raise. Sometimes straight-leg raise on one side gives rise to pain on the contralateral side due to a tug on the main dura.
(2) Pain on coughing or (less distinctly) on a deep breath.

Each of these signs can be specifically examined for, as set out in Table II.

The nerve roots

Thirty pairs of nerve roots project from the dura mater. Each nerve root draws out with it an investment of the dura mater[2] that extends, judging by clinical data, for at least 2 cm (see *Figure 10.2*).

Compression of the dural sleeve causes pain distributed on an accurate segmental basis – for example, from the C8 root to the third, fourth and fifth fingers, and from the L4 root down the leg and big toe.

Mobility

In addition, the dural sleeve is mobile at lumbar levels and any interference with mobility may be detected by unilateral pain on stretching by passive movements –
straight-leg raise and prone-lying knee flexion. These are the tests for nerve root mobility.

Each root also possesses an internal aspect – the parenchyma – which serves conduction only. Mild pressure on the dural sheath may not be great enough to hamper the conduction of the parenchyma. In this case the tests show:

(1) Interference with mobility of the dural sleeve (i.e. pain increased by stretching).
(2) No impedence of conduction (i.e. neither paraesthesia nor weakness on resisted movements nor absence or sluggishness of jerks).

Conduction

Greater pressure disrupts nerve root mobility and conduction giving positive results for both tests.

Interference with sensory conduction produces pins and needles or numbness, generally located at the distal end of the dermatome. Weakness (motor conduction) will be detectable in the appropriate muscle groups and the reflexes absent or sluggish. Accordingly, the function of the parenchyma is assessed by tests for sensation, power and reflexes.

Extreme pressure may result in ischaemic root atrophy.

Mobility and conduction

The clinical picture at different spinal levels does not always permit examination for both mobility and conduction.

At the cervical spine the nerve roots are tethered to the transverse processes and therefore cannot be stretched by any arm movements; they are immobile. Consequently, examination at cervical levels is limited to the parenchyma (although gently forced sustained neck flexion may reproduce brachialgia). Any weakness detected by resisted arm movements should be monoradicular (see below).

At the thoracic spine, root pain is not uncommon and is a particularly deceptive symptom as pain is only felt anteriorly. However, no practicable way exists of testing the nerve roots for mobility although neck flexion provides an occasional indicator. Conduction is very rarely affected.

At lumbar levels, a disc lesion could, theoretically, affect any nerve root(s) between L1 and S4. In fact, displacements at L1 and L2 are extremely rare, L3 is relatively uncommon and a protrusion here attacks only the third lumbar nerve root. Fourth or fifth lumbar disc lesions are the norm and may give rise to monoradicular or polyradicular root signs as discussed below. So the parenchyma is examined by resisted movements for weakness. Nerve root mobility at L3 is tested by prone-lying knee flexion and at L4, L5, S1 and S2 by straight-leg raise.

Polyradicular and monoradicular symptoms

At cervical levels, the nerve roots are aligned almost horizontally. Hence any symptoms emanating from impingement on a nerve root by a cervical displacement will be monoradicular. Theoretically, any root between C3 and T2 is at risk. In practice, the clinician is most often concerned with the roots at C5, C6, C7 and C8.

At lumbar levels, the nerve roots project obliquely. This downward slope has an important practical bearing: it enables a herniated disc to compress two roots simultaneously (*Figure 10.6*). Furthermore, a displacement at a particular level is not necessarily paired with one particular root. Thus a protrusion lying almost centrally at the fourth level can pinch the fifth root or, by inclining a little more to one side, compress only the fourth root. A larger protrusion could, of course, affect both. Thus symptoms may be polyradicular.

The findings from this section are incorporated in the table on the following page.

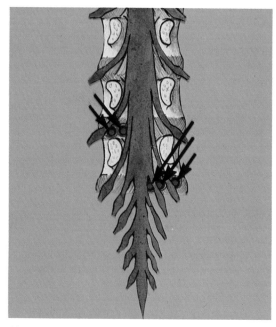

10.6 *Lumbar nerve roots, posterior view. The exact site of a displacement determines the root(s) compressed. An L4 protrusion (left) can affect either the L4 or the L5 root, or both simultaneously. L5 disc lesions (right) have an even wider choice.*

EXAMINATION FOR A SPINAL DISPLACEMENT: SUMMARY III

Spinal level	CERVICAL	THORACIC	LUMBAR
History *Always characteristic*	Usually unilateral scapular pain, almost always referred extrasegmentally. Any nerve root pain felt in appropriate dermatome	Posterior trunk pain, often referred extrasegmentally. Any nerve root pain felt anteriorly (sometimes the only symptom)	Pain in lumbar region, buttocks, legs, often referred extrasegmentally. Nerve root pain felt in lower limb in appropriate dermatome(s)
Joint Signs			
Dural Signs *Sometimes present*	Painful neck flexion (ambiguous; stretches thoracic extent of dura)	Painful neck flexion (ambiguous, see left) Check for pain on moving shoulder girdle backwards, forwards and upwards Ask if deep breath or coughing painful	Test for bilateral limitation on SLR Ask if deep breath or coughing painful
Nerve Root Signs: Mobility *Sometimes present*	No test – nerve roots tethered to transverse processes (but see right for T1 and T2)	Mobility of T1 and T2 roots tested by scapular approximation during cervical examination. No test for other thoracic roots	Test for unilateral limitation on SLR (L4, L5, S1 and S2 roots) Test for unilateral pain on prone knee flexion (L3 root)
Nerve Root Signs: Weakness and paraesthesia *Sometimes present*	Any signs monoradicular. Test upper limb for muscle weakness (revealed on resisted movements) and absent or sluggish jerks. Test lower forearm and hand for sensory changes. T1 and T2 included in this examination	No test for T3–T12; weakness not detectable. For T1 and T2, see left. Paraesthesia is rare and of little localizing value	Signs may be polyradicular. Test lower limb for weakness (revealed on resisted movements), sensory changes and absent or sluggish jerks
Cord Signs			

The posterior longitudinal ligament

This runs the length of the spinal canal, being attached to the vertebral bodies and, by weak lateral fibres, to each disc. The ligament narrows as it runs caudally and affords some protection to the dura from intervertebral disc prolapse. But although the ligament occupies the mid-line, it is deficient at each side; it does not span the full width of the vertebrae.

Hence disc material initially protruding centrally runs into the barrier of a tough ligament (*Figures 10.7* and *10.8*). The ligament may bulge out enough to compress the dura, resulting in extrasegmental pain. But its

10.7

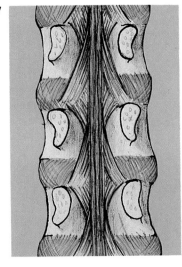

10.8

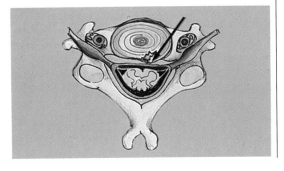

10.7, 10.8, 10.9 *The posterior ligament is strong centrally (Figure 10.7) but can be bulged backwards by a central displacement to interfere with the dura (Figure 10.8). The ligamentous deficiency at the sides allows direct access to the nerve roots (see over, Figure 10.9)*

resistance tends to contain the displacement, a process accounting for the regular occurrence of spontaneous reduction in lumbago.

After repeated attacks, the protrusion is apt to shift posterolaterally where the ligament is weaker. There it threatens the nerve roots (*Figure 10.9*), and thus as the protrusion enlarges it usually becomes unilateral. As a result, central pain in the back is replaced by root pain in the lower limb, and unilateral scapular pain exchanged for brachial symptoms. This is reflected in the history.

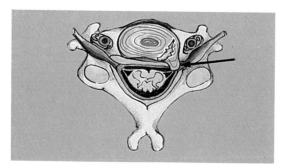

10.9

The disc

Between the bodies of each two vertebrae (except C1 and C2) lies a disc, the largest avascular structure in the whole body. Each disc is separated from the dura's anterior aspect by the posterior longitudinal ligament.

Being of cartilage, the disc:

(1) Lacks the capacity to transmit pain (despite recent *in vivo* findings of innervation).
(2) Is radiotranslucent (although it may show alteration in CT or NMR reflectivity).
(3) Has very limited potential for repair.

A wide capsule of fibrocartilage (*annulus fibrosus*) composed of various criss-crossing layers encases a soft water-absorbent *nucleus pulposus* which distributes pressure hydrostatically. The nucleus consists of a softish gelatinous polysaccharide. In the young it is quite distinct from the annulus, less so in adults and by middle age has disappeared completely, degenerating into fibrous tissue.

When time and the multiple traumata of ordinary active life have initiated damage, the cartilage becomes slightly, and then more, cracked. In the end, a fragment forms that is either completely detached within the joint or lies hinged.

Sometimes the nucleus pushes past the annulus. If so, pure herniation of pulp with an intact annulus results. Alternatively, a cartilaginous displacement of sufficient size may become aggravated by secondary herniation of nuclear material.

Thus a displacement of disc material may consist either of a cartilaginous loose fragment or of nuclear material or both. Any of these may move posteriorly to compress the dura mater centrally via the posterior longitudinal ligament or laterally to impinge on the nerve roots. Either way, pain will result.

Cartilage is hard and such a displacement is often susceptible to manipulative reduction. Nuclear material is soft and cannot be nudged back into place. Sustained heavy traction is the treatment of choice.

A lateral protrusion of disc material indenting the nerve roots lies outside the joint, and its extra-articular position deprives the fragment of its nutrients. Hence the protrusion slowly shrinks.

At the neck, spontaneous recovery from nerve root impingement giving brachial pain may be expected four months after the pain shifts into the arm. For some unknown reason, spontaneous recovery does not occur at thoracic levels. But at the lumbar spine the corresponding period is recovery within a year.

However, this mechanism is not brought into play when the displacement remains central, causing pain chiefly in the back. Thus backache or neckache may persist or recur indefinitely.

Onset of backache from a cartilaginous displacement is rapid and often immediate. Pain from a nuclear displacement tends to come on over some hours or overnight, intensifying bit by bit as the pulp herniates and the bulge enlarges. At the neck nuclear displacements are rare, at the thoracic spine they are even more unusual, but at the lumbar spine clinical experience suggests they contribute about one case in three in patients under 60. Patients over 60 no longer have a nucleus.

Displacements at the spine, as elsewhere, give rise to the characteristic history of sporadic attacks. Cartilage is an avascular structure and has little capacity for regeneration.

In common with other structures, cartilage degenerates with the passage of time, but this causes no pain of itself. In old age the discs crumble away, an individual sometimes losing two inches or more in height. Disc trouble then ceases and although spinal mobility is often minimal the limitation is nearly always painless. In fact, the highest incidence of back trouble is in the age group 40–49, tailing off thereafter[3]. It should therefore be abundantly clear that degeneration of any tissue in the spine cannot provide the explanation for back trouble.

The findings from this section are tabulated incrementally on page 149.

EXAMINATION FOR A SPINAL DISPLACEMENT: SUMMARY IV

Spinal level	CERVICAL	THORACIC	LUMBAR

History
Always characteristic
	Usually unilateral scapular pain, almost always referred extrasegmentally. Any nerve root pain felt in appropriate dermatome
	    Brachial symptoms may follow scapular pain. Pain in upper limb recovers spontaneously within four months from onset
	    Discs radiotranslucent.
	History of recurrent attacks
		Posterior trunk pain, often referred extrasegmentally. Any nerve root pain felt anteriorly (sometimes the only symptom)
		    No spontaneous recovery from root pain
		    Discs radiotranslucent.
		History of recurrent attacks
			Pain in lumbar region, buttocks, legs, often referred extrasegmentally. Nerve root pain felt in lower limb in appropriate dermatome(s)
			    Root pain in leg comes on as pain in back fades. Spontaneous recovery from pain in lower limb within one year from onset
			    Discs radiotranslucent. Cartilaginous displacements characterized by rapid onset; nuclear displacements (confined to those under 60) by slow onset. History of recurrent attacks

Joint Signs			

Dural Signs
Sometimes present
	Painful neck flexion (ambiguous; stretches thoracic extent of dura)	Painful neck flexion (ambiguous, see left)
		    Check for pain on moving shoulder girdle backwards, forwards and upwards
		    Ask if deep breath or coughing painful
			Test for bilateral limitation on SLR
			    Ask if deep breath or coughing painful

Nerve Root Signs: Mobility *Sometimes present*	No test – nerve roots tethered to transverse processes (but see right for T1 and T2)	Mobility of T1 and T2 roots tested by scapular approximation during cervical examination. No test for other thoracic roots	Test for unilateral limitation on SLR (L4, L5, S1 and S2 roots) Test for unilateral pain on prone knee flexion (L3 root)
Nerve Root Signs: Weakness and paraesthesia *Sometimes present*	Any signs monoradicular. Test upper limb for muscle weakness (revealed on resisted movements) and absent or sluggish jerks. Test lower forearm and hand for sensory changes. T1 and T2 included in this examination	No test for T3–T12; weakness not detectable. For T1 and T2, see left. Paraesthesia is rare and of little localizing value	Signs may be polyradicular. Test lower limb for weakness (revealed on resisted movements), sensory changes and absent or sluggish jerks
Cord Signs			

The joints

In principle, the joints at the spine are examined by the normal routine of resisted and passive movements. Although muscular lesions are rare, the findings on resisted movements are valuable in assessing the patient both for neurosis and malingering.

At the thoracic and lumbar spine active movements are substituted for the passive, as body weight ensures that the active movements (although instigated by muscular action) are largely passive in their diagnostic import.

As at other joints the findings may be of:

(1) The capsular pattern (uncommon).
(2) The non-capsular pattern, nearly always of a kind compatible with internal derangement (common).

The intervertebral joints have no capsule, and thus the capsular pattern at all spinal levels results from an affection of the facet joints.

Internal derangement of the intervertebral joints produces the partial articular pattern. Movement about the joint painfully forces any protrusion against the dura mater;

the pain is then present on some, but not all, movements. Additionally, a displacement obstructs free movement at the joint giving rise to limitation. So a displacement produces pain and limitation in the non-capsular pattern characteristic of internal derangement. This is in addition to dural signs previously discussed where the dura is stretched by traction exerted from a distance by, for example, straight-leg raising.

In fact, often a disc lesion is evidenced only by its history and the limitation of spinal movements in the pattern of internal derangement. Examination of the dura mater, nerve root sleeve and parenchyma often prove negative.

Zygapophyseal hypertrophy can threaten the nerve at the intervertebral foramen giving rise to root pressure. If this occurs together with a disc it puts the emerging nerve root in double jeopardy.

The zygapophyseal joints

The facet joints are non-load-bearing joints which contribute to stability and, at the lumbar spine, prevent rotation. They possess both a capsule and a small intra-articular cartilage, but at lumbar levels, Nachemson's 1962 research shows that for loads of less than 200 kg in the mid-position, no facet compression strain is apparent. The menisci are positioned so that they can be pinched on extension but never on flexion.

The facets are often cited as a source of spinal pain but, excluding the acknowledged capsular conditions, the evidence is less than persuasive. First, the arguments supporting the proposition are often inconclusive. Thus there may well be local tenderness around the facets, but this is consistent with dural extrasegmental tenderness. Nor is the phenomenon of the temporary abolition of tender spots by massage or even steroid injection conclusive. If the relief is short lived and the tender spots reappear elsewhere, this has all the hallmarks of referred symptoms; similar but lasting relief may be obtained by, for example, manipulative reduction. It is possible that the steroid therapy functions through the acupuncture effect. Likewise, the fact that some back pain produces discomfort only on extension does not of itself prove facet involvement; it is equally likely that extension pinches or impels an intervertebral protrusion posteriorly, particularly if nuclear.

Second, many clinical and anatomical considerations militate against facet involvement in partial articular lesions. In the neutral position at least, the facets are well protected against traumatic strain which is likely to be previously

absorbed by (primarily) the intervertebral disc and (secondarily) the vertebra itself. Further, individual cases with undisputed facet joint disorientation are often symptomless. The gross disc degeneration attendant on ageing (with its knock-on effect on facet loading) is marked by a statistical decrease in backache; and similarly, degenerative spondylolisthesis is often undiagnosed (because pain-free) until an X-ray is taken for another reason.

Third, once the cases on which there is agreement that the facets could not be involved are excluded from overall caseload, little remains. Thus the facets cannot be responsible for root signs, pins and needles, painful arcs, pain that is precisely central, pain that moves markedly from or to the centre, or pain brought on by neutral-position sitting or by bending forwards into semi-flexion.

While it is true there remain instances of backache which pose difficult diagnostic problems, to date there are no verifiably reported cases – dissection or otherwise – in orthodox medicine of non-capsular conditions (including a displaced meniscus) of the facets. The facets can and do suffer various capsular disorders (many painless) from which the spinal capsular pattern results, the vertebral joints themselves lacking a capsule. In some capsular cases, in the absence of systemic or gross pathological signs, they may benefit from an injection of steroid suspension, but both the diagnostic criteria and the results are uncertain, and the injection impossible to accomplish accurately with any certainty in the absence of X-ray control.

Intervertebral pressure

The thoracic kyphosis is compensated for by the secondary neck and lumbar lordoses. Both neck and lumbar flexion open the posterior aspect of the joint and close the anterior. So the tilt of the vertebral surfaces during flexion subjects the disc, by the parallelogram of forces, to pressure directed posteriorly towards the dura mater. By contrast, a healthy degree of lordosis generates anterior pressure (*Figure 10.10*). Moreover, the experimental findings of Nachemson[4] show it

is during flexion that intervertebral pressure reaches its peak. If the pressure within the disc while an individual is standing is taken as 100, then on lying supine it is 25, while lying on the side it is 75 and while sitting it is 140. When standing slightly bent forwards it reaches 150; sitting slightly bent forwards, 180; standing bent well forwards, 210 and sitting bent well forwards, 270.

Flexion of the spine thus:

(1) Exerts strong pressure on the disc.
(2) Exerts pressure directed posteriorly, engendering 'disc creep' which can produce pain a few hours later.

Not surprisingly, many attacks of disc trouble are triggered off by bending and lifting, a fact which likewise has important implications for prophylaxis.

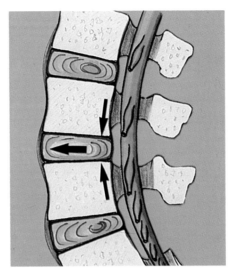

10.10 *Lordosis of the lumbar spine subjects the disc to anterior pressure, directing it away from sensitive structures.*

The spinal cord

A major disc lesion may threaten the integrity of the spinal cord. Whether at cervical, thoracic or first lumbar levels this affords the strongest possible contraindication to manipulation. Examination for cord signs is mandatory.

Spinal cord compression is not painful. At the cervical spine, pins and needles (unaccompanied by pain) in both upper limbs or all four limbs may result. These symptoms may possibly be elicited only by neck flexion.

Encroachment on the spinal cord at thoracic or first lumbar levels may give rise to a tingling sensation in both lower limbs.

Irrespective of the spinal level at which the lesion is expected to lie, the plantar response is always tested.

Summary

Examination
The examination described in the previous sections will:

(1) Show disc lesions constitute by far the largest category of spinal disorders.
(2) Differentiate the other spinal disorders, as they do not conform to the known characteristics of a disc lesion.

Treatment
Examination, diagnosis and treatment at each spinal level are elaborated in the ensuing chapters. In brief:

(1) At cervical levels nearly all displacements are cartilaginous and respond to manipulation (although osteophyte formation may limit the eventual attainment of full range).
(2) At thoracic levels the pattern is similar but with a greater tendency to relapse, which may be countered by injections of sclerosant material.
(3) At lumbar levels, nuclear displacements can be dealt with by sustained traction[5] and cartilaginous displacements by manipulation. Sclerosants diminish the tendency to relapse, and epidural local anaesthesia may permanently abolish the pain from an otherwise irreducible displacement[6]. Surgery or discolysis is only very seldom required.

EXAMINATION FOR A SPINAL DISPLACEMENT: SUMMARY V

Spinal level	CERVICAL	THORACIC	LUMBAR

History
Always characteristic
	Usually unilateral scapular pain, almost always referred extrasegmentally. Any nerve root pain felt in appropriate dermatome
	   Brachial symptoms may follow scapular pain. Pain in upper limb recovers spontaneously within four months from onset
	   Discs radiotranslucent. History of recurrent attacks limiting spinal mobility
		Posterior trunk pain, often referred extrasegmentally. Any nerve root pain felt anteriorly (sometimes the only symptom)
		   No spontaneous recovery from root pain
		   Discs radiotranslucent. History of recurrent attacks limiting spinal mobility. Onset of pain often during bending/lifting
			Pain in lumbar region, buttocks, legs, often referred extrasegmentally. Nerve root pain felt in lower limb in appropriate dermatome(s)
			   Root pain in leg comes on as pain in back fades. Spontaneous recovery from pain in lower limb within one year from onset
			   Discs radiotranslucent. Cartilaginous displacements characterized by rapid onset; nuclear displacements (confined to those under 60) by slow onset. History of recurrent attacks limiting lumbar mobility. Onset often during bending and/or lifting

Joint Signs *Always characteristic*	Test for pain and limitation on passive cervical movements in some but not all directions	Test for pain and limitation on thoracic movements in some but not all directions	Test for pain and limitation on lumbar movements in some but not all directions (except lumbago, where all movements asymmetrically limited)

Dural Signs
Sometimes present
	Painful neck flexion (ambiguous; stretches thoracic extent of dura)	Painful neck flexion (ambiguous, see left)
		   Check for pain on moving shoulder girdle backwards, forwards and upwards
		   Ask if deep breath or coughing painful
			Test for bilateral limitation on SLR
			   Ask if deep breath or coughing painful

Nerve Root Signs: Mobility *Sometimes present*	No test – nerve roots tethered to transverse processes (but see right for T1 and T2)	Mobility of T1 and T2 roots tested by scapular approximation during cervical examination. No test for other thoracic roots	Test for unilateral limitation on SLR (L4, L5, S1 and S2 roots) Test for unilateral pain on prone knee flexion (L3 root)
Nerve Root Signs: Weakness and paraesthesia *Sometimes present*	Any signs monoradicular. Test upper limb for muscle weakness (revealed on resisted movements) and absent or sluggish jerks. Test lower forearm and hand for sensory changes. T1 and T2 included in this examination	No test for T3–T12; weakness not detectable. For T1 and T2, see left. Paraesthesia is rare and of little localizing value	Signs may be polyradicular. Test lower limb for weakness (revealed on resisted movements), sensory changes and absent or sluggish jerks
Cord Signs *Rare*	Check plantar response. Never manipulate if cord signs present	Check plantar response. Never manipulate if cord signs present	Check plantar response (L1 only). Never manipulate if cord signs present

NB Although this mode of examination is specifically geared towards detection and classification of a displacement, it also serves to differentiate other causes of spinal pain.

Spinal manipulation

At joints containing a meniscus it has long been accepted that manipulation acts to abolish symptoms caused by a displacement.

However, the same logic is not always extended to intra-articular displacements at the spine. Spinal manipulation is sometimes denigrated as an unorthodox procedure.

The principal reason for its reluctant acceptance appears to be diagnostic. Pain from a spinal disc lesion is often misascribed to strained back muscles, osteoarthrosis and so on, through, for example, failure to test the patient's movements against resistance or excessive reliance on the X-ray. Many such cases nevertheless respond readily to manipulation because the original diagnosis was incorrect and the relief is brought about by reduction of the undiagnosed displacement.

This creates many apparent complications. Medical men are understandably reluctant to concede that rotating the vertebrae has healed a sprained muscle or abolished osteophytes still visible radiographically. The picture is further complicated by the claims of laymen, who undoubtedly achieve many manipulative successes irrespective of any underlying theoretical deficiency.

This confusing picture can be reduced to orthodoxy by a single non-controversial proposition: at the spine, as elsewhere, manipulation reduces displacements. Clinically both its *modus operandi* and effect are clear: a loose body is identified, the joints are rotated, the displacement shifts, the pain eases and mobility returns. Objective confirmation of this clinically demonstrable hypothesis has been afforded by an East European paper of 1978. Although imperfectly structured and reported, its import is clear. A trial was conducted on a sequence of 50 patients with the 'one-sided sciatic syndrome'. Forty-six had disc lesions visible on the epidurogram, all of whom were manipulated, with epidurograms taken immediately before and after treatment. Eighteen patients were rendered pain-free immediately, 12 of them with the second epidurogram showing reduced or negative disc herniation[7]. It is to be hoped this research can be further consolidated in future controlled trials.

Technique

Manipulation is an outstandingly simple out-patient technique. Although substantial improvement comes with experience, it can be undertaken from the first with both confidence and successful results, often obtained immediately. Tolerable competence can be gained with extreme rapidity.

The objective is to move a loose body between the vertebrae, a result hard to achieve if the process is undertaken gingerly. Controlled vigour is required. Similarly, where manual traction forms part of the manipulation it must be sufficiently strong to bring about separation of the joint surfaces. This sometimes needs the full strength of the operator and his assistant.

Manipulation is not an uncontrolled wrench. As set out on page 27, the joint is first taken to its maximum attainable range. Then the over-pressure is applied. What gives the treatment finesse is the continual recourse to re-examination, allowing each successive manoeuvre to be fine-tuned.

This reappraisal is an integral part of each manipulation. After every manipulation the patient is asked if his pain has altered and the operator checks whether range has improved. Thus the patient performs the movements previously restricted and reports on any alteration in the pain. Any change is immediately apparent.

Clinical judgement, based on reassessment of the patient, provides guidance on what to do next – whether to abandon the session or repeat the same manipulation as before with equal strength, greater strength or in the opposite direction, or whether to try some different manipulation altogether. The underlying principle is that if something has made the patient better it should be repeated.

At lumbar and thoracic levels there are two basic procedures – extension strains and rotation strains. On the whole the sessions will start with the weaker methods before building up to those deploying greater purchase. Likewise, each new technique is first applied well below its maximum to establish the appropriate force.

TREATMENT OF AN INTERVERTEBRAL DISC LESION: SUMMARY

Cervical Displacement	Thoracic Displacement	Lumbar Displacement
Manipulative reduction	Manipulative reduction	Manipulative reduction if cartilaginous
To forestall relapse: 1. Postural education	To forestall relapse: 1. Postural education 2. Sclerosants	Traction if nuclear
		Epidural local anaesthesia if irreducible
		To forestall relapse: 1. Postural education 2. Corset 3. Sclerosants
		Only a tiny proportion of cases go to operation

Note that signs or symptoms may strongly contraindicate manipulation or traction

At the cervical spine there are a variety of different approaches. As well as extension and rotation, the neck can be side-flexed or glided anteroposteriorly. Each produces a slightly different effect and generally each is suitable for a particular purpose.

Even so it is impossible and ill-advised to be categoric about the order in which the manipulations should be tried. During the original examination the clinician notes which movements are limited and which are painful. Guided by his findings on re-examination he makes up his own mind as to the next step. Fifteen or twenty minutes per session is probably about as much as the patient can stand, during which half a dozen techniques of varying vigour may be tried. Very often, in cases of partial improvement, the patient may have to attend a couple of days later to dispose of the residual symptoms. Three sessions would be the

maximum; by then, the patient should be as well as he can be made by any form of effective manipulation.

By trial and error and relying on a growing body of experience, the clinician strives to achieve full reduction. The methods set out in the ensuing pages evolved over the years and are tried and tested, but the reader need not feel bound by them: the most effective technique is the best. By contrast, the continual recourse to reappraisal is indispensable. It makes spinal manipulation both productive and safe.

It follows that manipulation under anaesthetic is a dangerous waste of time, the more so since the procedure should be painless.

Occasionally re-examination shows manipulation has made the patient not better but worse. Normally the first recourse is the same manoeuvre but in the opposite direction.

Diagnostic aids and misleading phenomena

X-ray

The disc is cartilaginous and does not show on the X-ray. As elsewhere with soft-tissue trouble, a number of misleading inferences may be drawn from radiographic appearances, not least the presence of fractures, stress fractures, micro-fractures, spondylolisthesis, spina bifida occulta and the like. These can and do cause pain, but their mere detection on the X-ray is far from conclusive evidence that they are the cause of the present pain. Additionally:

(1) Osteoarthrosis/osteophytosis are usually symptomless. Radiological surveys have shown that, by the age of 50, lumbar osteophytosis is present in 90% of normal men. Osteophytes (with very rare exceptions) protrude anteriorly away from the dura mater.

(2) A narrowed joint space is immaterial of itself. It merely proves the disc is thinned. But many discs atrophy with advancing age without herniation, and a normal disc space by no means excludes gross displacement of disc material. By discography, Collis[8] showed that 56% of herniations arose at intervertebral spaces of normal thickness.

(3) Osteoporosis is normally symptomless[9]. Elderly patients, usually women, with marked generalized rarefaction of the spine may sustain a pathological fracture of one or more vertebrae. It is more frequent in the thoracic than the lumbar region. The wedging may evolve slowly. It is then painless (unless a secondary disc lesion develops on account of the upper lumbar kyphosis at the joints above and below the collapse). However, if the wedging comes on abruptly, bone pain results. It may be severe for a week or two but fades in two or three months. The kyphosis is visible and palpable. Osteoporosis does not appear to cause aching unless fracture supervenes, but frequent bouts of lesser pain may well be caused by

repeated micro-fractures. Symptomless osteoporosis visible on the radiograph may occur simultaneously with a disc lesion.

(4) Spondylolisthesis – particularly if posterior – does not necessarily cause symptoms[10]. It may result in no more than instability of the lateral joints (see page 200).

(5) Scoliosis and lordosis are the names of shapes and, unless severe, are not painful of themselves. Schmorl's nodes produce no symptoms.

(6) Scheuermann's disease is not a disease but a ring epiphysitis of the developing vertebrae. It may be painful for several years. Posture is important; manipulation and traction give little help.

Myelography/radiculography

When a neuroma is suspected, contrast myelography is obviously indicated. For disc lesions, it may be highly unreliable diagnostically, but can be used in conjunction with CT or NMR scanning.

If a disc protrusion passes laterally, the dural tube is not indented and the displacement is not disclosed. Findings[11] for invisibility of disc lesions are 11.9% at the fourth lumbar level and 23.8% at the fifth. Hence a negative finding does not exclude herniation. Nor, for that matter, is a positive finding necessarily relevant. Both cervical and lumbar filling defects may be entirely inconsequential, as Hitselberger and Whitten[12] found in 1968 when investigating patients with suspected acoustic tumour. They extended their observations to the spinal canal. Even when all patients with a past history of back troubles were excluded, they detected myelographic defects indicating disc abnormality in no less than 37%. Clinical judgement is a surer arbiter of a displacement's presence and severity.

Computer assisted tomography

CT retains its place because of good bone imaging. It also shows certain elements of the soft tissues. CT is a cross-sectional imaging technique; reformatting the anatomical information in other planes is not very satisfactory and the production of three-dimensional images tends to be complicated and costly. A lateral or central disc herniation will be displayed, but as with any technique, experience is required to interpret the results. There are indications that patients who have had disc lesions displayed on CT and who become pain-free may still show protrusions on follow-up examination.

Magnetic resonance imaging

MRI is probably the best imaging technique for showing soft tissues in detail. It is useful both for detecting tissue abnormality and for accurate localization, including for example the precise tendon affected. Importantly, it can image in any plane. Although expensive in capital terms, MRI is an out-patient procedure increasingly acceptable as an alternative to arthroscopy, which is invasive and carries well-recognized morbidity. Unlike CT, MRI produces no ionizing radiation and for this reason alone is preferable.

MRI shows disc protrusions and is particularly useful in excluding the difficult central cervical protrusions. It also displays the abnormal synovium of rheumatoid arthritis. The advent of the contrast medium gadolinium DTPA has opened up the potential to explore joint disease more fully, as any inflammatory disease is likely to be hypervascular.

Clearly, statistical work correlating MRI findings with the results of clinical diagnosis is now an important possibility.

Bone scintigraphy (technetium^{99m} phosphate compounds)

A highly sensitive but very non-specific technique. Sportsmen may produce stress fractures and early bone changes which are visible on bone scan before they are noted on X-ray. A blood-pool image will indicate blood flow, and a three-hour scan, bony activity. A combination of images enables assessment of soft tissue lesions, fractures, shin splints or avascular necrosis. A bone scan provides indications of increased activity suggesting pathology.

Muscular pain

At the spine the proliferation of diagnostic attributions is particularly broad. Not all theories of back pain are well thought through. Possibly the concept combining the least evidence with the broadest support relates to the role of muscular strain and muscle spasm. If the patient's trunk and/or neck movements are tested against resistance it hardly ever increases the pain, thus excluding muscular lesions. That is, no diagnosis of muscular trouble in the spine should be accepted unless it has first been put to the proof by means of this simple test. This applies even where exercise, exertion or sport precede the onset of pain; the recent performance of these activities does not necessarily entail a finding of sprained muscles. It follows that treatment directed at the muscles, whether in the form of heat, massage, muscle relaxants, muscle strengtheners or exercises – including machine-based regimens – is misconceived.

In severe cases, muscle spasm will be evident. But as elsewhere this is a painless secondary phenomenon brought into play to guard the joint and does not require treatment.

Lumbago, sciatica, fibrositis and rheumatism are of course not diagnoses but names of symptoms.

Exercises

These are not justified, except as symptomatic help after the underlying cause has been rectified. No matter how sophisticated or alluring the exercise equipment, its use is not warranted in the absence of a muscular lesion. Well-developed musculature does not diminish the liability to displacements[13].

However, postural education and exercises that build up postural control may help prevent recurrence.

Spinal stenosis

This does not produce backache of itself, but patients with too small a spinal canal are apt to suffer from encroachment on its space by, for example, a disc lesion, zygapophyseal (facet joint) hypertrophy, ligamentum flavum kinking or hypertrophy and any cause of bone enlargement. Symptoms include spinal claudication. Imaging is not always reliable and the best results are probably obtained by radiculogram done in the supine position and also erect with the spine extended.

References
1. Edgar, M.A. and Nundy, S. (1966) Innervation of the spinal dura mater. *Neurol. Neurosurg. Psychiat.*, **29**, 530
2. Frykholm, R. (1951) Lower cervical nerve-roots and their investments. *Acta Chir. Scand.*, **101**, 457
3. Leavitt, S.S., Johnson, T.L. and Beyer, R.D. (1971) Patterns in industrial back injury. *Industry Med. Surg.*, **40**, 8
4. Nachemson, A. (1960) Measurement of intradiscal pressure. *Acta Orthop. Scand.*, Suppl. 43,1
5. Mathews, J.A. (1968) Dynamic discography: a study of lumbar traction. *Ann. Phys. Med.*, **7**, 275
6. Coomes, E.N. (1963) Comparison between epidural local anaesthesia and bed rest in sciatica. *Br. Med. J.*, i, 20
7. Szechery, F., Csispo, L. and Kiss, E. (1978) *Psychopathology, Szentes. Psychiatric Theory*, **31**, 436-440
8. Collis, J.S. (1963) *Lumbar Discography,* Charles C. Thomas, Springfield, Ill.
9. Ross, E. (1962) Ergebnisse einer Reihenröntgenuntersuchung der Wirbelsäule bei 5000 Jugendlichen. *Fortschr. Röntgenstr.*, **97**, 734
10. Key, J.A. (1945) Intervertebral disc lesions are the commonest cause of low back pain with or without sciatica. *Ann. Surg.*, **121**, 534
11. Gurdjian, E.S. and Thomas, L.M. (1970) *Neckache and Backache*, Charles C. Thomas, Springfield, Ill.
12. Hitselberger, W.E. and Whitten, R.M. (1968) Abnormal myelograms in asymptomatic patients. *J. Neurosurg.*, **28**, 204
13. Nachemson, A. and Lind (1969) Measurement of abdominal and back muscle strength with and without low back pain. *Scand. J. Rehab. Med.*, **1**, 60

CHAPTER ELEVEN

THE CERVICAL SPINE

The great majority of soft-tissue symptoms at the neck originate from different stages of the same disorder: degenerative conditions of the disc. Manipulative reduction is the treatment in all but a few cases.

A disc lesion at cervical levels as elsewhere will block the joint, resulting in extrasegmentally referred dural pain – familiar as the colloquial stiff neck – with or without nerve root symptoms and signs. Patients with limited cervical range and cervical pain suggest the appropriate diagnosis, but the discomfort may be confined to the scapular area. The first issue to settle with shoulder pain is thus whether it originates from the neck.

As at other spinal levels, dural pain is often attributed to muscular disorders since that is where the pain is felt. But assessment by function will show this is not the case. Although a collar may be prescribed to prevent the neck jolting into painful range, this is a secondary measure since cervical discs trouble is particularly susceptible to immediate manipulative reduction. The great majority of cases can be dealt with satisfactorily in one or two swift sessions.

Nevertheless, the examination is thorough because a number of alternative causes of pain (some serious and/or strongly contraindicating manipulation) must be recognized.

In particular, the arm is examined for weakness to establish if any neurological deficit is consistent with a disc lesion.

The dura mater

A central disc lesion impinges on the dura mater via the posterior longitudinal ligament, most often giving rise to unilateral scapular pain or, less frequently, pain in the head and neck (*Figure 11.1*). Displacements are common at the C4, C5, C6 and particularly the C7 level.

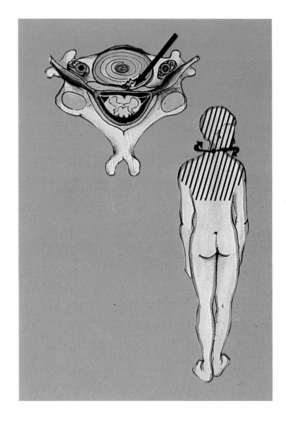

11.1 *Possible areas to which pain can be referred by pressure on the dura mater at cervical levels. Normally the symptoms are unilateral.*

The nerve roots

A posterolateral disc protrusion may compress the dural sleeve and nerve root (*Figure 11.2*). Pressure slight enough to affect the sleeve alone engenders pain in the relevant dermatome. Greater pressure results in conduction losses, making for weakness in the appropriate muscles, absent or sluggish jerks and paraesthesia in the distal end of the dermatome.

Symptoms of a disc lesion may thus be dual. First, the displacement may block the joint, leading to pain and limitation of movement in the non-capsular pattern of internal derangement. Second, the protrusion may produce root signs.

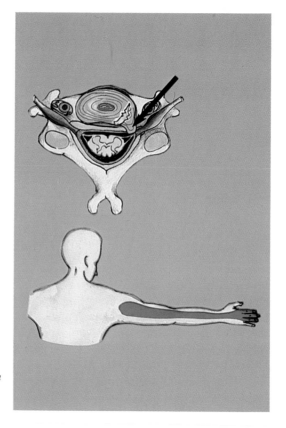

11.2 *A lateral displacement affecting a nerve root gives pain down the arm. C7 dermatome illustrated.*

History

Displacements

A displacement has a characteristic history. The attacks are usually recurrent, sometimes accompanied by sudden fixation of the joint; milder symptoms accompany minor limitation. The condition may settle over a week or continue inter-mittently for years, and the patient complains of a stiff neck.

The slightest jolt may be sufficient to account for onset, so much so that the patient may be at a loss to remember the cause. Many displacements occur through no more than maintenance of postural asymmetry at night. Whiplash injuries are a common cause of disc displacement but evoke central pain; they are tackled by a special manipulation (see page 174).

Root pain and weakness from a displacement are highly unusual in those under 35. Recovery – which cannot be expedited – usually follows within four months of the pain shifting to the arm.

Examination

Joint signs

The neck can move in many directions, but for purposes of examination these are reduced to the six primary ranges. If these prove full and painless, the lesion must be sought elsewhere.

First the active movements are assessed, starting with extension (*Figure 11.3*).

The two side flexions follow (*Figures 11.4* and *11.5*).

The patient then rotates her head first in one direction and then the other (*Figures 11.6* and *11.7*).

Active flexion (*Figure 11.8*) is the last to be tested,

since it is frequently the most painful/restricted and is thus the movement to cause the patient apprehension. More important, it is the most likely to shift the displacement posteriorly. It stretches both the cervical and thoracic extent of the dura mater, so pain on this cervical movement alone may originate from a thoracic disc lesion.

Pain and limitation on each active movement are noted for subsequent correlation with symptoms elicited by passive movements, which immediately ensue.

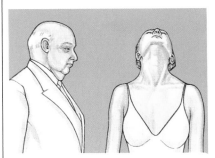

11.3 *Pain on active cervical movement suggests a cervical lesion. Active extension.*

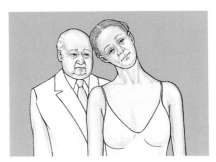

11.4 *Active side flexion.*

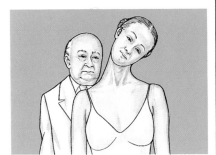

11.5 *Active side flexion.*

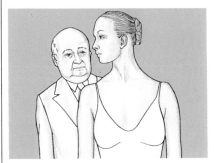

11.6 *Active rotation.*

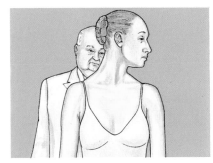

11.7 *Active rotation.*

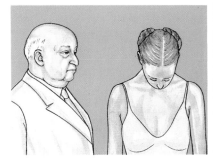

11.8 *Active flexion. Usually the patient finds this the most uncomfortable and worrying movement, so it is tested last.*

The first passive movement is extension (*Figure 11.9*). For the passive side flexions (*Figures 11.10* and *11.11*), care must be taken to limit the movement to the neck by counter-pressure to the thorax, otherwise trunk movements will complicate the clinical picture.

When the passive rotations (*Figures 11.12* and *11.13*) are tested, rotation of the patient's trunk is precluded by the examiner's elbows, one placed in front of the shoulder and the other behind, against the opposite scapula.

Passive flexion is normally omitted as any disc lesion may be exacerbated. The end-feel should be noted throughout, particularly on passive rotation. Vertebral metastases are signalled by the sudden twang of muscle spasm, and early rheumatoid arthritis by a characteristic boggy end-feel.

Passive movements should hurt in the same pattern as the active, but slightly more so because the joint is taken slightly further towards any painful limitation by the operator.

The capsular pattern is limitation of all movements except flexion, which remains relatively full. The non-capsular pattern of internal derangement is pain and limitation of two, three or four movements.

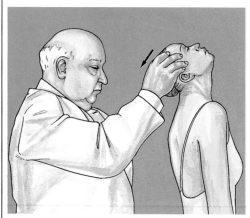

11.9 *The previous movements are now performed passively, for correlation with the active movements. Passive extension.*

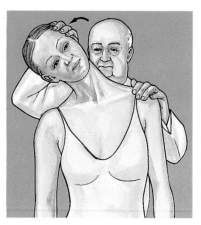

11.10 *Passive side flexion.*

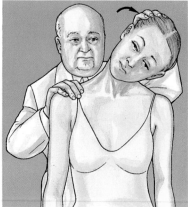

11.11 *Passive side flexion.*

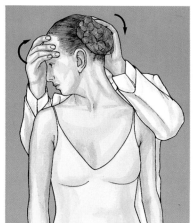

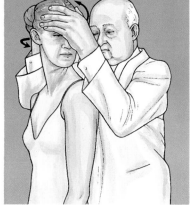

11.12, 11.13 *Passive rotations. Since it is never safe to force flexion, it is not tested passively.*

Next, the six resisted movements are tested. Muscular lesions occur around the cervical spine, and the aetiology is usually either:

(a) a severe whiplash injury (strain of the sub-occipital muscles) or
(b) contractures in the splenius capitus following skull traction for a broken neck.

For the first, an accompanying disc lesion is a certainty and, for the second, a possibility. A muscular lesion following a whiplash injury is relatively unusual. In either case, treatment should be directed initially at the disc.

Additionally, cervical resisted movements may produce pain in severe disc lesions (especially if nuclear) through increase in the intra-discal pressure. With a muscle lesion alone, there will be pain only on the appropriate resisted movement.

First, the examiner resists extension, preventing all movement at the joint so that only the neck muscles are brought into play (*Figure 11.14*). If the patient is not adequately restrained by counter-pressure, the extensors of the entire trunk will be used. Both the side flexions are resisted, with counter-pressure at the opposing shoulder (*Figures 11.15* and *11.16*).

Both resisted rotations (*Figures 11.17* and *11.18*) are tested. If weakness is found (rare), a C1 root palsy – probably the result of serious disease – may be present and would be accompanied by limitation in the capsular pattern. The elbows are used to prevent trunk movement.

Flexion is resisted (*Figure 11.19*) with the free hand applying counter-pressure to the thorax.

Muscular lesions at the neck are extremely rare, so the resisted movements normally prove painless, although occasionally acute torticollis can be aggravated.

Other causes of pain on resisted movement are fracture of the first rib, anginal glandular fever, vertebral metastases, neurosis or sterno-clavicular capsulitis.

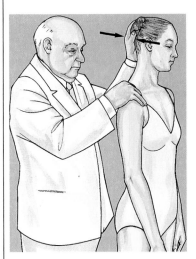

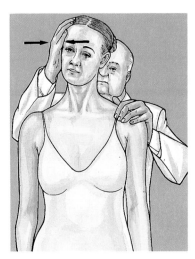

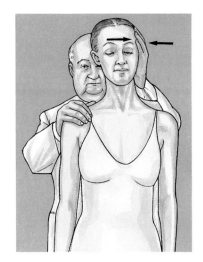

11.14 *The previous movements are again tested, this time against resistance, following the same order. Pain from genuine cervical lesions is rarely aggravated. Resisted extension.*

11.15, 11.16 *Resisted side flexions.*

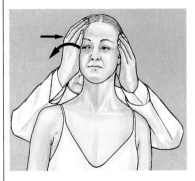

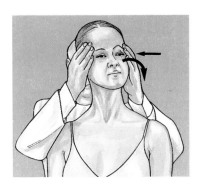

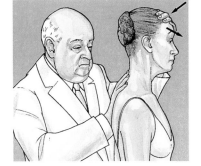

11.17, 11.18 *Resisted rotations.*

11.19 *Resisted flexion.*

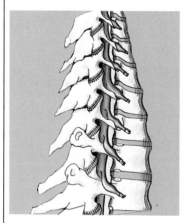

11.20 *The cervical nerve roots. A disc lesion compresses the root one higher in number. Thus the C6 disc impinges on the C7 root.*

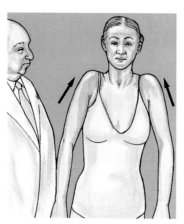

11.21 *Active shoulder girdle elevation. Immobility of the scapula or ostensible weakness of the trapezius suggests either neurosis or serious disease.*

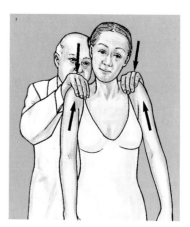

11.22 *Resisted shoulder girdle elevation.*

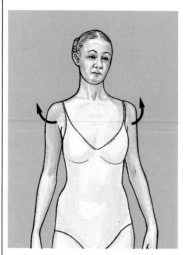

11.23 *T1 and T2 stretch. These two thoracic roots can cause brachial pain; their dermatomes run down the arm.*

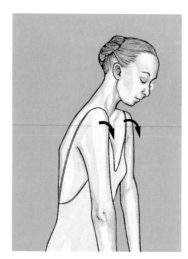

11.24 *Dural stretch.*

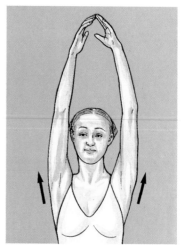

11.25 *Active arm elevation. If full and painless, this rules out capsular lesions of the shoulder; muscular lesions are checked by examination of the nerve roots – see next page.*

The thorax and scapula: dural and nerve root signs

Introduction

The examination now turns to the thorax, scapula and arm. No tests exist for mobility of the nerve roots as each adheres to a transverse process (*Figure 11.20*). However, any weakness of the upper limb from interference with conduction can be detected by painless weakness on resisted brachial movements.

Brachial symptoms fall broadly into three categories. The first is monoradicular signs consistent with a disc lesion. Second, there may be polyradicular signs (rare) inconsistent with a disc lesion and this suggests serious disease. For the significance of mono- and polyradicular signs the reader is referred to pages 146 and 177. Third, a finding of pain on resisted arm movement(s) incriminates a contractile structure at the shoulder as an alternative source of brachial symptoms.

It may well be that examination of the arm draws a blank. In that case the diagnosis is based on the neck movements and history alone.

Examination

Shoulder girdle elevation (*Figure 11.21*) demonstrates whether the scapula – as is usually the case – possesses normal mobility in relation to the thorax. Pulmonary neoplasm, contracture of the costocoracoid fascia, secondary malignant deposits or advanced ankylosing spondylitis in the acromioclavicular joint may limit range.

The trapezius and levator muscles are tested against resistance (*Figure 11.22*). A root palsy at C2 (never a disc) or C3 or C4 (both unlikely to be a disc) would produce weakness.

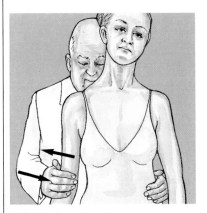

11.26 *Resisted brachial movements are primarily tests for nerve root signs, but also serve to pick out any muscular lesion. Resisted abduction: C5 root.*

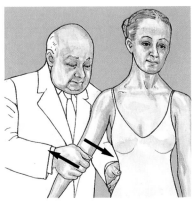

11.27 *Resisted adduction: C7 root.*

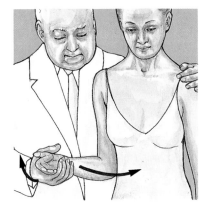

11.28 *Resisted medial rotation.*

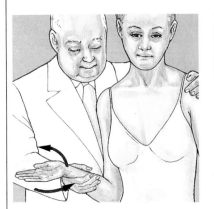

11.29 *Resisted lateral rotation: C5 root.*

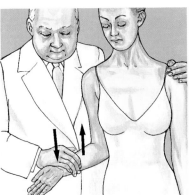

11.30 *Resisted elbow flexion: C5 or C6 roots.*

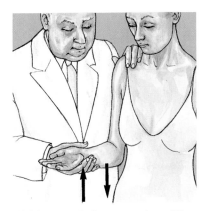

11.31 *Resisted elbow extension: C7 root.*

Active scapular approximation/retraction (*Figure 11.23*) tugs on the first and second thoracic nerve roots, thereby lifting the whole thoracic (but not the cervical) extent of the dura.

Protraction (*Figure 11.24*) similarly shifts the thoracic extent of the dura. Pain on both or either of these movements suggests a thoracic dural lesion.

Examination now passes to the shoulder. The patient elevates both arms (*Figure 11.25*). Full elevation through 180° is to be expected and would exclude a capsular lesion of the shoulder. Limitation unaccompanied by subsequent pathological findings is attributable to neurosis. For the mechanism of arm elevation, the reader is referred to page 35.

Nerve root signs
The examiner now runs through a series of resisted movements, primarily to check for weakness caused by nerve root pressure. A protrusion large enough to hinder conduction is too large to be shifted by manipulation and thus contraindicates successful treatment. If weakness is found, the good side is compared. But pain on resisted movement suggests a lesion of the appropriate contractile structure.

Abduction is resisted (*Figure 11.26*). Pain indicates a defect of the deltoid (rare) or supraspinatus (common), or sometimes the sub-deltoid bursa, and painless weakness a C5 root palsy or a suprascapular neuritis. To detect weakness here and elsewhere the examiner must be correctly positioned, applying counter-pressure to the far side of the patient's body. Neglect of this injunction will activate other muscle groups.

If resisted adduction (*Figure 11.27*) proves weak and painless, a C7 palsy is present.

Painless weakness on resisted medial rotation (*Figure 11.28*) is rare and normally attributable to a partial rupture of the subscapular tendon.

Painless weakness on resisted lateral rotation (*Figure 11.29*) incriminates the C5 root, although suprascapular neuritis again is a possibility. Pain suggests a lesion of the infraspinatus (common) or the teres minor (rare). The counter-pressure is applied at the opposite shoulder.

Elbow flexion is resisted (*Figure 11.30*). Painless weakness points to the C5 or C6 root. Pain indicates a lesion of the biceps or brachialis.

If resisted elbow extension (*Figure 11.31*) is weak, the C7 root is at fault and in fact the great majority of nerve root palsies caused by cervical disc lesions occur here. If the movement is painful, a lesion of the triceps (rare) is suggested.

163

If resisted wrist extension (*Figure 11.32*) proves weak, the C6 root is at fault. If painful, the extensores carpi radialis longus and brevis are incriminated.

Weak resisted wrist flexion (*Figure 11.33*) implicates the C7 root. If painful, the common flexor tendons are responsible.

Painless weakness on resisted ulnar deviation (*Figure 11.34*) denotes involvement of the C8 root and pain suggests a lesion of the ulnar deviators.

For resisted thumb adduction (*Figure 11.35*) the patient presses her thumb inwards. Painless weakness is attributable to a palsy of the C8 root as is weakness on resisted thumb extension (*Figure 11.36*).

Thumb abduction is resisted (*Figure 11.37*). Theoretically any weakness is attributable to the C8 root but in practice the cause is far more often a cervical rib.

The fingers are squeezed together for resisted finger adduction (*Figure 11.38*). Painless weakness suggests a lesion of the T1 root but in fact a disc lesion is never

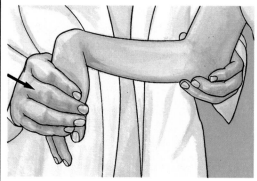

11.32 *Resisted wrist extension: C6 root.*

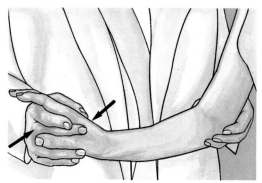

11.33 *Resisted wrist flexion: C7 root.*

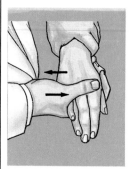

11.34 *Resisted ulnar deviation: C8 root.*

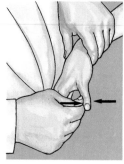

11.35 *Resisted thumb adduction: C8 root.*

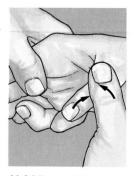

11.36 *Resisted thumb extension: C8 root.*

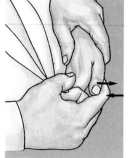

11.37 *Resisted thumb abduction: cervical rib, C8 root.*

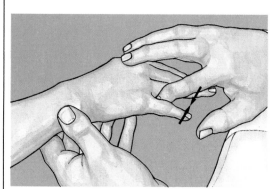

11.38 *Resisted finger adduction.*

responsible; serious disease is more probable.

Next the reflexes are tested. A sluggish brachioradialis jerk (*Figure 11.39*) points to a defect of the C5 root.

A sluggish or absent biceps jerk (*Figure 11.40*) incriminates the C5 or C6 root, and sluggish or absent triceps jerk (*Figure 11.41*) the C7 root.

Cutaneous analgesia is sought at the hand and lower forearm.

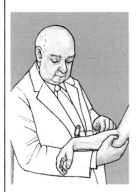

11.39 *Brachioradialis jerk: C5 root.*

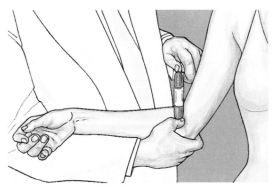

11.40 *Biceps jerk: C5 or C6 root.*

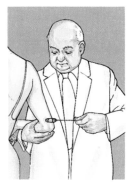

11.41 *Triceps jerk: C7 root.*

Cord signs

Evidence of an upper motor neuron lesion is sought by assessing the patient's plantar response (*Figure 11.42*).

A spastic gait and inco-ordination and clonus of the lower limbs are also diagnostic of cord compression. A central posterior protrusion at cervical (or thoracic) levels may compress the spinal cord and is an absolute bar to manipulation.

Paraesthesia in hands and/or feet is a cord symptom calling for great circumspection.

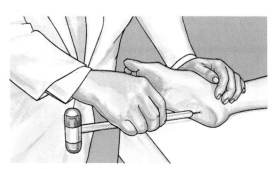

11.42 *Plantar response: cord sign.*

Root signs

The roots emerge from the cervical spine horizontally, so any palsy from a cervical protrusion is monoradicular. The root indented by a disc lesion is one greater in number than the disc. Thus the C2 disc impinges on the C3 root, and so on, with nine out of ten disc lesions concentrated at the sixth cervical level compressing the C7 root.

Root signs (i.e. weakness) indicate that treatment by manipulation will fail, whereas root symptoms (i.e. pain without weakness) indicate that manipulation may fail.

The discovery of brachial symptoms is a prime diagnostic consideration, and before progressing to treatment for a disc lesion the clinician must be assured his diagnosis is correct and that history and joint signs tally. Although disc lesions far outnumber other disorders at the cervical spine, differential diagnosis is of paramount importance and error could prove dangerous.

During examination, root signs are tested for in a logical order, working down the arm for the patient's convenience. On pages 177–179 the maximum root signs are grouped together root by root. In addition to pain in the dermatome, the symptoms may be preceded or accompanied by scapular pain brought on by pressure on the dura mater. Alternative causes of cervical and brachial symptoms are found on page 176.

Findings

Capsular lesions

The capsular pattern is pain and equal limitation of all movements apart from flexion, which is scarcely restricted. End-feel on all the other movements is liable to be hard, except in early rheumatoid arthritis where it is soggy or empty, that is, the movement ceases at a point the examiner can tell is far short of its structural limit.

The capsular pattern occurs with fracture, ankylosing spondylitis, cervical myeloma, chordoma and rheumatoid arthritis. Secondary neoplasm is characterized by rapid onset with polyradicular signs if the invasion is at the fourth to seventh level. At the upper vertebrae, detection is more difficult, but resisted movements will be both painful and weak. All these disorders fall outside the orthopaedic physician's scope and rarely come his way. The commonest cause of capsular limitation is painless loss of mobility attendant on ageing.

Osteoarthrosis of the facets does not produce symptoms except in advanced cases where painless limitation in the capsular pattern is apparent. A disc lesion at an osteoarthritic joint will superimpose painful non-capsular limitation on the painless capsular limitation and should be treated as a disc lesion at a non-osteoarthritic joint. This means that anterior osteophytes may be safely disregarded as they are themselves painless and do not interfere with sentient structures.

Displacements

A disc lesion is characterized by pain and limitation of two, three or four movements, the others retaining full painless range. Limitation is asymmetric (cf. the capsular pattern) and the pain usually unilateral, felt anywhere in the neck or scapular area. Very occasionally a central displacement (often a whiplash injury) will cause pain and/or paraesthesia in both upper limbs.

Brachial pain from a cervical disc lesion hardly every occurs before the age of 35 and disappears (although scapular pain may remain) within four months of onset. Nor – with rare exceptions – will neck movements either cause or accentuate pain down the arm unless passive pressure is maintained by the examiner.

If only one movement is painfully limited by a disc lesion, it is nearly always rotation towards the painful side.

A finding of no painful movements except side flexion *away* from the painful side may indicate an apical lung tumour.

Treatment

Treatment for a minor disc lesion (i.e. in the absence of a root palsy, pain down the arm on cervical movements or other contraindications) is immediate manipulative reduction, practicable even in cases of acute torticollis provided the appropriate method is followed (see Restrictions on Technique 2(4), over).

Manipulation should cease immediately if it brings on or increases brachial pain.

If manipulation is impracticable, alternatives include:
(1) Neck traction. Indications include cervical movements causing/increasing brachial pain, root pain of more than two months and primary posterolateral protrusions. It is valueless with a root palsy.
(2) Cervical epidural, a highly specialist procedure.

Conversely, cervical manipulation is contraindicated where the diagnosis is not of a cervical displacement.

During the acute phase a neck collar may help by stabilizing the neck to prevent jolting into painful range, but should not be considered an alternative to treatment.

Bars to manipulation

A comprehensive history and examination will readily sift out conditions where manipulation could prove dangerous. For further information on differential diagnosis see page 176.

The three types of contraindication are set out below.

(1) Outright contraindications
(1) Cord signs and symptoms.
(2) Adherent dura (provoking extrasegmental paraesthesia).
(3) Drop attacks suggest momentary occlusion of one or both vertebral arteries. The cause may be vascular, degenerative or vertebral instability, the latter coming to light during the first application of manual traction when excessive longitudinal mobility or vertigo are encountered.
(4) Basilar artery insufficiency characterized by vertigo on changes of position; tinnitus and momentary blurring of vision may also occur.
(5) Rheumatoid arthritis of any joint, whether or not the cervical spine appears affected.
(6) Blood clotting disorders.
(7) Anticoagulants (aspirin is a potent anticoagulant).
(8) A destructive lesion.
(9) Other lesions unassociated with discs, including T1 weakness when associated with pain on contralateral side flexion (often a tumour) and ankylosing spondylitis.

Manipulations which rely on rotation during traction are dangerous in any posterocentral disc protrusion.

(2) Restrictions on technique

(1) Central lesions (giving rise to central pain or central pain radiating bilaterally and sometimes marked by postural vertigo) should only be treated by the straight pull. Other manoeuvres (e.g. rotation, side flexion, anteroposterior glide) may bruise the vertebral artery by pressing it against the body of the atlas. If spasm results in a patient with basilar ischaemia, the consequence may be cerebral ischaemia leading to death.

(2) Bilateral lesions: straight pull only.

(3) Patients with gross cervical deformity (e.g. with chin on chest, or ear on shoulder) must first be given half a session of repeated pulls of manual traction in the line of deformity until this has been overcome.

   If other manipulations are used first, damage to the spinal cord may result.

(4) Acute torticollis should be treated by the special method noted on page 175.

(3) Manipulation will not help

(1) Cervical movements cause or aggravate brachial pain. If this emerges during treatment, it is stopped forthwith. Await spontaneous recovery or consider cervical traction. The reason for manipulation's lack of success with these and the succeeding categories is most probably that the displacement is too large for reduction.

(2) Root pain (without a root palsy) of over two months' standing. Await spontaneous recovery or consider cervical traction.

(3) Root palsy. Minor pins and needles do not count. Await spontaneous recovery (four months from onset of pain in the arm) or consider cervical traction.

(4) Primary posterolateral protrusions, that is, where the symptoms arrive in the reverse of the usual order, commencing with paraesthetic fingers with the brachial and scapular pain appearing subsequently. Await spontaneous recovery or consider cervical traction.

Summary

Nearly all displacements can be manipulated, a high proportion with immediate success.

   In the long term the consequence of not reducing a cervical disc lesion can be serious. A displacement may draw out the intervertebral ligaments, and because bone grows until it meets its lining membrane, over the years posterior osteophytes form. Eventually the spinal cord is menaced and paraplegia may ultimately ensue. This train of events could be aborted decades previously by manipulative reduction.

Other conditions benefited by manipulation

Manipulation occasionally helps disorders other than displacements. These include tinnitus, migraine, and old man's matutinal headache, set up by ligamentous contracture at the upper two joints. The patient wakes with a headache that normally passes off by lunchtime and is lastingly relieved by stretching out the contracted ligaments.

Manipulation

The sessions, which follow immediately after diagnosis, may last some 20 minutes. Using one manoeuvre can occasionally secure complete reduction, but more likely a sequence of techniques will be employed during each treatment. Most relief is obtained during the first two sessions and a fourth is a great rarity. The principles are simple:

(1) Manual traction is applied throughout. Neglect of this injunction may lead to aggravation.

(2) The over-pressure is then administered during continued traction.

(3) The patient is then re-examined, and manipulated again if necessary in the light of any change in her symptoms.

   The importance of really strong manual traction cannot be overestimated. It distracts the joint surfaces, tautens the ligaments and creates reduced and centripetal pressure within the expanded joint space. This facilitates reduction and, by ensuring that if the loose fragment moves it moves centrally, makes it safe. Audible clicks during the manipulation, although gratifying, are not significant.

   In the absence of a special manipulation couch, a high couch will serve, with an assistant to hold the patient's feet and supply counter-pressure to the operator's traction. Add-on equipment to the couch by way of 'Cyriax horns' and a lean-back bar will obviate the need for the assistant.

   The neck should never be manipulated in flexion; the head must be held either in the neutral position or in slight extension.

   Before the manipulative attempt starts, neck movements are noted so the operator knows which hurt and which do not and the approximate degree of limitation – this allows the monitoring of progress after each manoeuvre. If one method produces improvement, it is repeated and/or repeated more strongly; if not, another is tried.

   With the experience of years it may be possible to go straight to the appropriate manipulation, particularly on a second session, but if in any doubt it is sound policy to follow the sequences set out below. In due course, clinicians evolve their own rules-of-thumb; for instance, that in clear annular lesions rotation *towards* the painful side is the most effective, and *away* in nuclear lesions. Such a consideration would be balanced against the standard procedure of first gaining the patient's confidence by rotating in the direction in which movement is painless, irrespective of which side the pain is felt.

The straight pull

The first manoeuvre consists of straight traction (*Figure 11.43*) held for no more than two or three seconds.

This helps secure the patient's confidence and often achieves reduction of itself. Thus it is always employed at the beginning of a new session, performed gently at first, as it is not only a therapeutic manoeuvre but also diagnostic. It is only during a first straight pull that contraindications such as an adherent dura occasionally emerge.

The patient lies supine, shoulders level with the top end of the couch and her feet grasped by an assistant. The initial pull is extremely gentle. The operator supports the patient's occiput with one hand, while the other is hooked under the jaw with the little finger clear of the trachea and the head maintained in the neutral, i.e. non-flexed, position. The traction is delivered by the operator leaning backwards while the pull is maintained.

The manoeuvre may be repeated with progressive increase of strength several times, but after each attempt – as for all the manipulations – the patient is re-examined. If indications are good, it is likely the session will progress to rotation during traction.

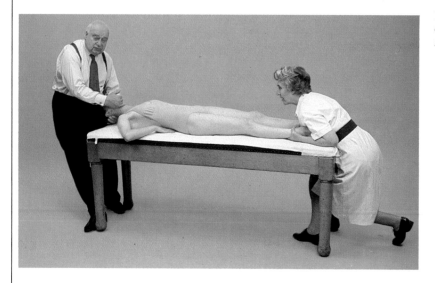

11.43 *A straight pull is the first manoeuvre. Care must be taken to keep the head in the neutral position.*

Re-examination: an example

After each manipulation the patient is re-examined to confirm that movements previously full and painless remain normal. At the same time the previous limitations of, say, flexion and rotation may be found to have eased (*Figures 11.44–11.47*).

On the basis shown, there has been improvement sufficient to warrant the original manipulation's repetition. Each manipulative attempt is followed by re-examination. A sound rule-of-thumb is the harder the end-feel, the less likely that repetition will do any good. When maximum benefit is obtained after a couple of attempts then, unless the patient is well, a different manipulation is used, most probably a stronger rotation strain.

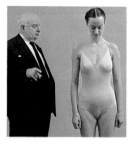

11.44, 11.45 *Re-examination. Flexion before the manipulation (left) and after (right). Any improvement will be clearly detectable.*

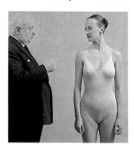 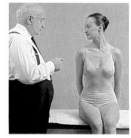

11.46, 11.47 *Rotation, before and after. The operator's next move is determined by his findings on re-examination.*

Rotation during traction – 1

This is the same as the straight pull, but with the added element of rotation. The head is rotated in the direction that does not hurt, while an assistant grasps the patient's ankles, bracing her thighs against the couch (*Figure 11.48*).

The operator's grip makes strong traction easy to maintain. The hand grip is as for the straight pull; one hand supports the occiput, while the other is hooked under the jaw with the little finger clear of the trachea (*Figure 11.49*).

The operator increases the traction by leaning back heavily until his arms are straight, and stays pulling for a second or two (*Figure 11.50*). Then, during continued traction, he turns the head smoothly until the resistance that heralds the approach of full range (*Figure 11.51*).

Finally, a quick thrust of low amplitude is delivered by pulling downwards with the hand at the jaw. This forces a few more degrees of rotation. On the first attempt it may be best to take the head no more than, say, two-thirds of the way towards full range before the high-velocity/low-amplitude thrust. Then, following a favourable re-examination, the patient's head can first be taken to the end of comfortable range.

Here, as elsewhere, traction must be maintained throughout the manoeuvre and not released until the head is returned to the mid-line.

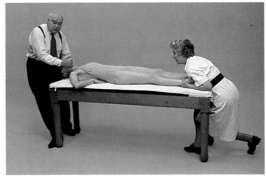

11.48 *The starting position is as for the straight pull. Traction is a vital safety factor.*

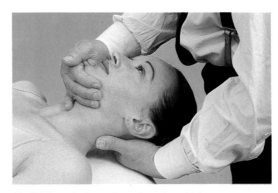

11.49 *The grip (seen from the other side).*

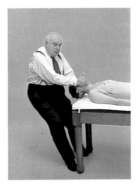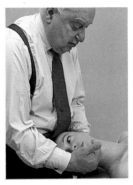

11.50, 11.51 *Manipulation to the right. The operator leans back, rotates the head and gives the over-pressure.*

Rotation during traction – 2

This technique (*Figure 11.52*) is used when the previous manipulation ceases to benefit. It resembles its predecessor, but a different grip gives greater power at the extreme of rotary range because it is the uppermost hand that thrusts downwards. Again an assistant anchors the feet.

The operator's motive hand is applied to the patient's cheek, pressing on her maxilla with his thenar eminence while the other hand supports the occiput. A solid grip is thus secured (*Figure 11.53*).

The operator leans back (*Figures 11.54* and *11.55*) and during considerable traction turns the head in the painless direction until he feels the gathering tissue resistance.

A further thrust is now given (*Figure 11.56*). The patient is re-examined and, if there has been additional improvement, the manoeuvre is repeated and the results reappraised. If not, the rotation may be attempted in the direction that hurts.

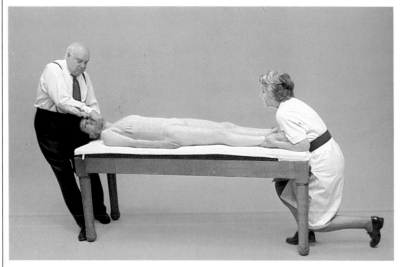

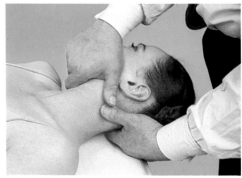

11.52, 11.53 *The starting position. The method differs from its predecessor in that reversal of the operator's upper hand gives stronger purchase. Figure 11.53 demonstrates the grip in detail, seen from the other side.*

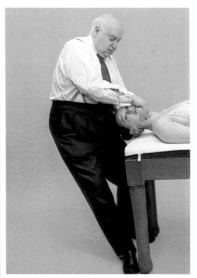

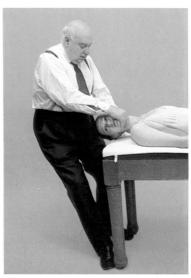

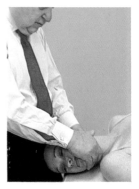

11.56 *The final thrust.*

11.54, 11.55 *Manipulation to the right. The patient's head is taken smoothly to the extreme of comfortable range. Note flexion is avoided throughout.*

Side flexion during traction

If full reduction has not been accomplished by the previous manipulations, side flexion during traction is the next measure (*Figure 11.57*).

The assistant's role is twofold. First, by placing her abdomen against the patient's arm she stops the patient from slipping sideways. Second, she braces her forearm against the patient's shoulder to prevent her riding up the couch.

The operator will pivot on one leg through a right angle, thereby side flexing the cervical spine.

Side flexion is always performed *away* from the side on which the pain is felt, thereby opening the affected side of the joint. It is immaterial which side flexion produced that pain. The operator's forearm, pressing against the skull just above the ear, is used to force side flexion at the last moment. The web of his other hand is pressed in the gap between the C6 and C7 transverse processes to concentrate the side flexion at this part of the spine.

For side flexion to the left, the operator braces his left leg against the couch and then leans back to apply traction. He kicks backward and to the left with his right leg using the momentum to swivel his body on the left leg (*Figure 11.58*). As he swings round, the patient's head is side flexed until the approach of tissue resistance.

The overthrust is given by the operator drawing his elbow – which has been allowed to lag behind – crisply into his side (*Figure 11.59*). The patient is re-examined and, if improvement is noted, the manipulation repeated. Should side flexion towards the painful side be the only movement which remains uncomfortable, manipulation in this direction may be cautiously attempted.

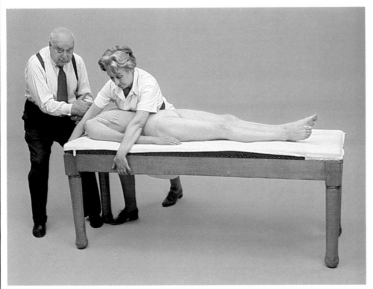

11.57 *Starting position. The operator will swing round to side flex the patient's neck while the assistant prevents trunk movement.*

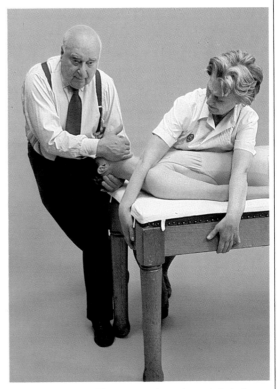

11.58 *Mid-action. The operator's entire weight is borne by his left leg which remains in the starting position. But his trunk has already swivelled round, following the backward sweep of his right leg (scarcely visible behind the leg of the couch).*

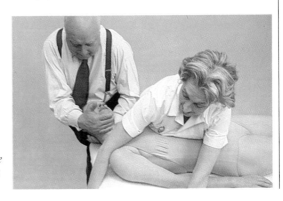

11.59 *Finishing position. The final impulse is delivered by the operator's forearm, as he pulls his elbow sharply into his side.*

Anteroposterior glide during traction

This method is useful if limitation of extension remains the only painful movement. An assistant grasps the feet. The patient's head is maintained in the neutral position throughout, that is, neither in flexion nor extension (*Figure 11.60*). The operator fixes his lower leg against the couch and leans heavily backwards. Traction is applied via the hand at the occiput which also furnishes support for the patient's head

(*Figure 11.61*). As the chin bears the brunt of the manipulation it can be protected by rubber padding or similar.

Strong downwards pressure is exerted momentarily on the chin, not by movement of the hands so much as by the operator flexing his knees (*Figure 11.62*). This achieves backward gliding of each cervical vertebra on the next. The patient is re-examined.

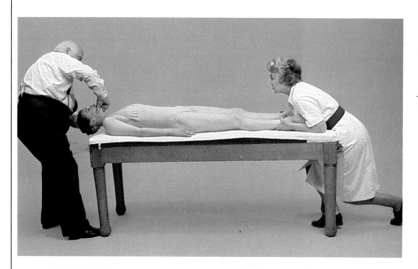

11.60 *Starting position. As with other cervical manipulations, the traction engenders centripetal force. This ensures that if the loose fragment moves at all, it moves centrally.*

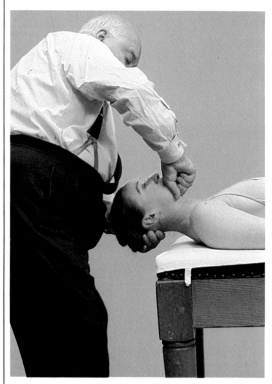 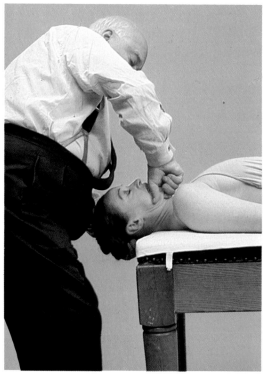

11.61, 11.62 *Starting and finishing positions. The manipulator's hands are above each other in the vertical plane; the patient's head remains horizontally aligned throughout. The manipulation consists of a single downwards thrust.*

Lateral gliding

Lateral gliding (*Figure 11.63*) serves principally to remove any residual ache after otherwise complete reduction. An assistant clasps the patient's trunk hard against her trunk to maintain it immobile.

The head is held in the neutral position. The operator's thumbs (with the thumb nail horizontal) are aligned on the patient's mandibles to keep the head in line with the body and prevent side flexion (*Figure 11.64*).

There is no traction. The operator presses sideways with one thumb and maintains the patient's head in line with her body by pressing in the opposite direction with the thenar eminence of his other hand. By simultaneously swinging his body at the hips he achieves a pure gliding movement from side to side (*Figures 11.65* and *11.66*), repeated several times each manipulation.

Re-examination ensues.

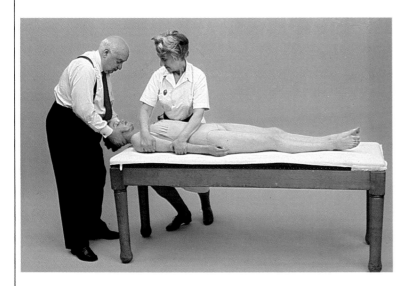

11.63 *Starting position, group. Traction is not required; the physiotherapist prevents the patient's trunk from side-flexing.*

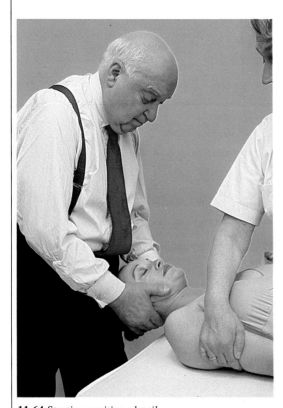

11.64 *Starting position, detail.*

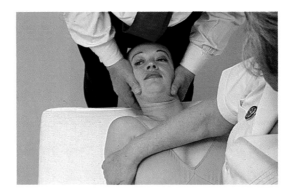
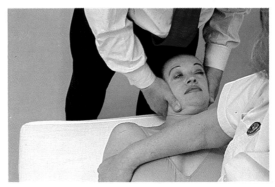

11.65, 11.66 *The movement is repeated a number of times. Note the operator swings his hips. Despite appearances, it is a relatively gentle manoeuvre.*

Traction with leverage

This is a useful technique (*Figure 11.67*) for central cervical disc protrusions setting up central pain which may be referred bilaterally, sometimes accompanied by pins and needles in hands and/or feet. As well as abolishing the immediate pain, reduction forestalls osteophytic growth which may, in the long run, threaten the spinal cord. It is strongly contraindicated by signs (but not symptoms – see page 165) of spinal cord interference.

An assistant holds the patient's feet, and a layer of sponge is placed under the patient's occiput. With both feet against the legs of the couch, the operator holds the patient's head marginally flexed; he then leans backwards, the traction sustained by the hand under the mandible (*Figure 11.68*).

He bends his knees, extending the patient's neck to the neutral position with a jerk, his lower hand acting as a fulcrum (*Figure 11.69*). In this way the distracting force is doubled.

The patient is re-examined.

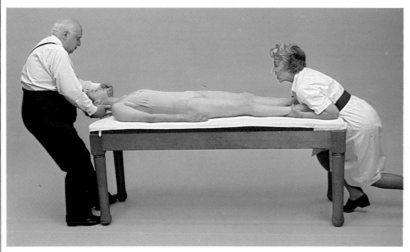

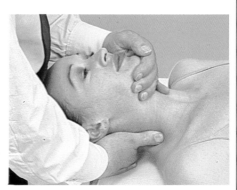

11.68 *Starting position, detail. The right hand acts only as a fulcrum; the left hand does all the work.*

11.67 *Starting position. A safe manipulation if cord symptoms (but not signs) are present. Distraction is the strongest possible; there is no rotation.*

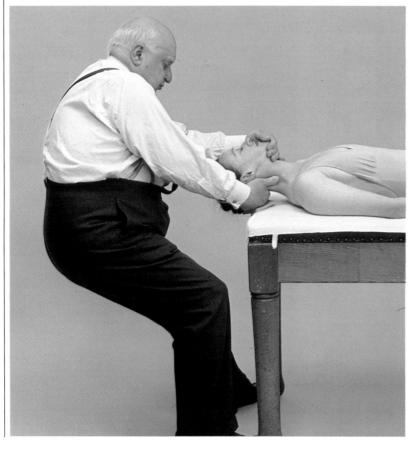

11.69 *The operator all but sits down, achieving immense distraction.*

Acute torticollis

A special tactic must be adopted where a young patient (generally under 30) suffers the acute torticollis brought on by a nuclear protrusion. The patient cannot bring her head up to the vertical, far less rotate it in the direction that hurts and, typically, the pain has developed over some hours. First, the standard manipulations, the Straight Pull and Rotations 1 and 2 (see pages 168–170), are used until she can get her head back to the neutral position. Then the technique, known as 'Bateman's' in honour of the first patient, follows to encourage full range.

The head is rotated in the painful direction until it hurts a little (*Figure 11.70*) and is then supported in this position for some five minutes (*Figure 11.71*). It will then transpire that further range is attainable (*Figure 11.72*) so the patient's head is supported in the new position (*Figure 11.73*) with full rotation progressively achieved in this manner in about an hour. The method may be modified (*mutatis mutandis*) for any restriction of side flexion.

Partial relapse frequently sets in by the next day, in which case the procedure is repeated, most probably with lasting benefit. Alternatively, reduction may now be practicable in the normal way.

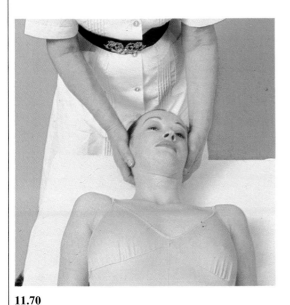

11.70

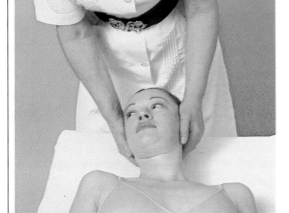

11.72

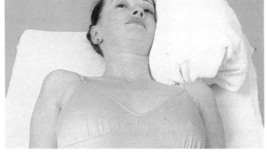

11.71

11.70–11.73 *Full rotation (shown limited to the right) can be restored step-by-step in the course of an hour. Acute torticollis in patients over 30 is treated in the ordinary way.*

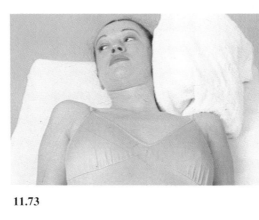

11.73

Differential diagnosis

Numerous conditions other than disc displacements produce cervical, scapular or brachial symptoms. Each disorder of itself is rare and may readily be distinguished from a disc lesion. Manipulation is at best useless and at worst dangerous for these cases.

Capsular conditions have been briefly noted on page 166. Other possibilities include the following:

(1) Pancoast's tumour should be considered if the only painful movement is side flexion away from the painful side. Horner's syndrome and a first thoracic palsy are present and elevation of the scapula is limited. An X-ray is required.

(2) A neurofibroma should be suspected in any patient who seems to have had a disc lesion causing root pain in the limb for longer than six months. The patient's age, a cough hurting down the arm, primary posterolateral onset, duration of brachial pain, extent of weakness, bilateral development, cord symptoms and cord signs may all prove diagnostic.

(3) Basilar ischaemia. Temporary ischaemia without thrombosis can be the consequence of pressure on the vertebral arteries. Vertigo on neck extension is a common complaint. Manipulation with rotation could cause traumatic spasm where the atlas compresses the vertebral artery and may end in death. In the younger age group, symptoms are associated with anatomical variations including a cervical rib. They result in compression of vascular structures and are altogether more severe. Most reported cases of occlusion have occurred following specific high-velocity thrusts to the upper cervical joints (cf. the preceding techniques). A number of tests for ischaemia have been described, usually involving sustained cervical extension and rotation away from the affected side. Unfortunately these cannot be relied on to be positive in relevant cases.

(4) Drop attacks result from congenital ligamentous laxity or a deformed odontoid process. They may permit such instability that both vertebral arteries can be momentarily occluded and the patient is apt to fall to the ground for no apparent reason. On no account must the patient be manipulated.

(5) An osteophyte may occasionally grow obliquely over the course of years to transfix a nerve root at the foramen. The resultant osteophytic root palsy is attended by little pain; in severe cases, the osteophyte should be drilled away with a dental burr.

(6) Neuralgic amyotrophy follows a distinctive progression. It begins as a central pain succeeded by bilateral and then unilateral brachial pain. The muscles are affected regardless of root derivation. Spontaneous recovery occurs within six months of onset; the full neck movements coupled with violent pain provoke a marked diagnostic contrast.

(7) In addition to nerve root impingement or an upper motor neuron lesion, pins and needles in the hand may result from:

(a) Acroparaesthesia – pins and needles occupying all 10 digits in elderly patients. The symptoms come and go in erratic fashion day and night without actually lasting more than an hour at a time. A bilateral displacement may be responsible. In default of cord signs, manipulation sometimes gets rid of the symptoms (see page 174).

(b) Thoracic outlet syndrome – pins and needles, which may be bilateral, recur around 2 am followed by matutinal numbness lasting a few minutes. The syndrome is due to a pressure neuropathy of the lower trunk of the brachial plexus, not the nerve roots, and is associated with a cervical or first rib squeezing the T1 and C7 roots during the day (*Figure 11.74*) as they pass under the clavicle. No symptoms are evoked at the time. The pins and needles are a release phenomenon, occurring after the pressure is removed. The treatment is to educate the patient to keep the shoulder elevated at all times.

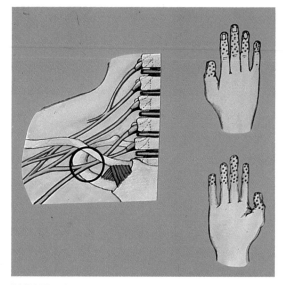

11.74 *The thoracic outlet syndrome. Daytime pressure on the nerve roots (ringed) produces nocturnal pins and needles in both aspects of all five digits. By day the clavicle drops; at night the brachial plexus is freed from compression, evoking the symptoms.*

(c) Carpal tunnel syndrome – unilateral pins and needles in the anterior aspect of three-and-a-half digits. There is no paraesthesia above the wrist, although the pain may move centrally up the forearm. Treatment is dealt with on page 69.

Appendix II summarizes other conditions capable of producing pins and needles in the hand.

Root signs

During the examination, root signs are looked for in logical order, working down the arm for the sake of completeness. Here they are marshalled together root by root and in each case it is the *maximum* signs that are given, that is, all the signs that could be caused by a fully developed root palsy. In practice it is unlikely all will be encountered simultaneously; even one of the listed symptoms is indicative.

It will be remembered that in addition to pain in the dermatome, the symptoms may be preceded or accompanied by scapular pain referred from the dura mater.

C1 root pressure
Rare. No disc at this level. Cancer is the probable cause, producing pain in the dermatome (*Figure 11.75, top*) and weak, painful and limited neck rotation.

C2 root pressure
Rare. No disc at this level. Cancer is the probable cause, producing pain in the dermatome (*Figure 11.75, upper centre*) and numbness at mid-neck.

C3 root pressure
Rare. Pain in the dermatome (*Figure 11.75, lower centre*). Numbness in the cheek.

C4 root pressure
Rare. Pain in the dermatome (*Figure 11.75, bottom*). Numbness at point of shoulder.

A C2, C3 and C4 root palsy weakens scapular elevation.

C5, C6, C7 and C8 root pressure
Displacements at these levels are commonplace and the maximum root signs are dealt with in detail on the next two pages.

T1 root pressure
Rare. Most patients with symptoms apparently attributable to interference with this root are, in fact, the victims of some other disorder such as a cervical rib, a pulmonary sulcus tumour, secondary vertebral neoplasm or pressure on the median or ulnar nerve trunk.

T2 root pressure
In practice never occurs.

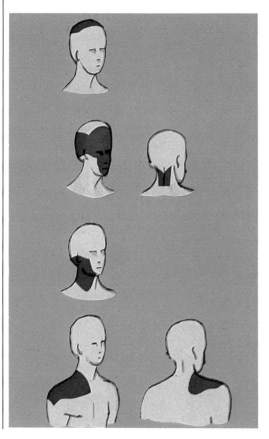

11.75 *The cervical dermatomes. C1 (top), C2 (upper centre), C3 (lower centre), C4 (bottom). There are no discs to cause C1 or C2 root pressure; disc lesions compressing the C3 or C4 roots are rare. But dural extrasegmental reference can and frequently does produce pain in these areas.*

C5 root pressure

Disc lesions fairly common. Pain in the dermatome (*Figure 11.76*). Pins and needles are normally absent.

Weak deltoid, supraspinatus – resisted abduction.
Weak biceps – resisted elbow flexion.
Weak infraspinatus – resisted lateral rotation.
Biceps jerk – absent or sluggish.
Brachioradialis jerk – absent, sluggish or inverted.

Differential diagnosis

In addition to a C4 disc lesion, consider:
(1) Lesion at the shoulder (e.g. supraspinatus tendinitis etc., see page 43).
(2) Rupture of the infraspinatus or supraspinatus tendon. The latter is the more common; weakness and no pain result.
(3) Palsy of the axillary nerve after dislocation at the shoulder (weakness but no pain).
(4) Traction palsy of the fifth cervical root.
(5) Neuritis of the spinal accessory, long thoracic or

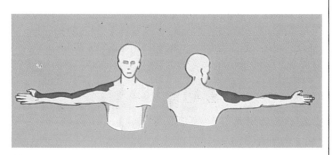

11.76 *The C5 dermatome, front and back.*

suprascapular nerve (pain and weakness – see page 49).
(6) Myopathy deleteriously affecting the serratus anterior and both spinatus muscles complicated by capsular pain from the shoulder.
(7) Secondary malignant deposits in the humerus.
(8) Diaphragmatic pleurisy.

C6 root pressure

Disc lesions fairly common. Pain in the dermatome (*Figure 11.77*). Pins and needles in the thumb and index finger.

Weak extensores carpi radialis – resisted wrist extension.
Weak brachialis and biceps – resisted elbow flexion.
Weak subscapularis (occasionally) – resisted medial rotation.
Biceps jerk – sluggish or absent.

Differential diagnosis

In addition to a C5 disc lesion consider:
(1) The carpal tunnel syndrome (see page 69).
(2) The thoracic outlet syndrome (see page 176).

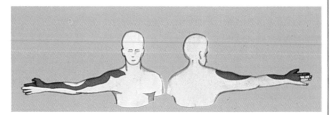

11.77 *The C6 dermatome, front and back.*

(3) Tendinitis or partial rupture of the biceps muscles (see page 48).
(4) Radial nerve pressure palsy at mid-humerus.
(5) Tennis elbow (see page 58).

C7 root pressure

Disc lesions extremely common. Probably 90% of cervical disc lesions causing a root palsy are at the sixth level compressing the seventh root. Pain in the dermatome (*Figure 11.78*). Pins and needles are usually felt in the index, long and ring fingers.

Weak latissimus dorsi – resisted arm adduction.
Weak triceps – resisted elbow extension.
Weak common flexor muscles–resisted wrist flexion.
Triceps jerk – rarely affected.

Differential diagnosis

In addition to a C6 disc lesion consider:
(1) Lead poisoning (always bilateral).

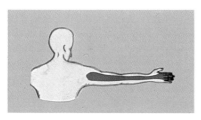

11.78 *The C7 dermatome.*

(2) Carcinoma pf the lung.
(3) Golfer's elbow (see page 61)
(4) Tricipital tendinitis.
(5) Fracture of the olecranon.

C8 root pressure

Disc lesions fairly common. Pain in the dermatome (*Figure 11.79*) and also in the lower scapular area and the back or inner side of the arm and the inner forearm. Pins and needles in the long, ring and little fingers.

    Weak thumb adduction.
    Weak thumb extension.
    Weak ulnar deviation.
    Weak adduction of the index finger.

Differential diagnosis

In addition to a C7 disc lesion consider:
(1) Cervical rib.
(2) The thoracic outlet syndrome (see page 176).
(3) Malignant deposits at the seventh cervical or first thoracic vertebra. Weakness is severe, pain is slight.

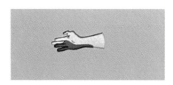

11.79 *The C8 dermatome.*

The seventh cervical and first thoracic root are often also involved.
(4) Pancoast's tumour (see page 176).
(5) Angina, normally characterized by pain in the pectoral area spreading down the upper limb to the ulnar aspect of the hand.
(6) Traction palsy of the lower two roots of the brachial plexus.
(7) Frictional ulnar neuritis at the elbow (see page 62).
(8) Pressure on the ulnar nerve at the wrist.
(9) Thrombosis of the subclavian artery.

CHAPTER TWELVE

THE THORACIC SPINE

Disc lesions account for a higher proportion of thoracic pain than is often realized.

Clinically the thoracic spine is divisible into three sections, the first consisting of T1 and T2 which is examined with the cervical spine because the nerve roots serve the upper limbs. This leaves from T3 to T6, where displacements are unusual, and from T6 to T12, where they occur relatively frequently, often producing anterior pain aggravated by inhalation. Reduction is easy, relapse is commonplace.

The dura mater

As at other spinal levels, the mechanism of pain is primarily dural. A protrusion may compress the dura centrally, giving rise to unilateral extrasegmentally referred pain (*Figure 12.1*).

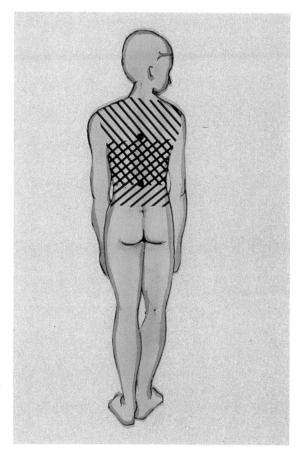

12.1 *The maximum extent of dural extrasegmental reference. A T6 protrusion (upper marker) can produce pain up to the base of the neck and down to the waist. T12 (lower marker) can refer pain up to T6 and down to the sacrum.*

The nerve roots

A posterolateral displacement produces root pain referred anteriorly. At T1 and T2 (both rare) the symptoms may be felt in the arm; root pain at lower levels causes symptoms experienced at the side or front of the trunk (*Figure 12.2*).

A cervical disc lesion is the routine cause of pain felt at upper thoracic levels. Discomfort below the sixth thoracic dermatome might arise from a thoracic disc lesion. At these levels diagnosis is often difficult and best approached from two aspects, the absence of visceral disease balancing and confirming signs of articular disorder.

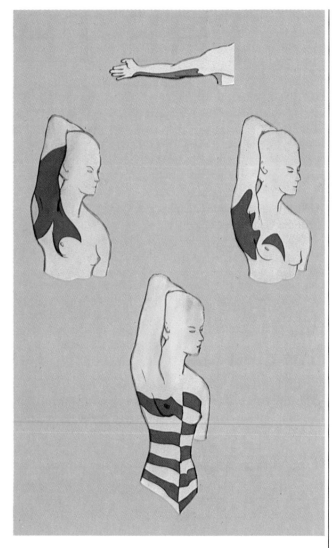

12.2 *The dermatomes. T1 (top), T2 and T3 (centre left and centre right), T4–T12 (bottom).*

History

Displacements
The mode of onset of a disc lesion is various, ranging from sudden ('thoracic lumbago') to posterior thoracic backache coming on slowly. In cases of primary posterolateral protrusion, the unilateral pain will be confined to the front of the chest or the abdomen – a highly misleading phenomenon. Compression of the T11 or T12 roots provokes discomfort in the iliac fossae, perhaps radiating to the testicles. Root pain may linger on indefinitely (cf. cervical and lumbar spines).

A deep breath usually hurts more than coughing. But symptoms of pleural, intercostal, costal and muscular provenance will also be increased so that respiratory exacerbation serves to exclude cardiac pain only.

Articular signs are seldom obvious and neurological signs conspicuous only by their absence. There are no tests for either conduction (i.e. weakness) or mobility of the nerve roots, and analgesia is not often encountered. As at other levels, pain from a disc lesion will be dependent on posture and activities.

Rowers are prone to thoracic displacements but can also develop stress fractures in the ribs.

Examination

The upright spine is scrutinized in a good light for any bony irregularity and will, at the end of the physical examination, be palpated prone for deformity and the stiffness of ankylosing spondylitis.

Dural signs

The spine is examined for dural signs. Neck flexion (*Figure 12.3*) stretches the dura mater at both cervical and thoracic levels. Pain on neck flexion is therefore common to a defect at either level, but if other neck movements are full and painless, attention is directed to the thoracic joints. However, scapular approximation (*Figure 12.4*) pulls only on the dura's thoracic extent via the first and second thoracic nerves and may elicit pain from both a central or lateral thoracic disc lesion.

Pain from stretching the first thoracic root (*Figure 12.5*) via the ulnar nerve incriminates only the T1 or T2 root. In practice, displacements at either level are great rarities and are never accompanied by neurological signs. Thus the possibility of serious disease should be investigated if weakness is also present.

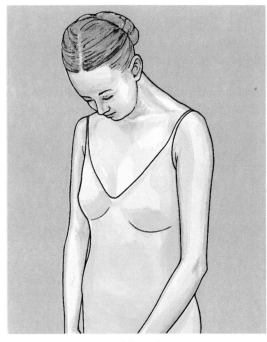

12.3 *Neck flexion: painful whether the lesion is at cervical or thoracic levels.*

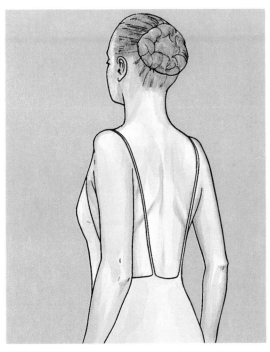

12.4 *Scapular approximation: painful if the lesion is thoracic.*

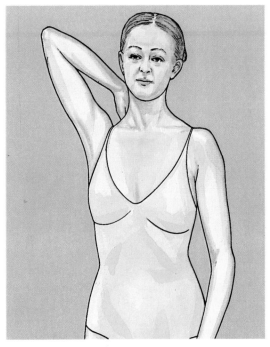

12.5 *T1 stretch; painful if the lesion is at T1 or T2.*

Joint signs

Articular signs are now sought by a series of active movements, largely passive in their diagnostic significance because of the effect of body weight. Extension is tested first (*Figure 12.6*).

The two side flexions follow (*Figures 12.7* and *12.8*). Bilateral limitation in the young suggests serious disease but in the elderly may be attributable to no more than mobility fading with the passage of time.

The patient rotates one way, then the other (*Figures 12.9* and *12.10*) and finally flexes (*Figure 12.11*) her thoracic spine.

A displacement generally causes asymmetrical pain and/or limitation on two, three or four movements.

The movement most likely to hurt with a disc lesion is at the extreme of passive rotation (*Figures 12.12* and *12.13*), achieved by holding the patient's knees between the examiner's to fix the pelvis; indeed, in a minor protrusion, this may be the only painful movement.

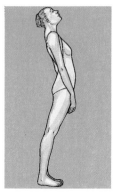
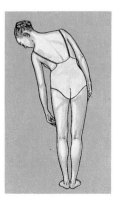
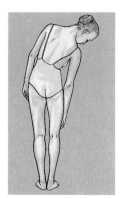

12.6 *Extension.*   **12.7, 12.8** *The active side flexions.*

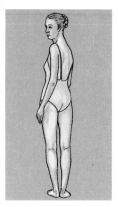
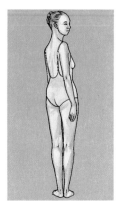
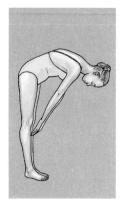

12.9, 12.10 *The active rotations.*   **12.11** *Active flexion.*

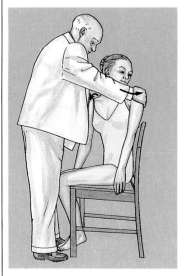
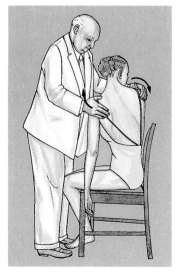

12.12, 12.13 *The passive rotations, with the patient's knees fixed.*

Resisted movements

At the thoracic spine, resisted movements have particular significance as the muscles of the abdomen can and do suffer strain. For the resisted rotations (*Figures 12.14* and *12.15*), the examiner grasps the patient's shoulders and inhibits movement of the pelvis by clamping her knees between his.

The side flexions are resisted (*Figures 12.16* and *12.17*) by the patient bending outwards against the operator's arm while counter-pressure is applied at her hip.

Movement must be prevented at both sternum and knee when testing resisted flexion (*Figure 12.18*). The final resisted movement is extension (*Figure 12.19*).

Contractile structures that may be affected include:

Pectoral muscles – pain on resisted adduction felt at the front of the chest.
Intercostal muscles – pain on breathing.
Latissimus dorsi – pain on resisted adduction felt at the back of the chest.
Inferior posterior serratus – rare; pain on resisted rotation.
Rectus abdominis – pain on resisted flexion.
Oblique abdominal muscles – pain on resisted rotation.

All respond well to deep transverse massage.

Note that muscular lesions do not radiate pain from the posterior thorax to the anterior (or vice versa); such distribution on its own constitutes a sufficient negative diagnosis.

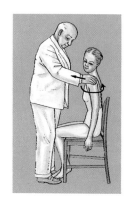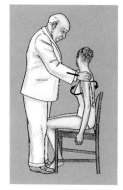

12.14, 12.15 *The resisted rotations.*

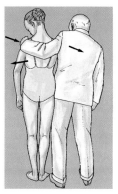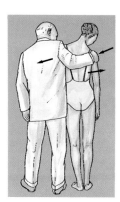

12.16, 12.17 *The resisted side flexions.*

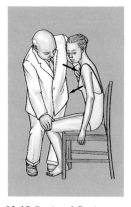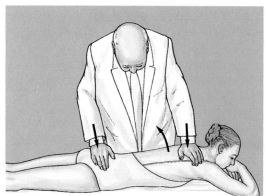

12.18 *Resisted flexion.*   **12.19** *Resisted extension.*

Cord signs

Finally, the patient's plantar response is tested (*Figure 12.20*). Sometimes the only signs of cord interference are pins and needles in both lower limbs on neck flexion. Such cases do not always progress and may remain unaltered for decades.

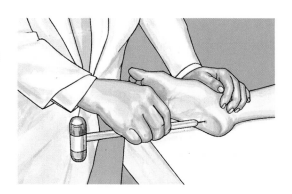

12.20 *Plantar response.*

Findings

Differential diagnosis

A disc lesion must be differentiated from the many other sources of thoracic pain. Some are noted briefly below. Visceral disorders are not influenced by thoracic movements.

(1) A neuroma on one side of the spine will painfully limit side flexion away from that side. That is, side flexion away from the painful side hurts, the opposite of the expected finding with a disc lesion. A spreading patch of cutaneous analgesia also arouses suspicion. The initial symptoms may be confined to the posterior thoracic area and the condition is usually diagnosed late.

(2) Adolescent osteochondritis is normally painless but produces mounting kyphosis at the affected joint. It may precipitate a disc lesion.

(3) Adult osteochondritis is painless but limits extension.

(4) Senile osteoporosis is painless until pathological wedging takes place. This may cause symptoms lasting three months (see also page 235).

(5) Ankylosing spondylitis produces a pain that comes and goes, continuing for years irrespective of what the patient does. Often the ache is at its worst on waking. Normally the lumbar spine becomes rigid before the thoracic joints stiffen, and a flat lumbar spine associated with an upper thoracic kyphosis is suggestive. Treatment consists of non-steroidal anti-inflammatory drugs or occasionally steroids. The HLAB-27 test is positive and posture is vital. For athletes, non-contact games should be encouraged.

(6) Osteitis deformans, aortic aneurysm, tuberculous caries and secondary malignant deposits set up pain arising from diseased bone with skeletal rather than articular signs.

(7) Fracture of a rib or a stress fracture in rowers results in localized pain lasting six weeks at most. Symptoms from fracture of a vertebra cease at the end of three months.

(8) Neuritis of the spinal accessory, long thoracic or suprascapular nerve produces constant unilateral scapular pain for three weeks; the weakness (much more pronounced) continues for four to eight months (see page 49).

(9) Initially, neuralgic amyotrophy causes bilateral upper thoracic pain. Subsequently the symptoms spread down one or both arms (see page 176).

(10) The diaphragm is derived from C3, C4 and C5 with pain normally confined to the C4 dermatome.

(11) Pain arising from the part of the pleura not in contact with the diaphragm is felt in the chest. A Pancoast's tumour invades the chest wall. In epidemic myalgia the pain is bilateral and accompanied by fever.

(12) The heart is mainly derived from the first, second and third thoracic segments.

(13) Pain from early thrombosis of the lower aorta is occasionally felt in the lower thorax.

Visceral embryology

For the convenience of those faced with thoracic or abdominal pain, a list of approximate segmental derivations of the viscera follows:

Diaphragm	C3–5
Heart	C8–T4 (left)
Lungs	T2–5
Oesophagus	T4–5
Stomach and duodenum	T6–8
Liver and gall bladder	T7–8 right
Pancreas	T8 left
Small intestine	T9–10
Appendix and ascending colon	T10–L1
Epididymis	T10
Ovary, testis and suprarenals	T11–L1
Bladder fundus)	
Kidney)	T11–L1
Uterine fundus)	
Colonic flexure	L2–3
Sigmoid colon and rectum)	
Cervix) S2–5	
Neck of bladder, prostate and urethra)	

Caution

A finding of painful and limited side flexion away from the painful side with both rotations free should always arouse suspicion of serious trouble, since rotations are the movement most likely to hurt with a disc lesion. The discrepancy of full and painless rotary range coupled with another movement hurting should put the physician on his guard. Neoplasm or neuroma are possibilities.

Capsular lesions

The capsular pattern is equal and severe limitation of movement in every direction. This indicates tuberculosis (rare), ankylosing spondylitis or mid-line destructive lesions.

Displacements

Thoracic disc lesions respond well to manipulation – success is almost invariable. It is the predisposition to recurrence that constitutes the problem (countered by sclerosants – see page 195), although many patients are kept continuously comfortable by attending for manipulative reduction on each relapse.

Posture at work with the thoracic spine straight, a higher table/lower chair ratio and avoidance of undue rotation and flexion movements will help. Some clinicians have obtained particularly good results in re-educating posture with micro-pore strapping applied paravertebrally from the root of the neck to the sub-costal margin.

Treatment

All the findings that, at cervical and lumbar levels, show manipulation will fail have no bearing at the thoracic spine. All thoracic disc lesions are manipulated. Two assistants are required and a low couch is used. The only contraindications are:

(1) Signs of spinal cord pressure. However, traction may be attempted in cases marked merely by paraesthetic feet. The procedure is as for the lumbar spine (see page 221).
(2) A patient on anticoagulants (including aspirin).

The general remarks on manipulation in Chapters 2 and 10 should be noted. Sessions last 20 minutes or so and varying techniques of increasing intensity may have to be tried. Maximum benefit normally accrues in one or two sessions.

The manipulations parallel those at lumbar levels save that two assistants apply manual traction.

Before the session begins, passive extension is tested with the patient prone. Each joint is pressed towards extension with a slight jerk, in the hope that it hurts more at one level than another or that greater resistance is encountered. This identifies the exact level of the lesion.

But often similar stiffness is detected at several adjacent levels, in which case for the first manipulation pressure is brought to bear on the one in the middle. By contrast, rotation strains involve the entire thoracic spine and not just one joint. For the rare upper thoracic lesions, see page 194.

Extension during traction – 1

The first manipulation consists of no more than a sharp downwards thrust delivered, for maximum impact, at the moment of the patient's full exhalation. Traction is supplied by two assistants, one grasping the patient's hands and the other the feet (*Figure 12.21*). They pull strongly in opposite directions for a few seconds before and during the manipulation.

The ulnar border of the operator's palm is angled so that the centre of the fifth metacarpal bone presses on the spinous process at the affected joint (*Figure 12.22*). Reinforcement is now given with the other hand (*Figure 12.23*).

After a few seconds of traction, the patient is asked to take a deep breath and exhale fully. A sharp downwards jerk of small amplitude is then imparted towards extension by the operator thrusting downwards while keeping his arms straight (*Figure 12.24*). The patient is re-examined.

With the elderly, it is not difficult to fracture a rib using this method, and rotary techniques (see pages 190—193) should be preferred. If the lesion lies at the upper thorax, considerably greater force is required.

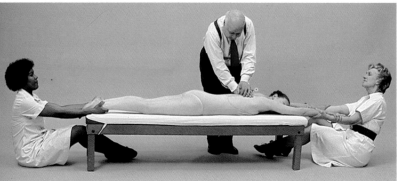

12.21 *The two assistants pull in opposite directions.*

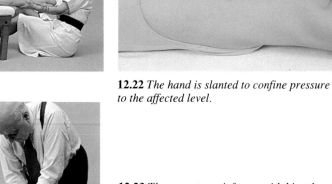

12.22 *The hand is slanted to confine pressure to the affected level.*

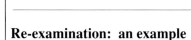

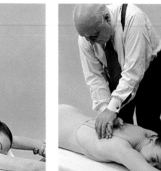

12.23 *The operator reinforces with his other hand and presses gently while the traction takes effect.*

12.24 *The overthrust, delivered as the patient exhales. A downwards jerk is transmitted via the arms.*

Re-examination: an example

After each manipulation the patient must be re-examined to check she is no worse and to register any improvement (*Figures 12.25–12.28*). Movements previously of full painless range should still be normal. But if, say, the original limitation of extension and rotation has diminished, then the manipulation has helped and, as a general rule, should be repeated more strongly a couple of times until reappraisal shows no further improvement. In the absence of such improvement, the manipulation is tried again at an adjacent joint and the patient re-examined before progressing as necessary to the next manoeuvre, which adds an element of rotation.

12.25, 12.26 *Extension before the manipulation (left) and after (right). Any changes in the signs are readily apparent.*

12.27, 12.28 *Rotation, before and after. The patient reports on any change in symptoms, including on taking a deep breath.*

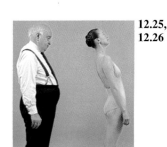

12.25, 12.26

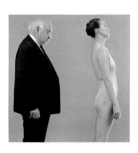

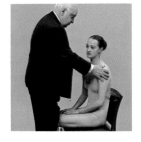

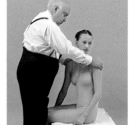

12.27, 12.28

Extension (with rotation) during traction – 2

This manipulation exerts a different thrust – the two pertinent vertebrae are rotated, again during traction applied by two assistants (*Figure 12.29*). Often reduction can be accomplished by use of this and the previous method. The object is to press down (the extension) while moving the hands applied against the lateral processes in opposite directions (the rotation).

The operator extends the wrist of one hand, bringing the pisiform bone into prominence and placing it to the near side of the spinous process just above the site of the displacement. The thumb of his other hand is abducted, driving it backwards to make the trapezio-first-metacarpal joint stand out. Then this is laid on the far side of the spinous process just below the affected level (*Figure 12.30*). The more cephalically-placed hand always rests on the patient's painless side. The operator now presses down with a sharp jerk, pushing the hand which is further away from him distally and his near hand proximally (*Figure 12.31*). The patient is re-examined and if improvement has resulted the manipulation is repeated.

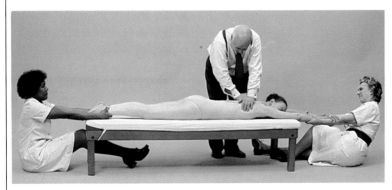

12.29 *The operator's hands are crossed to produce a rotation thrust. Note one assistant has braced her knee against the couch and the other wedged her foot against its leg.*

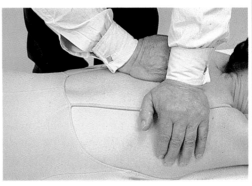

12.30 *Both hands are motive; they are simultaneously pushed downwards and in opposite directions.*

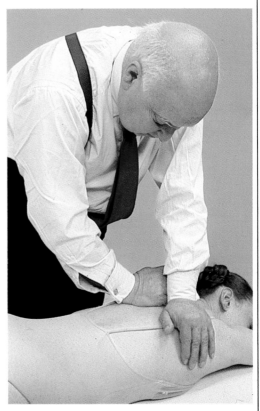

12.31 *The overthrust. The operator leans right over the patient.*

Rotation strains

For the rotations, the exact site of the displacement (provided that it is not an upper thoracic lesion) is of academic interest as the entire extent of the thoracic spine is manipulated with the strain falling on the blocked joint. The manipulations are arranged in order of increasing force.

The painful side must always be uppermost, because that is the side where the joint is to be opened, and the rotation is first in the direction that does not cause pain. Sometimes rotation into pain may follow.

Thus in Rotation 1 (see below), it is assumed that the patient's pain is right-sided and the patient's most comfortable rotation is to her right. Rotation 2, as shown, is appropriate for the same sided pain, but with the least painful rotation to the left. Thus in appropriate cases a session would start on Rotation 2 rather than 1.

Rotation during traction – 1

This is employed when the extensions cease to afford benefit or in the unlikely event that they prove excessively painful. The patient lies with the painful side uppermost and the trunk is rotated in the direction that does not bring on the pain, irrespective of which side the pain is felt. This consideration dictates the choice between this manipulation and the next.

The assistant at the feet grasps only the uppermost leg and, at the moment of over-pressure, participates by swinging it in the same direction as the manipulator forces the pelvis. The assistant at the upper end pulls on both arms, again in the direction of the manipulation (*Figure 12.32*).

The manipulator uses a downward thrust of his body weight to force one of his arms backwards and the other forwards. One hand is placed on the patient's buttock and the other against the prominent border of her scapula (*Figure 12.33*). The patient's thorax is then twisted as far as possible before the traction starts, and is maintained in this position for a couple of seconds until it takes effect (*Figure 12.34*).

The operator then rotates his thorax utilizing his body weight to impel the patient's thorax towards, and her pelvis away from, himself with a strong jerk (*Figure 12.35*).

The patient is re-examined and if improvement is apparent the manoeuvre is repeated.

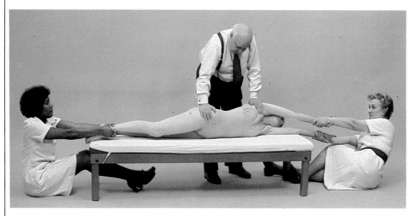

12.32

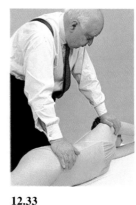

12.33

12.32–12.34
Starting position. The thorax is twisted as far as possible before the traction begins. In both Rotation 1 and Rotation 2 the distal assistant holds only the uppermost leg.

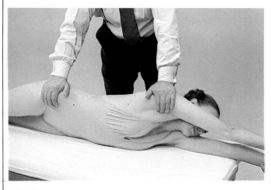

12.34

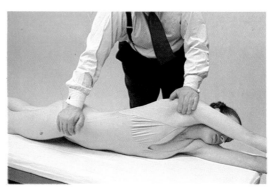

12.35 *Finishing position. Further rotation is forced. Note how the patient's axilla has come up while the pelvis is now flat on the couch.*

Rotation during traction – 2

This manipulation is the reverse of its predecessor and, as shown, is appropriate for a right-sided pain with rotation towards the left the least painful. The pelvis is pulled towards the operator and the thorax thrust down and away. The assistant at the foot takes the uppermost leg only and, as before, pulls it in the same direction as the operator forces the pelvis (*Figure 12.36*).

The fingers of one hand are hooked about the anterior superior spine of the patient's ilium. The heel of the other hand is lodged against the lateral aspect of her thorax; it is over this arm that the body weight is poised (*Figure 12.37*).

The operator twists the patient's thorax as far as it will go (*Figure 12.38*) and then waits a few seconds for the traction to open the joints.

The hand on the pelvis is then drawn sharply upwards and towards the operator, while the thoracic hand is pushed downwards and away (*Figure 12.39*). The movement is assisted by rotation of the manipulator's thorax, thus taking full advantage of his body weight. The patient is re-examined.

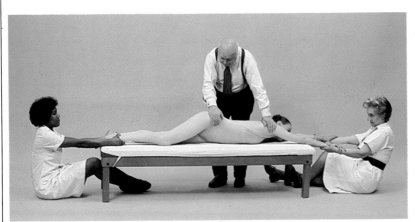

12.36 *The pelvis is to be lifted while the shoulder is held down.*

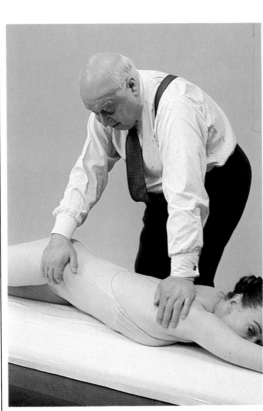

12.37

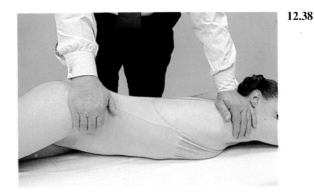

12.38

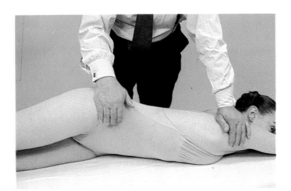

12.37, 12.38 *Starting position. The operator's body weight keeps the upper thorax flat on the couch.*

12.39 *The over-pressure. Rotation is clearly seen; note the expanse of abdomen, with both thighs now visible.*

Rotation during traction – 3

Rotations 3 and 4 enable the operator to increase rotary power at the slight expense of traction by using the patient's thigh as a lever. These techniques are seldom called for, but are useful if one rotation remains obstinately painful. The assistants apply the traction (*Figure 12.40*). One hand keeps the patient's upper trunk flat on the couch while the other holds her knee off the couch, rotating the thorax (*Figure 12.41*). The assistants pull.

After a couple of seconds the patient's knee is drawn sharply upwards (in the painless direction) while the thorax is maintained stationary by the operator's body weight (*Figure 12.42* and *12.43*). The upwards pull on the thigh is accomplished by arm strength alone.

The patient is re-examined. This method pays particular dividends when a small operator has to deal with a large patient.

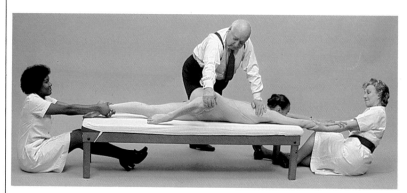
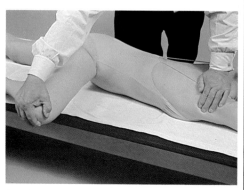

12.40–12.42 *Starting position. Again the body weight is over the scapula, pinning the upper thorax in the sagittal plane.*

12.41

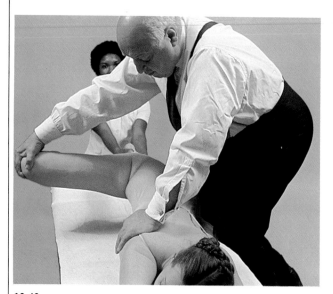
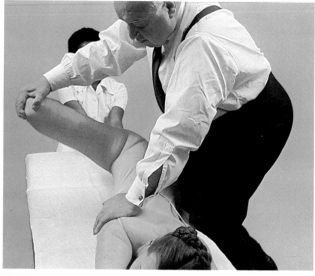

12.42

12.43 *The over-pressure.*

Rotation during traction – 4

Maximum mechanical advantage is obtained by this manipulation which lengthens the thoracic lever. The patient lies face upwards while two assistants apply strong traction for the few seconds preceding and during the manipulation (*Figure 12.44*).

The projecting lateral edge of the patient's scapula is pinned to the couch while her knee is flexed to a right angle. Her trunk is rotated until the resistance that heralds the end of range (*Figure 12.45*).

The patient's knee is smartly pressed (in the painless direction) towards the floor (*Figure 12.46*). During the manipulation, the operator's body weight is balanced over the patient's shoulder to keep her immobile on the couch. The patient is re-examined.

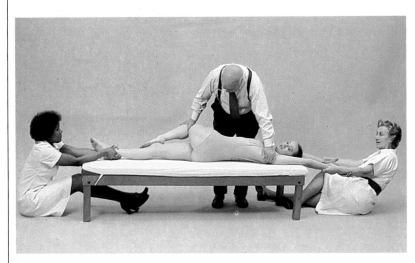

12.44, 12.45 *Starting position. This is the strongest rotation strain. The force is greatly enhanced both because the hands are applied to opposite extremes of the patient's body and because the thrust is downwards.*

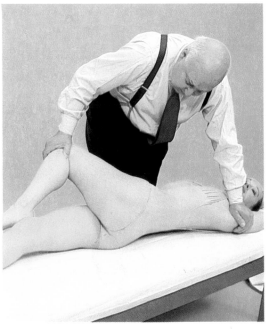

12.45

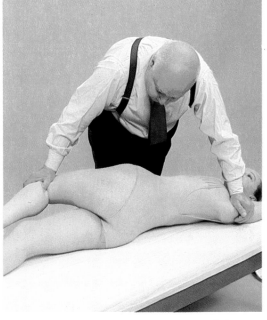

12.46 *The over-pressure is strong but controlled.*

Upper thoracic rotation during traction

Before resorting to this method, suited only to the rare upper thoracic protrusions, it is always worth while attempting a long straight pull identical to the cervical procedure set out on page 168. This is often sufficient to produce recovery. In default, the session progresses to upper thoracic rotation.

Traction is applied by the assistants, with one physiotherapist grasping the patient by the head (*Figure 12.47*). The patient's forearm is placed behind her back, and keeping the distal hand applied to the affected level, the rotation is obtained by forcing the cephalically-placed forearm in the direction of the patient's feet.

Thus the manipulator's hands are clasped through the circle formed by the patient's arm. The heel of his near hand presses down on the sixth to eighth thoracic levels; the other forearm is exerted against her shoulder, raising it off the couch (*Figure 12.48*)

The operator then side-flexes his thorax, lifting the patient's shoulder girdle up while delivering a rotary extension thrust with his lower hand (*Figures 12.49* and *12.50*). This simultaneously rotates and extends the patient's upper thoracic joints during traction.

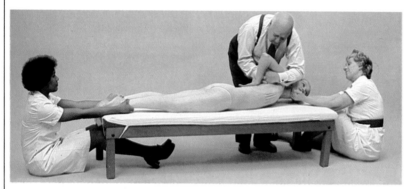
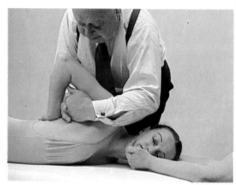

12.47–12.49 *Starting position. The operator links his hands through the circle of the patient's internally rotated arm.*   **12.48**

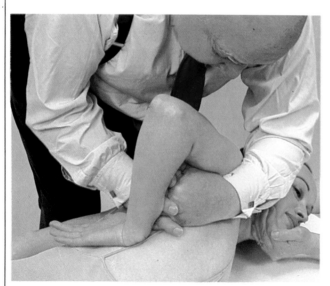
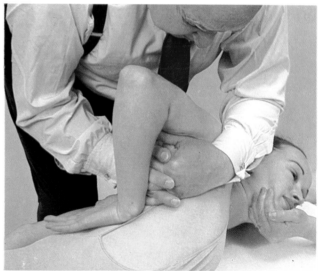

12.49

12.50 *The over-pressure. The operator presses down on the rib cage with his distal hand, while adducting his proximal elbow to raise the front of the thorax. The movement is best noted by diminution of background area between the operator's left arm and chest, representing the combination of arm extension and rotation of the upper thorax.*

Recurrence

Recurrence at regular intervals must be expected and normally requires no more than renewed manipulative reduction. A corset at the thoracic spine is seldom effective, but repeated relapses can be countered by sclerosant therapy.

Sclerosants

Ligamentous sclerosis is effective in preventing relapse, although the mechanism of its action is unclear. It has been postulated that the solution, by producing ligamentous sclerosis, reduces the range of movement at the affected joint. But this has never been adequately demonstrated. It is possible that the injection diminishes afferent inflow at the relevant segment by producing a destructive lesion. Whatever the mechanism, the injections are certainly effective in cases of persistent relapse, and are often sufficient to avoid the looming possibility of semi-continuous disability. The displacement should be reduced prior to the injection. The solution (1 ml) is injected into:

(1) Each ligamento-periosteal junction at both ends of the supraspinous ligaments.
(2) The facet joints to either side of the affected joint.

The solution, known as P2G, consists of:

phenol 2–2.5%
dextrose 20–25%
glycerine 20–25%
pyrogen-free water to 100%

In the syringe, 4 ml of this fluid is mixed with 1 ml of 1:50 procaine solution in saline.

A 5 ml syringe is used. Considerable pressure is required to force the fluid into the tough ligamentous attachments. Localization prior to manipulation will generally have indicated the level, but normally two – or, in cases of doubt, three – ligaments are injected for good measure.

After injection the patient is sore for at least the rest of the day. A total of three injections are given to each ligamento-periosteal site at weekly intervals and the patient is warned not to flex the thoracic spine for the next two months.

The patient lies prone and a grid is drawn on her back. One line runs down the mid-line and is intersected by three others at the mid-points between the spinous processes. The lateral boundaries of the grid overlie the facet joints about 1.5 cm from the mid-line.

The ligamento-periosteal junctions of the supraspinous ligament are infiltrated first. The needle is thrust vertically downwards where the cross-bar intersects the mid-line.

After 1 cm, the needle is turned and angled proximally until it touches bone and P2G 1 ml is deposited along the underside of one spinous process (*Figure 12.51*). The needle is then partially withdrawn and the tip tilted distally to complete the injection along the superior ridge of the other spinous process (*Figures 12.52* and *12.53*).

The supraspinous ligaments at the adjacent levels are now similarly infiltrated.

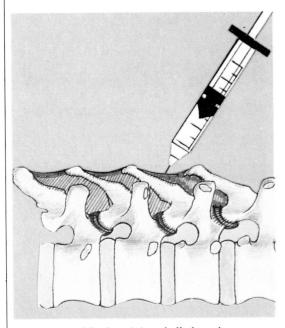

12.51 *Beads of fluid are injected all along the ligamento-periosteal junction. The outer intersections of the grid overlie the facet joints.*

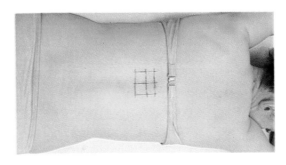

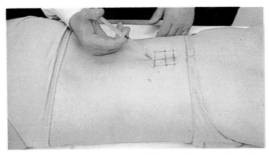

12.52, 12.53 *The cross-bars of the grid are at the mid-point between the tips of the spinous processes. To infiltrate the supraspinous ligaments, the angle of insertion must be varied in the course of the injection.*

Attention then turns to the facet joints. The insertion is made vertically at the intersection of the grid's cross-bar and the lateral line (*Figure 12.54*).

The needle hits bone at a depth of about 3 cm and the edges of the joint are sought. A series of droplets is injected along its length, and the procedure repeated at the other side (*Figures 12.55* and *12.56*) and then at the adjacent joints.

Patient and physician reconvene the next week and the week after for re-injection. If examination shows a displacement is present, it is reduced by manipulation before infiltration.

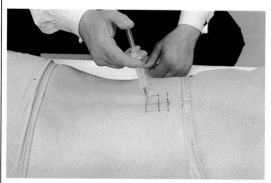

12.54

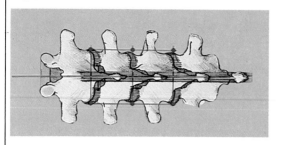

12.55

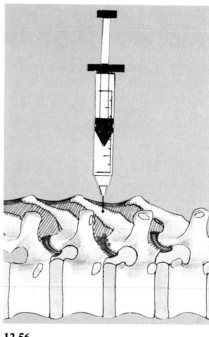

12.56

12.54–12.56 *Injection to the facet joints on both sides is difficult but not impossible. A series of droplets is delivered to each of the six intersections.*

CHAPTER THIRTEEN

THE LUMBAR SPINE

Clinical examination shows that the great preponderance of lumbar disorders are attributable to mechanical lesions, the commonest and best documented of which is the prolapsed intervertebral disc. Often this diagnosis is considered applicable only to severe cases with pain down the leg and neurological deficit. But in fact intervertebral displacements can be responsible for the mildest backache as well as for intermediate and severe symptoms. Here, as elsewhere at the spine, a displacement of disc material may move either posteriorly to compress the dura mater (*Figure 13.1*), giving rise to extrasegmental pain, or laterally to compress the dural sleeve of a nerve root, precipitating pain in the appropriate dermatome and weakness in the relevant muscle group.

At the cervical and thoracic levels treatment is simple: by and large, most displacements are manipulated. But at the lumbar spine the patient may need manipulation, traction, epidural local anaesthetic, sclerosants, a sinuvertebral block, a corset or, as a last resort, surgery. In addition, a great deal can be achieved by way of prophylaxis. The correct response to each case depends not only on examination but also on the patient's history which is of paramount importance. Only a tiny proportion of cases go to operation.

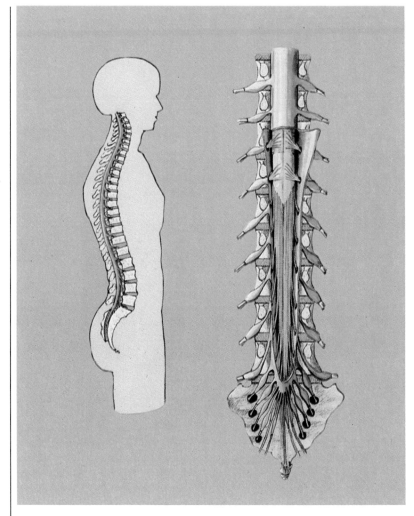

13.1 *The dura mater is a sensitive structure. The dural sheath to the nerve roots continues to the distal end of the intervertebral foramen; hence the phenomenon of root pain from disc pressure.*

The dura mater

A displacement of disc material compressing the dura mater causes pain felt anywhere from the back of the trunk to the scapulae; anteriorly at the abdomen or groins; at the side of the sacrum or upper buttock; at the coccyx or down both legs to the calves (*Figure 13.2*). Dural pain (in contradistinction to root pain) does not extend to the ankle or foot. Note that with extrasegmental reference the perception of pain in any particular location has no necessary bearing on the level of the articular lesion, although often the pain can be felt locally.

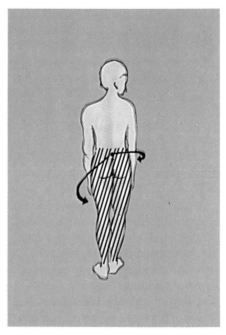

13.2 *Dural pain can be referred anywhere in this area, but is less common down the legs. If from a disc, it will be central or unilateral. Note the feet are excluded.*

The nerve roots

A lateral displacement may interfere with the dural sleeve of the nerve root only or with the parenchyma as well. The former produces pain in any part of the dermatome, the latter weakness and/or paraesthesia. The roots commonly affected are L4, L5, S1 and S2; the corresponding dermatomes are illustrated in *Figure 13.3*.

As the nerves emerge obliquely, root signs may be polyradicular. The joint itself is insensitive to internal derangement, although the annular ligaments are theoretically sensitive to pressure from disc creep and may produce pain.

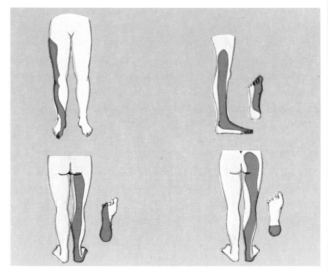

13.3 *The dermatomes of the commonly affected nerve roots. L4 (top left). L5 (top right). S1 (lower left). S2 (lower right).*

The disc

A displacement may be composed of cartilage or part of the nucleus pulposus. Nuclear material typically engenders pain of slow onset over some hours as the nucleus herniates through the weakened annulus; since the displacement is semi-liquid and cannot be clicked back by manipulation, the treatment of choice is traction. However, pulpy herniation may well accompany the abrupt fixation of a cartilaginous displacement. These mixed displacements may call for a dual therapeutic approach.

By the age of 60 the disc is uniform in substance throughout and the nucleus has disappeared. Thus in the elderly the question of whether a displacement is nuclear or cartilaginous does not apply. At that age and after, all appropriate displacements are manipulated. Annular protrusions are about twice as common as nuclear lesions.

History

Displacements

An exhaustive chronological history is taken, ascertaining when the pain started and whether this is the first attack, what brought it on, what the symptoms were then, what they are now, whether they spread, if so to where, whether the pain is constant or intermittent, whether a cough hurts, and whether the pain and disability are slight, moderate or severe.

Based on this information it can be decided:

(1) Whether a disc lesion or some other disorder is present.
(2) The type of any disc lesion present (hard/soft, large/small, central/unilateral, stable/unstable, primary posterolateral onset, etc.).
(3) The type of patient and whether the described degree of pain and disablement tallies with her appearance and known daily activities.

History affords the clearest indications on how to treat a disc lesion. It also differentiates backache from other conditions, as only a few disorders (e.g. internal derangement) give rise to episodic pain and only intermittent internal derangement repeatedly fixes a joint within its range of movement. Such a pattern makes, for instance, osteoarthrosis an improbable cause of pain and, further, a lengthy history running back over years of itself excludes serious progressive disease.

Pain from a disc lesion arises only from pressure exerted on the dura mater or the nerve root. So there is a limit to the different events which can take place in the closed cavity lying in the mid-line of the lumbar area. 'All discs are alike and all other disorders are different' is a sound working maxim.

Pain from a disc lesion is connected with posture, activity and exertion. It can be brought on by, for example, digging or, at the other end of the spectrum, by merely coughing while brushing the teeth.

In due course a central protrusion tends to shift posterolaterally to the nerve root(s), producing symptoms in the limb. The initial minor protrusion interferes with the movement of the joint and not the nerve root, so local pain and articular signs are thus at their most obvious when neurological signs are lacking. But when the protrusion has passed posterolaterally it interferes little with joint movement. Thus root pain and clear neurological signs supervene as the articular symptoms fade.

The mode of onset varies from a gradual ache to the abrupt fixation of lumbago and reflects the nature of the protrusion (cartilaginous/nuclear/mixed – see above). A cough is often painful.

Sciatica unaccompanied by backache recovers of itself in 12 months, but there is no such time limit to backache. If the pain came on first in the leg (i.e. primary posterolateral onset) this contraindicates manipulation and indicates traction.

In cases where the pain has spread down the leg, it must be established whether or not the pain in the back increased at the same time. If it did, this is a danger signal showing that the lesion is spreading (e.g. metastases) rather than shifting (e.g. a displacement). For other causes of pain see page 235.

Examination

This is conducted for:

(1) Bone signs.
(2) Joint signs.
(3) Dural signs.
(4) Nerve root mobility.
(5) Nerve root conduction.

After a careful history the patient undresses and the back is inspected in a good light. If an angular kyphosis is present, a vertebral body may have become wedge-shaped due to tuberculous caries, neoplasm or fracture. Localized osteitis deformans and senile osteoporosis are often symptomless.

Spondylolisthesis may be both visible and palpable as a bony shelf. If the shelf is constant, whether the patient is standing or prone, it may be due to either a stable spondylolisthesis (unlikely to give symptoms and generally only discovered when the patient eventually presents with discogenic pain) or merely an anomalous spinous process. But if the shelf is present on standing but disappears on lying, then an unstable spondylolisthesis (likely to give symptoms) is present. These defects are best displayed radiographically when the patient is standing.

A displacement of disc material can produce characteristic deviation (*Figure 13.4*); if gross, it is more likely to result from a fourth rather than a fifth lumbar disc lesion because of the stabilizing effect of the iliolumbar ligaments.

The posture of lumbago (*Figure 13.5*) indicates that the sacrospinalis muscles cannot be in spasm as the patient is fixed in flexion not in extension. However, the muscles do contract antagonistically to prevent the patient toppling further forwards into painful range.

Checks are made to see if the pelvis is horizontal (*Figure 13.6*) or oblique. Some 7% of the population have a difference of 1.2 cm or more in the length of their legs and usually this is nothing to worry about. All the same, if one leg is found to be shorter than the other, then the heel is raised by a series of thin platforms under the short leg until the pelvis is level. If this eases or abolishes the pain on standing, correction with a heel-raise will prove beneficial.

The patient points to the area of her pain. When a disc lesion results in local discomfort this is generally felt on a level with or just below the joint affected (generally L4 or L5). First and second lumbar disc lesions are extremely rare, so care must be exercised against ascribing pain felt at upper and mid-lumbar levels to a disc.

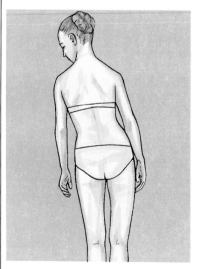

13.4 *A disc lesion at L4 may make the patient deviate. In genuine cases, the patient compensates by holding shoulders level and head upright.*

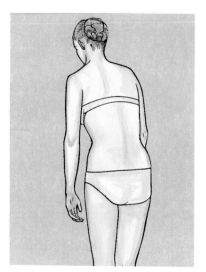

13.5 *Attribution of lumbago to spasm of the errector spine is remarkable in view of the patient's flexed posture.*

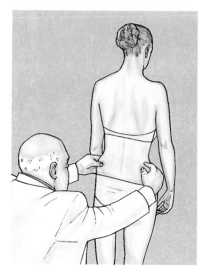

13.6 *Checking for lateral tilt of the pelvis. Inequality of leg length is not necessarily painful.*

Joint signs

The joints are now examined. There is no appreciable rotation at the lumbar spine and hence only four movements are tested; they are active but, because of the body weight, are passive in their diagnostic import. Passive extension (*Figure 13.7*) is the first.

Both side flexions are tested (*Figures 13.8* and *13.9*). All serious diseases of the lumbar spine result in equal limitations of both side flexions.

Flexion (*Figure 13.10*) is the movement most likely to be limited by a lumbar disc lesion. A painful arc may be noted, due to either a displaced piece of cartilage shifting during angulation of the joint surfaces or segmental instability. A patient suffering psychogenic pain is unlikely either to invent a transient deviation or to allege his pain disappears as flexion increases.

Alternatively, the patient may deviate during flexion.

The deviation, which materializes as the patient seeks to minimize traction on the dura mater or nerve root, is pathognomonic.

A displacement blocks part of the joint causing pain and/or limitation (unequal in different directions) on some but not all movements. However, in lumbago all four movements are apt to hurt, but the degree of pain and limitation still differ for each movement (cf. the capsular pattern).

The patient now moves to the couch. Her manner of so doing should correspond with her disablement. In suspected malingering she is enjoined to swing herself round with legs extended (*Figure 13.11*). If painless, this amounts to a finding both of 90° of painless trunk flexion and full painless straight-leg raise. A genuine patient will manoeuvre with caution (*Figure 13.12*).

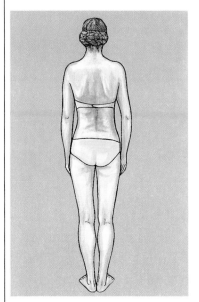

13.7 *Extension. Lumbar movements may evoke or alter the symptoms. Range may be full or limited.*

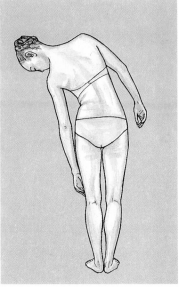

13.8, 13.9 *The side flexions. Consider if any limitation is capsular (symmetric) or non-capsular (asymmetric).*

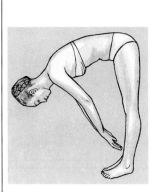

13.10 *Flexion is left till last, as an ache persisting afterwards might obscure the response to other movements.*

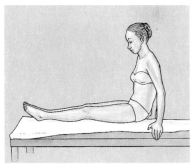

13.11 *Getting onto the couch. Postures achieved by the unsupervised patient can be revealing. The position above is inconsistent with severely limited flexion and constitutes full straight-leg raise.*

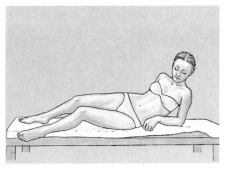

13.12 *A genuine patient may have to move very carefully.*

201

Dural signs: straight-leg raising

The patient lies supine and her straight-leg raise (SLR) is tested (*Figure 13.13*).

Raising the leg with the knee extended pulls on the dura mater via the sciatic nerve running down the back of the leg. SLR thus stretches the dura (*Figure 13.14*) and, if the membrane's normal mobility is impeded by a central disc protrusion, pain will result and range will be limited bilaterally.

Likewise, SLR pulls on the L4, L5, S1 and S2 nerve roots, one or two of which may be fixed by a lateral disc protrusion. There will then be pain and unilateral limitation.

Straight-leg raising is thus a test for dural mobility (bilateral limitation) and nerve root mobility at L4, L5, S1 and S2 (unilateral limitation). In practice, L4 root pressure sometimes gives rise to bilateral limitation.

Pain on full SLR suggests a small protrusion and is also common in elderly patients' sciatica and after laminectomy. Much backache (unlike lumbago) produces no limitation of SLR. A painful arc can be explained by a protrusion so small that the dura mater or nerve root merely catches against it and slips over. In doubtful cases, where the patient is unclear that SLR aggravates the pain, clearer signs may be elicited by full SLR coupled with dorsiflexion of the foot, flexion of the neck or both simultaneously. Some clinicians favour the 'slump test', where the patient slumps her neck back and forwards while sitting (back erect) on the couch during SLR, but this seems likely to confuse the clinical picture through involvement of other structures.

If neck flexion (*Figure 13.15*) increases pain, involvement of the dura is confirmed because the tissue with impaired mobility must run from neck to calf. Attention is thereby confined to the dura mater and its continuation as the sciatic nerve.

Limited SLR may be accompanied by neurological signs established subsequently in the course of the examination. This double finding indicates greater pressure involving the parenchyma as well as the nerve root sheath, and has important bearings on treatment.

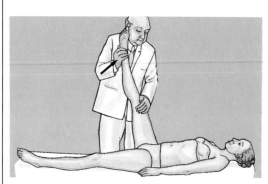

13.13 *Straight-leg raise. The larger the protrusion, the greater the limitation. Full range shown.*

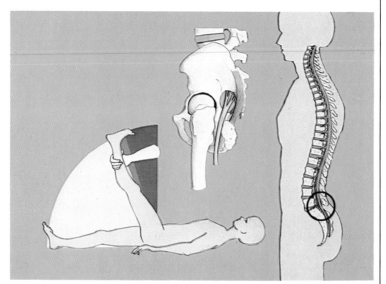

13.14 *Flexing the hip with the knee extended (left) pulls on the dura mater (right) via the sciatic nerve (centre).*

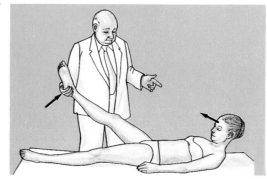

13.15 *Neck flexion pulls the dural tube upwards by an average of 3 cm. It may exacerbate pain.*

Root signs

Next the sacroiliac joint, the hip joint and the external aspect of the lumbar nerve roots are examined. A disc lesion interfering not just with mobility of the nerve root (i.e. painful limitation of straight-leg raising) but also with motor conduction of the parenchyma produces muscle weakness. So resisted movements of the leg prove weak rather than painful. Signs may be referable to more than one root.

The examination runs through the root signs in the order best suited to the patient's convenience, working progressively down the limb. The reader is referred to pages 236–239, where the signs are tabulated root by root in summary form. With the exception of acute lumbago, none of the following movements increases pain from a displacement.

The anterior sacroiliac ligaments are stretched (*Figure 13.16*) by downward and outward pressure applied to the anterior superior spines of the ilia. To prevent flattening of the lumbar spine during the downward pressure, the patient is asked to place her forearm in the small of her back, thus maintaining constant lordosis. The pressure may be further directed outwards by the examiner crossing his forearms to

deliver a contralateral thrust. If painful (cf. merely proving uncomfortable centrally), the sacroiliac joint is examined in detail (see page 78).

Resisted hip flexion (*Figure 13.17*) may be weak – the L2 or L3 root – or possibly painful, incriminating the psoas. The patient presses her thigh upwards with counter-pressure restraining her shoulder.

For resisted dorsiflexion the patient pushes her foot upwards (*Figure 13.18*); if weak, the L4 root is incriminated.

Impairment of conduction of the L4 or L5 root is indicated by painless weakness on resisted extension of the hallux (*Figure 13.19*).

Painless weakness on resisted eversion (*Figure 13.20*) suggests a lesion of the L5 or S1 roots.

The knee jerk (*Figure 13.21*) may be absent or sluggish in L3 lesions.

The patient turns over and her ankle jerk is tested (*Figure 13.22*). If absent or sluggish, this denotes involvement of the S1, S2 or occasionally the L5 root.

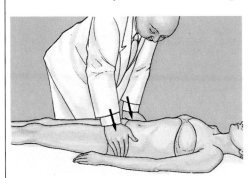

13.16 *The SIJ stretch.*

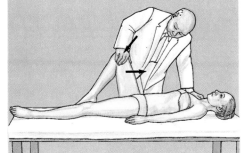

13.17 *Resisted hip flexion: L2 or L3.*

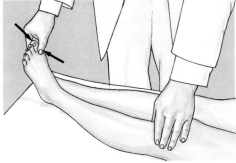

13.18 *Resisted dorsiflexion: L4.*

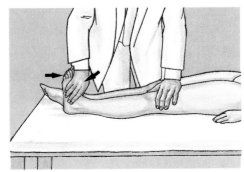

13.19 *Resisted toe extension: L4 or L5.*

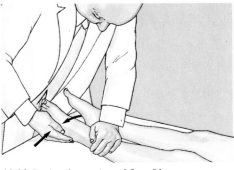

13.20 *Resisted eversion: L5 or S1.*

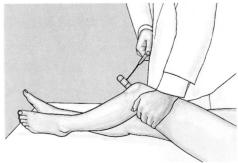

13.21 *The knee jerk:*

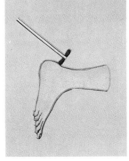

13.22 *The ankle jerk: S1 or S2.*

The mobility of the third lumbar root is checked by passive knee flexion in prone-lying (*Figure 13.23*), a procedure analogous to straight-leg raising. The root is stretched via the femoral nerve which passes to the front of the knee (and is thus relaxed by straight-leg raising itself). In L3 lesions, passive knee flexion tends to be painful at full range rather than limited. Minimal lumbar extension may be produced by this manoeuvre and therefore a spondylolisthesis or sacroiliac joint may produce pain. Painful structures anterior to the hip joint may also be compressed.

Weakness of the quadriceps is assessed by resisted knee extension (*Figure 13.24*). This tests the integrity of the L3 nerve root; the normal patient is stronger than the examiner.

Weak hamstrings show impaired conduction down S1 or S2, tested by resisted knee flexion; the patient presses her leg upwards (*Figure 13.25*). This time the examiner is stronger than the normal patient.

Next the patient is asked to squeeze her buttocks together and the bulk of the muscles is tested by pinching the gluteal mass (*Figure 13.26*). Some patients do this badly, and a straight-leg extension of the hip against resistance will confirm the gluteal mass. Wasting is attributable to involvement of the S1 or S2 roots.

The strength of the calf muscles is assessed by asking the patient to repeatedly stand on tiptoe one leg at a time (*Figure 13.27*). The nerve roots are S1 and S2. In practice this test is normally slotted into the beginning of the examination when the patient is still standing.

Analgesia is sought on the dorsum of the foot and toes. An L4 distribution occupies the big toe only, L5 the big toe and the two adjacent toes and S1 the outer two toes. The underside of the heel is S2.

Although the spinal cord itself terminates at L1, the plantar reflex (*Figure 13.28*) should be tested as a matter of course. Pulsation at the ankle is checked if intermittent claudication is suspected.

Finally an extension pressure is delivered in turn to the sacrum and centrally between each lumbar vertebra in order to establish whether pain or spasm are elicited.

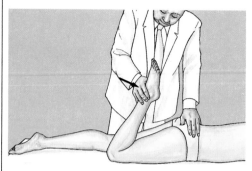

13.23 *Passive knee flexion: L3.*

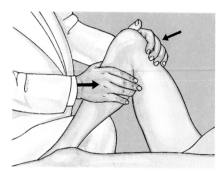

13.24 *Resisted knee extension: L3.*

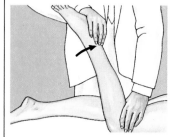

13.25 *Resisted knee flexion: S1 or S2.*

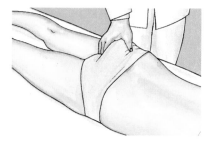

13.26 *Gluteal wasting: S1 or S2.*

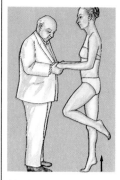

13.27 *Calf muscles: S1 or S2.*

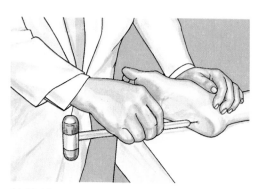

13.28 *Plantar reflex.*

Findings

Capsular lesions

All serious disorders of the lumbar spine result in limitation of movement in all directions. But because the amount of flexion and extension attainable by a normal individual are so markedly different, the capsular pattern is most easily recognized by equal limitation of both side flexions (*Figures 13.29* and *13.30*). Even with no flexion of the lumbar spine itself, the patient may still be able to touch her knees by bending at the hip (*Figure 13.31*).

Tuberculosis, neoplasm, chronic osteomyelitis, recent fractures, facet joint osteoarthrosis, ankylosing spondylitis and osteitis deformans all can produce the capsular pattern; all are visible radiographically and (with the exception of the facet joints) produce signs of gross pathology, and may or may not account for the patient's present symptoms.

A practised eye is required to detect the capsular pattern, since the range of side flexion ordinarily diminishes with age. Maximum side flexion attainable in youth can be favourably contrasted with that achieved by those of advancing years, even in the absence of any affection (*Figure 13.32*). Clinical judgement assesses the norm for any age group.

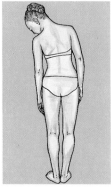 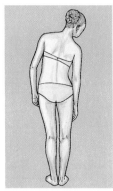 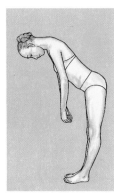 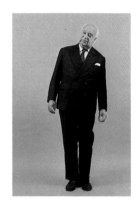

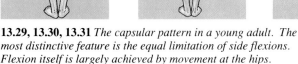

13.29, 13.30, 13.31 *The capsular pattern in a young adult. The most distinctive feature is the equal limitation of side flexions. Flexion itself is largely achieved by movement at the hips.*

13.32 *Limitation of side flexion is a normal finding in the elderly.*

The radiograph

It is common procedure when a patient presents with backache to call for an X-ray. This is not always productive since a number of conditions occur which, although visible radiographically, either never cause pain or only sometimes cause it. It is perfectly possible for united fractures, micro-fractures, narrowed joint spaces, osteoarthrosis and the like to exist silently. Schmorl's nodes, adolescent osteochondrosis, osteophytosis unless posterior, and numerous other conditions, are nearly always symptomless.

If osteophytes are present and accompanied by root symptoms, then as a highly specialist procedure a paravertebral block may be curative, although occasionally surgery is required to widen the lateral canal.

Spinal stenosis allows no room for minor disc protrusions and operation may be required.

Spondylolisthesis and osteoporosis sometimes produce symptoms of themselves. But the detection of these and any other X-ray findings should not lead to abandonment of the search for an alternative cause of pain until it is clear that the history and findings on clinical examination so warrant.

A large number of non-disc lesions give rise to back pain. These, including the above, are outlined on pages 235–236.

Displacements

A lumbar disc lesion may be characterized by any or all of:

(1) A history consistent with a displacement.
(2) Pain and limitation of the lumbar movements in the non-capsular pattern characteristic of internal derangement.
(3) Dural symptoms and signs.
(4) Nerve root symptoms and signs (impaired mobility).
(5) Nerve root symptoms and signs (impaired conduction).

Often (3), (4) and (5) will be absent, leaving the diagnosis founded on history and the partial articular pattern alone, reinforced by attendant congruous negative findings. In cases of extreme difficulty, diagnostic confirmation may be sought by radiculography or scan.

Clinical experience suggests that the propensity of the various spinal levels for disc lesions is, speaking very broadly, in the approximate proportions of:

L1: 1 : 10 000
L2: 1 : 1000
L3: 1 : 20
L4 and L5: Account for the remainder (i.e. nearly all disc lesions) about equally.

At L3 and above, a disc lesion (rare) protruding laterally will impinge on only the root of corresponding number.

A disc lesion at L4 may affect either the L4 or the L5 root or both (*Figure 13.33*).

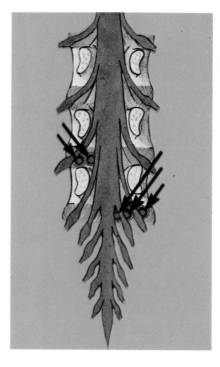

13.33 *The root(s) compressed at each level vary with the precise site of displacement.*

A disc lesion at L5 may compress one or two of the L5, S1 and S2 roots.

Both the S3 and S4 roots (dangerous) may be threatened by either the L4 or the L5 disc. The various combinations are tabulated on page 236.

Disc lesions: anomalies

Disc lesions at L1 and L2 (both very rare) are nearly all nuclear. The pain arises gradually when a certain posture is maintained and disappears when the posture is altered. Lesions at these levels do better with traction or stabilization with sclerosants than manipulation.

The so-called 'mushroom phenomenon' responds neither to traction nor to manipulation. The patient is elderly and the intervertebral disc largely eroded so that the gap between the vertebrae, originally about 1 cm, is now in the region of 1 mm. This makes the posterior longitudinal ligament extremely lax and any posterior protrusion of residual disc material bulges it out with ease to compress the dura mater.

The history is distinctive. The pain starts after the patient has stood for a while and the body weight has compressed the joints. The symptoms may consist of either backache with dural pain spreading to both limbs, or unilateral root pain without backache. The pain stops almost at once when the patient relieves the joint from weight-bearing by lying down.

Diagnostic confirmation may be obtained if the pain ceases immediately on bending forwards; this tightens the posterior ligament thus reducing the protrusion instantly. The patient is over 60.

The condition (pain on standing) must be differentiated from spinal claudication (pain on walking), caused by spinal stenosis which may fix the patient in flexion, unable to extend due to kinking of the spinal artery.

The 'mushroom's' central backache can be relieved by arthrodesis and the root pain by the specialist procedure of an injection of steroid suspension at the nerve root itself ('the paravertebral block').

Treatment

Summary

The main conservative treatments for a lumbar disc lesion are:

(1) Manipulation (see pages 207–220).
(2) Traction (see pages 221–225).
(3) Epidural local anaesthesia (see pages 226–230).

Relapse may be dealt with either by sclerosants (see page 231) and/or a corset (see page 234), both administered after reduction of the displacement and accompanied by postural education. Only a tiny proportion of cases require – or are appropriate for – the drastic remedy of surgery; an alternative is now provided by the two methods of percutaneous discectomy (discotome/chymopapain) which, in selected cases where the disc has herniated as a unit, may provide results comparable with more invasive surgical techniques.

Manipulation

Manipulation of the lumbar joints follows the same principles as elsewhere and, for those unfamiliar with this work, the general remarks in Chapters 2 and 10 must first be noted.

In contradistinction to the cervical and thoracic levels, the corset of muscles surrounding the lumbar joints is so strong that manual traction has no effect and accordingly is discarded. Hence there is no need for assistants. Sessions last 20 minutes or so and after each manoeuvre the patient is re-examined to assess progress.

The rotary manipulations aim to open the joint on the painful side (i.e. the side on which the lesion lies). Thus the patient is positioned with her painless side on the couch.

Although the manipulations are non-specific as to spinal level, it is always the joint with restricted range that receives the impact.

It is a sound principle to start off each new manoeuvre cautiously for observation, end-feel, response and the like. If manipulation – both the rotary and extension strains – shoot pain down the leg, manipulation is contraindicated and is abandoned as a method of treatment.

During a session, various techniques of increasing strength are tried, always in the light of the results of the previous manipulations. The procedure is empirical. Most benefit materializes during the first two sessions; it is rare that a fourth encounter yields further improvement.

A low couch about 15 inches (38 cm) high is required. It must be firm.

Absolute bars to manipulation

(1) Spinal cord signs (which in any case indicate the lesion lies above L2).
(2) Signs of impingement on the fourth sacral root. Sacro-perineal numbness or weakness of the bladder or anus are danger signals. Pain is felt in the perineum, rectum and scrotum. All these symptoms, which emerge during history, suggest that the posterior ligament is bulging considerably and is possibly partially ruptured. Manipulation might rupture it completely and allow massive extrusion of the entire disc.
(3) Bilateral sciatica unaccompanied by backache. The posterior ligament is attacked from both sides by a disc lesion and may be ruptured by manipulation.
(4) Spinal claudication implies considerable distortion of the posterior ligament; manipulation should be avoided. Walking causes pins and needles in both feet which cease as soon as the patient stops.
(5) Anticoagulant treatment (including aspirin during the preceding fortnight) contraindicates manipulation as intraspinal haematoma formation has been reported.
(6) Any non-discal condition and thus, by extension, recent vertebral fracture, etc.

Note also:
(1) Hyperacute lumbago renders manipulation intolerable. The patient is rigid with pain and
(a) when asked to lie prone takes some minutes to roll over
(b) gentle pressure to the patient's back sets up unbearable pain
Induction of epidural local anaesthesia should be carried out *stat* (see page 226). In the alternative, pain modulation (see page 231) may be attempted and, in these extreme circumstances, oscillatory techniques (such as Maitland's) may be helpful.
Reasonably severe lumbago responds well to manipulation, often with immediate relief.
(2) Pregnancy can be disregarded for the first four months. For the next four, supine and side-lying rotations may be used, but during the last month manipulation is best avoided.
(3) In cases of genuine organic symptoms coupled with psychogenic exaggeration, manipulation may be cautiously attempted having first warned the patient that a 'post-manipulative crisis' may strike briefly some hours after recovery as the patient adjusts to the shock of being well. Cases of pure neurosis should be left well alone.

Manipulation may not succeed

The sole indication for spinal manipulation is a cartilaginous prolapsed intervertebral disc. Roughly one-third of lumbar displacements are nuclear, except in patients over 60 where all are cartilaginous. The possibility of mixed protrusions has been considered on page 199. Primary posterolateral protrusions (i.e. sciatica without immediately preceding backache) all appear to be nuclear. Manipulation will not help the cases set out below which, with the exception of 5b and 6, all relate to sciatic pain:

(1) Pain down the leg with root signs (i.e. weakness, sluggish or absent reflexes or analgesia). The protrusion is too large.
(2) Root pain (unaccompanied by significant backache) which has been down the leg for six months or more in a patient under 60. There should, however, be spontaneous recovery within a year of onset.
(3) Sciatica with lumbar deformity. If there is root pain with little or no backache (cf. backache with slight sciatica), together with considerable lateral deviation at the lumbar spine when the patient stands normally, manipulation usually fails. The protrusion is too large. Side flexion barely reaches the vertical and shoots a pain down the lower limb.
(4) Sciatica without backache, with the patient fixed in slight flexion, normally proves intractable except by operation. Any attempt to stand erect sends twinges down the lower leg. The protrusion is too large.
(5) The patient is under 60 and:
   (a) Any trunk movement other than flexion increases or brings on the pain in the lower limb.
   (b) Side flexion in a patient with backache hurts on the side towards which the patient leans.
   In both cases the displacement is probably nuclear and will benefit from traction.
(6) Post-laminectomy. Manipulation seldom succeeds although there is no harm in having a go, particularly if there is a fresh protrusion at another joint. Traction is also worth trying.
(7) In cases of sciatic pain without backache where the reasonably intense root symptoms are subsiding, it is best to steer clear of both manipulation and traction. The patient is over the worst and the residual symptoms are best dealt with by epidural local anaesthesia.

Additionally, clinical experience suggests a proportion of unresponsive sciatic disc cases may benefit from a course of acupuncture (e.g. acupuncture/electro-acupuncture, acupuncture with moxibustion). The therapeutic mechanism has been extensively researched but the overall picture remains incomplete in terms of Western medicine. The number of reliable cases is small, but includes recovery in patients otherwise destined for surgery.

Rotation strains

Despite engagement of the articular processes at each facet joint limiting rotation, a rotation strain is a highly effective way of securing reduction at low lumbar levels. Manipulative sessions should always start with Rotation 1 (see page 210) and then, after maximum benefit has been imparted, progress as necessary to the stronger rotations. However, for a second session the operator may well – unless the patient has regressed – start where he left off.

With the elderly or those suffering minor protrusions, following incomplete reduction by the first manipulation, it may be judged better to move on to the milder extension strains.

For all rotation strains the patient lies on her painless side. This means the distracting force opens the joint on her bad side, thus allowing the displacement room to move.

If the pain is central, straight-leg raise usually elucidates the situation by proving painful unilaterally. In the absence of any indicator, the manipulator proceeds by trial and error. When maximum benefit has been afforded by any particular manoeuvre, another is tried and suggested routines are set out below.

Caution

If manipulation sets up pain in the lower limb, the rotary methods are dispensed with and the manipulations towards extension tried instead. If they too shoot pain down the limb, manipulation ceases altogether.

Re-examination: an example

After each manipulation, the patient is re-examined. Thus, if straight-leg raise was previously limited, it is now reassessed; increased range (*Figures 13.34* and *13.35*) indicates a corresponding diminution of the displacement and would encourage the operator to try the same manoeuvre again before progressing to stronger measures if necessary. Straight-leg raise is a highly sensitive indicator which may attain full painless range before reduction is complete. If this happens, or if straight-leg raise was full and painless to start with, the patient's lumbar movements are reassessed each time, checking both that the bad ones are better and the good no worse. If a cough was originally painful this too is checked.

As a rule, if the patient has improved, the manipulation is repeated and the patient re-examined. In due course, after maximum benefit has been attained, the session progresses to the next manipulation.

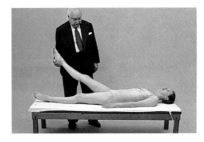

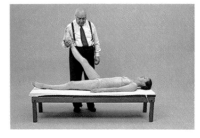

13.34, 13.35 *Re-examination. Straight-leg raising before (top) and after the manipulation (bottom) is a sensitive indicator of progress. Once it is full, the lumbar movements are tested instead.*

Rotation strain – 1

The patient lies on her painless side with her upper thigh flexed to bring the femoral trochanter into prominence (*Figure 13.36*). The manipulation consists of twisting the patient's trunk during distraction.

One hand is used to push the trochanter forwards and the other to force the front of the shoulder downwards: this preliminary measure rotates the patient's trunk in opposite directions.

As the manipulator leans forwards, his body weight is used to secure additional rotation and also to distract the lumbar joints; the distraction is achieved as one hand is impelled sideways towards the patient's head and the other hand towards her feet (*Figure 13.37*).

An operator of slighter build may have to lean forwards very considerably to achieve the same effect (*Figure 13.38*).

After a few seconds of sustained pressure, the overstrain is applied by the manipulator jerking his body forwards to increase momentarily both rotation and distraction (*Figures 13.39* and *13.40*).

The patient is re-examined and, if improvement has resulted, the manoeuvre is repeated. Once maximum benefit has accrued, the most likely successor may well be Rotation 3. In the unlikely event that this first rotation has made the patient worse, rotation in the opposite direction is instantly tried by using the Reverse Rotation Strain.

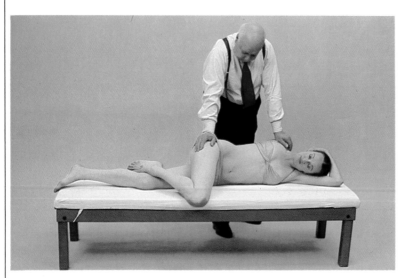

13.36 *Starting position. The patient's trunk will be rotated in opposite directions. Note the low couch and the absence of any assistants.*

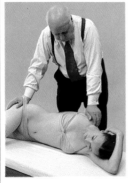
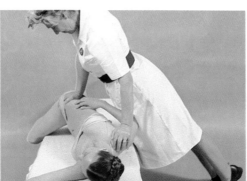

13.37   **13.38**

13.37, 13.38 *Starting position. The hands are in contact with the skin to avoid slippage. An operator of lighter build uses all her body weight.*

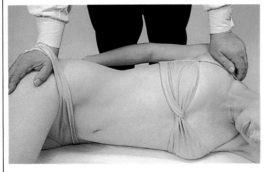
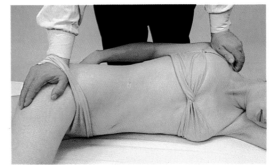

13.39, 13.40 *Starting and finishing positions as the trochanter is pressed forwards and the shoulder back.*

13.39   **13.40**

Reverse rotation strain

This is the reverse of its predecessor, in that during distraction the pelvis is forced towards, and the shoulder away from, the operator (*Figure 13.41*). The manoeuvre is reserved for cases aggravated by Rotation 1, which it should speedily rectify. Progressive amelioration can subsequently be imparted by the extension strains (see page 215). The patient lies on her pain-free side.

One hand is curved round the patient's anterior iliac spine and the palm of the other hand placed on her upper thorax against the spine of her scapula (*Figure 13.42*).

The operator leans forwards over the patient, stretching her thorax and pelvis apart by pushing outwards. Rotation is gradually increased (*Figure 13.43*).

To apply over-pressure the manipulator jerks his body downwards and simultaneously forces his arms further apart and into rotation, drawing the iliac spine in towards him and thrusting the scapula down and away (*Figure 13.44*).

The patient is re-examined and the manoeuvre repeated if improvement is apparent, with subsequent progression as necessary.

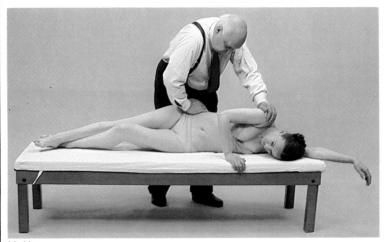

13.41

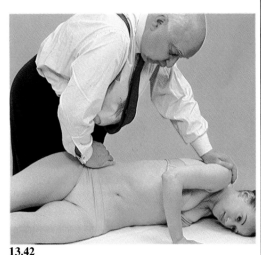

13.42

13.41, 13.42 *Starting position. The operator takes the patient to the extreme of comfortable range.*

13.43, 13.44 *Starting and finishing positions. The forceful overthrust momentarily pushes the patient's shoulder towards her ear and her pelvis towards supination.*

13.43

13.44

Rotation strain – 2

Both this manipulation and its successor, Rotation 3, are contraindicated in patients with arthritis of the hip and the elderly with whom the strength of the femur is unreliable. This is because the thigh is used as a lever, held horizontally and pulled into extension towards the manipulator while the shoulder is pinned to the couch. The patient lies on her painless side (*Figure 13.45*). Rotation 2 should be used if the Reverse Rotation Strain is indicated, but fails.

The operator's knee is wedged against the patient's lower buttock to steady her on the couch. One hand bears down on the shoulder. It is here that the body weight is applied while the other hand fully extends and adducts the hip joint (*Figure 13.46*).

The overthrust is applied by keeping the pressure on the shoulder while the manipulator rotates his thorax and jerks the patient's thigh sharply upwards (*Figure 13.47*). The patient is re-examined.

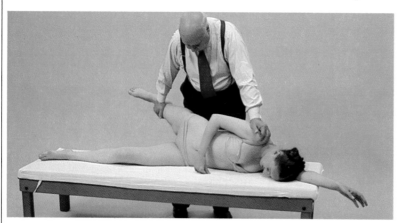

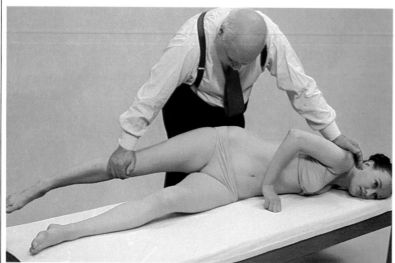

13.45, 13.46 *Starting position. Extension of the hip is most clearly shown in Figure 13.45. The operator's knee steadies the patient's lower back.*

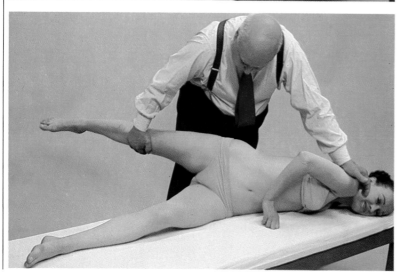

13.47 *Finishing position. Note how the movement is assisted by the operator leaning towards the patient's head; he swivels his thorax to achieve added extension of the patient's hip.*

Rotation strain – 3

Many practitioners regard this as the most effective of the lumbar manipulations. Like Rotation 2, it affords maximum rotation but little distraction and similarly should be avoided with the elderly or those with arthritis of the hip. Again the thigh is used as a lever, but this time it is forced downwards (*Figure 13.48*).

The patient lies face upwards, well towards the side on which the manipulator stands. He uses his knee to steady her trunk and keep her on the couch. Then he flexes her hip to a right angle and applies his other hand to her shoulder. It is over this arm that body weight is concentrated in order to ensure the patient's thorax is maintained flat on the couch (*Figure 13.49*).

Muscular force is used to press the knee sharply towards the floor and rotate the lumbar spine (*Figure 13.50*).

The patient is re-examined and the manipulation repeated if benefit has accrued. In patients who hold the spine vertical without lumbar deviation, it is often best to start with the hip flexed to rather less than a right-angle.

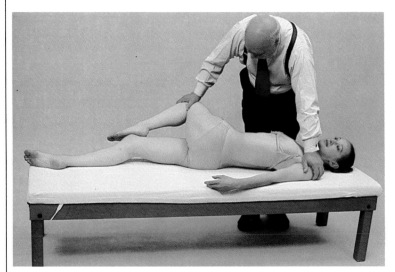 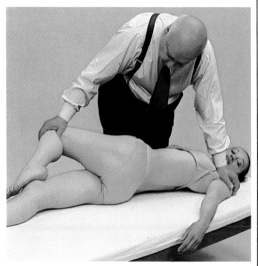

13.48, 13.49 *Starting position. The body weight is balanced over the patient's shoulder, clamping it to the couch.*

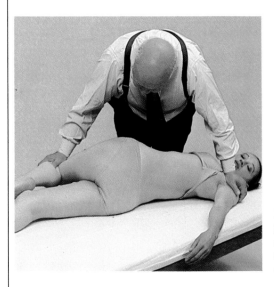

13.50 *Finishing position. The operator half-turns as his hands are thrust downwards and apart.*

Rotation strain – 4

This is a variation on Rotation 3. Downward pressure is again delivered to the thigh at the knee, but this leg is also used to achieve side flexion transmitted via the other leg hooked over it (*Figure 13.51*).

For the starting position the patient flexes her knees and crosses her legs, the leg on the painless side uppermost. The operator stands opposite the painful side and places his hand on the lower knee. The other hand is on the patient's shoulder, fixing the upper part of the trunk flat on the couch. It is over this arm that body weight is poised (*Figure 13.52*). The hand on the patient's knee is used to gradually ease the patient into maximum side flexion towards the operator.

Downward pressure on the knee is then increased until the tissue resistance, heralding the end of range. During this stage the patient's free knee is kept in position by pressure against the operator. Sharp overstrain then forces the knee further downwards, rotating the lumbar spine while simultaneously achieving side flexion towards the painless side (*Figure 13.53*).

The patient is re-examined. This manipulation is often successful for those with considerable lateral deviation; for other corrective methods the reader is referred to page 220.

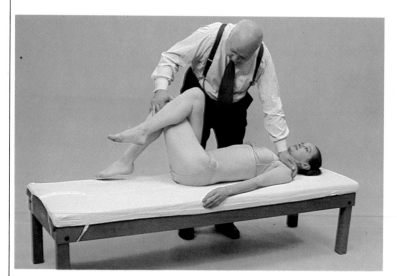

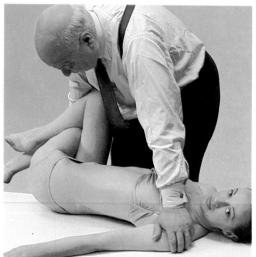

13.51, 13.52 *Starting position. This time it is the hip on the good side which is flexed over the painful leg, which is used as the lever.*

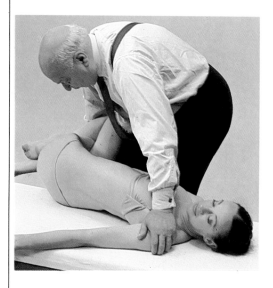

13.53 *Finishing position. The operator's body pressure against the good thigh fixes the lumbar spine in side flexion, while the rotation is imparted by a sharp thrust on the bad knee.*

Extension strains

The extension strains are best reserved for the elderly, those with a minor protrusion or as a follow-up to the corrective measure of the Reverse Rotation Strain. They are unlikely to bring about much improvement where the patient has already been through the rotary methods, but they may be useful for the new or more nervous patient.

If, altogether, the extension strains do prove fruitful, then the rotation strains – if not previously employed – are tried.

Even if the patient is no better, it is probably worth while trying the rotation strains nevertheless, although it may be necessary to reconsider the original diagnosis of a cartilaginous displacement.

Forced extension – 1

This manipulation consists of pressing down sharply at the site of the displacement as determined at the end of the examination (*Figure 13.54*).

One hand is placed so that the mid-shaft of the fifth metacarpal bone engages against the prominence formed by the spinous process of the relevant vertebra (*Figure 13.55*). This will almost certainly be L4 or L5.

The other hand is used for reinforcement (*Figure 13.56*). Only the ulnar border of the lower hand is in contact with the patient, thus localizing the pressure.

The manipulator leans on the patient's back for a few seconds to secure some extension and then bends his head and thorax abruptly forwards using body weight to give the final jerk. As he does so, each upper limb is kept rigid to transmit the downwards thrust of his trunk (*Figure 13.57*). The patient is re-examined.

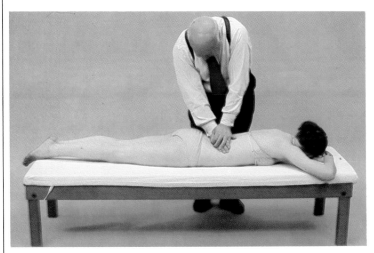

13.54, 13.55, 13.56 *Starting position. One hand is tilted; the other is cupped over it.*

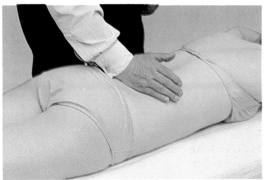

13.55

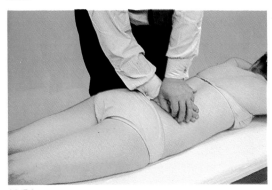

13.56

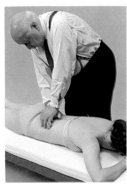

13.57 *The overthrust. The operator leans sharply forwards and downwards.*

Forced extension – 2

This manipulation is all but identical to the preceding one, except that the operator's hands are placed further over, beyond the patient's mid-line (*Figure 13.58*). This means that the weight of the thrust is medial as well as downwards and thus produces a significant amount of rotation.

The operator stands on the patient's bad side; it is this side of the joint which will be opened. Both hands are applied to the patient's good side, with the forearm just short of pronation. The other hand is again used for reinforcement (*Figure 13.59*) and the operator leans right over the patient and presses until all play has been taken out of the joint.

He then jerks his head and thorax downwards, keeping his arms rigid to apply the over-pressure which is directed towards himself (*Figure 13.60*).

The patient is re-examined. If some benefit has accrued, the procedure is repeated.

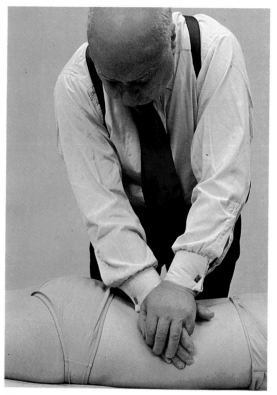

13.58 *Starting position. The hands are well to the side of the mid-line.*

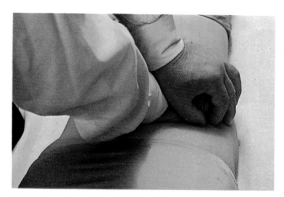

13.59 *Configuration of the hands.*

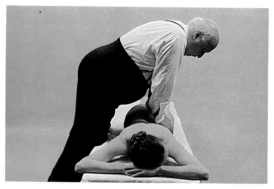

13.60 *The over-pressure. The operator uses all his body weight, pressing downwards and backwards towards himself.*

Forced extension – 3

A stronger extension strain can be obtained by using the thigh as a lever (*Figure 13.61*). This is particularly productive where partial reduction has already been achieved, but should not be attempted if previous extension strains have not resulted in improvement.

The operator stands on the side away from the patient's pain. The ulnar border of one hand bears down just above the posterior spine of the ilium, while her hip is extended and strongly adducted to open the lumbar joints (*Figure 13.62*).

The lumbar hand is pressed down and the knee hand pulled sharply up. The movement is assisted by simultaneously leaning heavily towards the patient's head (*Figure 13.63*).

The patient is re-examined and if some benefit has resulted the procedure is repeated.

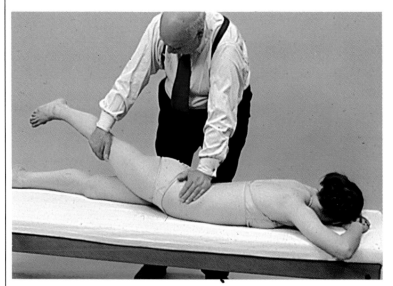
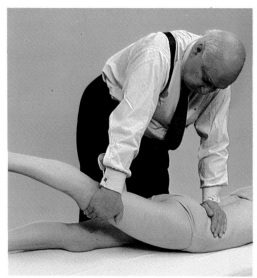

13.61, 13.62 *Starting position. The operator's distal hand pulls up, the proximal hand pushes down well lateral to the spine.*

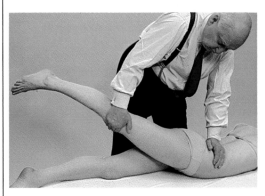

13.63 *Finishing position. The operator pulls the thigh up and towards himself.*

Forced extension – 4

This is a stronger version of the previous manipulation, suitable for dealing with a heavily-built patient. The added force is obtained by using the knee to apply downward lumbar pressure (*Figure 13.64*). Like its predecessor, this manipulation should be omitted if the previous extension strains have not helped.

The operator stands on the patient's painful side, and the hip is again strongly adducted and extended to its utmost, lifting the patient's pelvis off the couch (*Figure 13.65*).

The overthrust is applied by pressing down with the knee while raising the patient's thigh towards further extension and adduction (*Figure 13.66*).

The patient is re-examined and, if necessary, the final extension manipulation is employed.

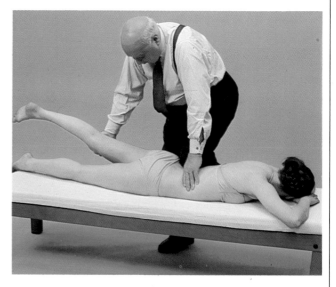

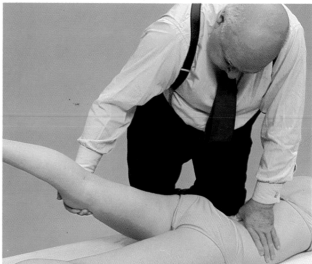

13.64, 13.65 *Starting position. Note that the operator's knee clamps the patient's trunk to the couch; his distal hand is in supination so the thigh can be adducted during extension of the hip.*

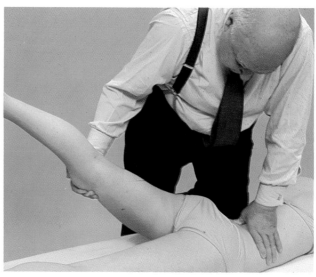

13.66 *Finishing position.*

Forced extension – 5

The patient lies prone with her trunk side-flexed as far over as possible towards the painless side: this opens the joint space on the affected side. The manipulation forces extension with further distraction (*Figure 13.67*).

The operator stands on the patient's good side, with his forearms crossed. The heel of his lower hand is on the iliac crest and the heel of the upper pushes, under the lowest ribs (*Figure 13.68*), towards the head.

The operator forces his hands in opposite directions by leaning his trunk forwards. Keeping his elbows rigid he then jerks his thorax downwards, imparting a sudden extension thrust at the fourth lumbar level together with momentary further distraction (*Figure 13.69*). The patient is re-examined.

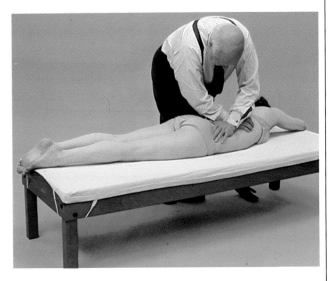

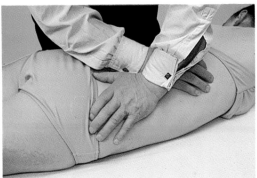

13.67, 13.68 *Starting position. The patient is side-flexed towards the operator. The hands are crossed and firmly applied to the patient's trunk.*

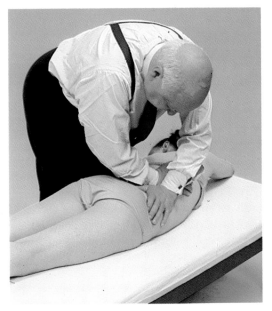

13.69 *Finishing position. The operator's hands are forced downwards and in opposite directions as he leans sharply forwards.*

Correction of lateral deviation – 1

This manoeuvre is indicated where manipulation has eased the pain but side flexion in one direction remains limited. Both this and its successor may also be useful in straightening up a badly deviated patient before progressing to the manipulations proper.

Deviation is made up of two components, a primary lumbar and secondary thoracic curve. For example, deviation to the left consists of side flexion to the left at the lumbar spine and side flexion to the right at the thoracic. It is the lumbar component that is the primary deviation requiring correction. In this instance, the patient's right thigh would be crossed over her left and the movement performed into right side flexion.

The patient lies on her back and flexes both hips. Her legs are crossed. If the lumbar deviation is towards the right, the right thigh is uppermost (*Figure 13.70*).

By simultaneously pulling on the near knee and pushing on the far, full lumbar side flexion is achieved in the previously blocked direction (*Figures 13.71* and *13.72*). The rotary movement is repeated several times to develop range; then on the fourth or fifth twist, the extreme of range is held for a good minute or so. This goes on a number of times for, say, 10 minutes until the spine stays vertical after the patient has stood for a while.

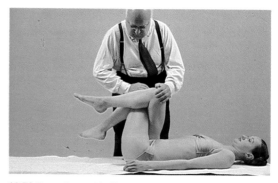

13.70 *Sometimes side flexion remains obstinately limited; the patient may stand crooked. The starting position for this corrective manipulation entails crossing the patient's legs with the thigh on the limited side uppermost.*

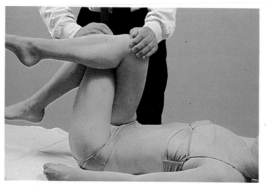 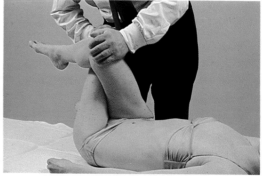

13.71, 13.72 *The legs are repeatedly swung from side to side; side flexion will gradually increase and the corrected position should be held to consolidate range.*

Correction of lateral deviation – 2

For this alternative measure, known as MacKenzie's, the patient stands and the manipulator puts his hands round the patient's pelvis, placing his chest against the patient's arm (*Figure 13.73*). He pulls the pelvis towards himself in the direction it will not go and repeats this movement several times (*Figure 13.74*). The patient is then kept in the laterally corrected position for a couple of minutes, during which time lordosis is restored by the patient repeatedly and increasingly extending her lumbar spine.

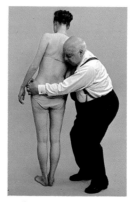 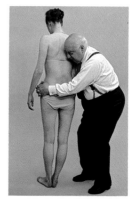

13.73, 13.74 *As the patient's pelvis is hugged towards the operator, his shoulder forces his spine upright. While in the corrected position, the patient actively achieves extension.*

Traction

Traction (*Figure 13.75*) is the treatment of choice for small nuclear protrusions. Whereas a fragment of cartilage can be clicked back into position by manipulation, the nucleus is soft and can be influenced only by suction.

To be effective the traction must conform to particular specifications:

(1) Distracting forces within the range of 20 kg (for a small woman) and 50 kg (for a large man) are normally adequate with modern friction-free couches. A cautious first treatment is recommended. The distracting force must be the greatest the patient can stand without discomfort and, in the case of the older manual equipment, higher readings are required as the equipment absorbs some of the pull: 35 kg/80 lb would be the minimum for a small woman and 80 kg/180 lb the greatest for a really large man.

Cautious resort to lesser poundage will, at best, fail to secure maximum distraction and, at worst, produce nothing at all; minimal poundage of the order in widespread conventional use often fails to overcome even body friction.

(2) The traction must be sustained for periods of half-an-hour. Intermittent traction will not achieve reduction (see below).

(3) The traction is best given daily, i.e. five times per week minimum. The object is to suck the intervertebral protrusion back further during one session than it comes out before the next.

(4) Two weeks' treatment are usual before full benefits are manifest. Only very seldom are more than four weeks necessary. The treatment may be supplemented by bodyweight traction at home using traction boots, back swing, etc.

Traction has three effects, all conspiring towards the same end:

(1) The lumbar vertebrae are separated. X-rays have shown an increase in width at each lumbar joint of 2.5 mm. This increase in distance between the articular edges allows more room for a displacement to return to its original site and may actually disengage a protrusion

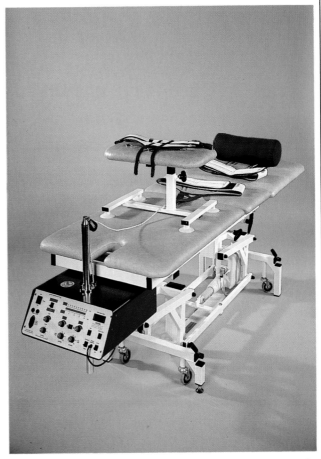

13.75 *Lumbar traction for nuclear displacements. Sessions must be daily and the traction must be sustained (not intermittent). On modern friction-free couches the pull should be within in the range of 20–50 kg. It is a comfortable treatment.*

just too large to shift during mere avoidance of compression by recumbency.

(2) The intradiscal pressure is greatly reduced when the bones move apart, with a resulting tendency to suck any protrusion back to the centre of the joint.

(3) The posterior longitudinal ligament is tautened. This pushes the protrusion anteriorly towards the centre of the joint.

These effects combine to reduce the displacement. Before each session, the patient is re-examined to see if any improvement has resulted from the previous day's treatment. In a suitable case some amelioration is evident after the first few sessions and should continue steadily thereafter. If no improvement is apparent after a week or 10 days, it is worth considering whether matters might be improved by altering the patient's posture on the couch (e.g. by flexing the hips or lying her face down) or by changing the position of the straps.

Traction and bed-rest

The aim of traction is to obtain rapid reduction of the protrusion by distracting the joint surfaces mechanically. This exerts substantial centripetal force, acting on the protruded part of the nucleus and greatly expediting recovery. This is a positive purpose. Bed-rest merely avoids the compression stress on the spine entailed by upright posture. This is a negative process. In patients under 60, bed-rest is usually successful in the end.

It achieves the same result as traction much more slowly but will of course complement the traction which brings the joint surfaces much further apart than just lying in bed. Bed-rest may be accompanied by postural manoeuvres such as pillows gradually introduced under the chest to encourage lumbar extension and disc reduction.

Bed-rest alone for patients with a nuclear protrusion is an unnecessary waste of time and money. But sometimes the harm done by travelling in a car to and from traction sessions can outweigh the benefit.

If the displacement is cartilaginous it should of course be manipulated.

In a combined lesion the patient is manipulated until maximum benefit has accrued. The remaining symptoms can then be eradicated by traction.

Intermittent traction

Continuous traction fatigues the muscles and after a while they relax. Only then does the pull fall on the joint and distraction commence – it is not until three minutes after traction begins that electromyographic silence is attained. Hence the pulls of shorter duration merely elicit the strength reflex and exercise the sacrospinalis muscles without separating the joint surfaces or contributing in any degree to reduction of the lesion. Such settings, albeit available on modern equipment, must be ignored.

Indications for traction

The sole indication is a small nuclear protrusion at lumbar levels. The patient is thus under 60 as after that age the nucleus no longer exists.

Nuclear protrusions are characterized by gradual onset of pain often brought on by sitting or stooping. The aggravation may mount overnight after, for example, a day's gardening.

The following symptoms also imply a nuclear protrusion.

(1) Side flexion towards the painful side increases the pain. This applies only to patients under 60 with backache as opposed to lumbago.
(2) Trunk movements other than flexion bring on or increase pain down the lower limb.
(3) Primary posterolateral onset, that is, the pain strikes first in the leg without previous backache. There is, however, a marked tendency in these patients to relapse following traction. In such cases it may be best to await spontaneous recovery assisted by local epidural anaesthesia.

Additionally, traction is more effective than manipulation in cases of:

(1) First and second lumbar disc lesions (very rare).
(2) Recurrence after laminectomy.
(3) Bilateral longstanding limitation of straight-leg raise in young adults (but up to three months, daily traction may be required).

In cases of doubt, that is, where the protrusion is of indeterminate nature, manipulation should be tried first as its effect is immediate. If manipulation fails, traction should not begin until the following day otherwise it may make the pain worse.

Contraindications

(1) Traction must be avoided in the presence of S4 root signs (see page 239).

(2) Acute lumbago strongly contraindicates traction. Severe backache is no bar, but lumbago with fixation in flexion or twinges in the back on trunk movement means traction must not be attempted.

   The traction itself will not hurt at the timeand indeed relieves the pain. However, the moment the pressure is eased even slightly, agonizing pain is engendered and it may take the patient some hours to get off the couch.

(3) Sciatica with gross lumbar deformity, whether fixation of flexion or side flexion, will be painful on traction. Operation is required.

(4) Patients with gross emphysema, heart disease, a thoracoplasty or any severe respiratory disorder may not be able to tolerate the band around the thorax.

Traction will not help

(1) Neurological deficit (as opposed to mere root pain). The protrusion is too large; manipulation will not work either and epidural local anaesthesia should be considered.

(2) Where sciatica (as distinct from backache with some leg pain) has lasted more than six months. Nor will manipulation prove effective unless the patient is over 60, in which case any displacement must be cartilaginous. The physician can either await spontaneous recovery or consider an injection of epidural local anaesthetic (also the treatment of choice where an attack of sciatica is already subsiding and the patient over the worst).

Equipment

Modern electronic couches, although expensive, greatly facilitate treatment. The sliding thoracic section eliminates body friction and thus poundage can be accurately set and maintained. Speed of wind-up and wind-down can likewise be preset, and the thoracic platform tilted to achieve alteration in the angle of pull. Velcro strapping is effective and much easier to apply than the old strap-and-buckle, but like its predecessor may require supplementary padding to avoid uncomfortable catching sub-costally.

   Nevertheless, equally effective results can be achieved (albeit with greater operator effort) by the old-fashioned manual couches (*Figure 13.76*) which can of course be adapted from any fixed couch by means of special attachments.

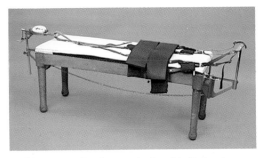

13.76 *Accessories that can be hand-bolted onto a standard couch are perfectly adequate.*

Technique

The patient is examined at each attendance before the treatment, since the physical signs immediately after traction are unreliable. Lumbar movement and straight-leg raise are assessed (*Figure 13.77*).

The straps are done up very tightly, with great attention paid to the positioning of the padding. Then the patient is covered with a blanket and the pressure is slowly raised over the course of some five minutes (*Figures 13.78* and *13.79*).

The distracting force is the maximum the patient can bear painlessly. Traction is a comfortable procedure and the patient should never feel pain. If it hurts, something is wrong: either the case is unsuitable or the treatment has been marred by bad technique.

The patient stays on traction for half-an-hour, but the operator remains within call. On the older manual machines some of the distracting force will be lost after the first few minutes and the poundage should be topped up.

At the end of the treatment, the patient is wound down very slowly, taking up to five minutes. Traction appliances with a ratchet releasing all the distraction at once are diligently avoided. Anything other than slow diminution of pressure can produce severe twinges.

The patient is left for some minutes to regain her normal length before compressing the joint by standing. She is shown how to get off the couch by rolling on to her side (*Figure 13.80*), putting her feet over the edge of the couch and then using her arms to rise sideways to a sitting position.

The patient must always bend at the knees when picking up her footwear. Use of a chair minimizes stooping when putting on shoes (*Figure 13.81*).

The first treatment should be cautious, particularly in patients with lumbago who have only just lost their twinges. For comfort's sake, the patient should not

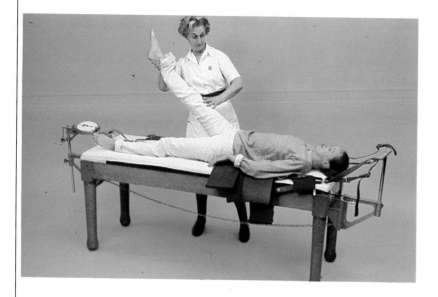

13.77 *Re-examination before treatment. After the traction, lumbar movements should be avoided while the spine settles down.*

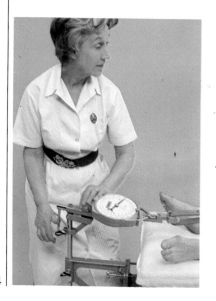

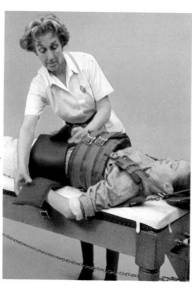

13.78, 13.79 *The high poundage demands plenty of soft padding under the thoracic and pelvic harness. Pressure is wound up slowly.*

consume a large meal before the session and should be encouraged to keep as relaxed and as still as possible during the stretch; coughing must be avoided.

Treatment is given daily until reduction has been secured. Normally this takes one to three weeks, although sometimes a fourth week is justified if improvement is

continuing. If 10 adequate sessions have done no good, traction should be stopped (except in cases of longstanding bilaterally limited straight-leg raise in young adults). When the patient is nearly well, a painful arc on straight-leg raising may become apparent. Many patients begin to get better only during the second week.

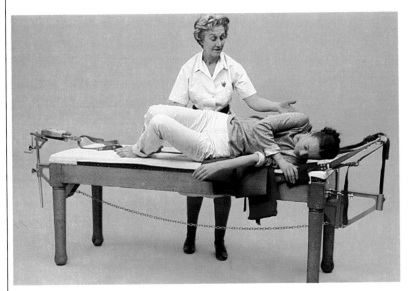

13.80 *After the treatment. The patient rolls into the sitting position, avoiding lumbar flexion.*

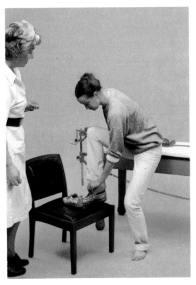

13.81 *Prophylactic education. No lumbar treatment is complete without cautioning the patient against unnecessary flexion strains.*

The patient's position

It is standard practice to start the treatments with the patient on her back. Unless re-examination shows this posture not to work, it is maintained for subsequent attendances. But if the traction has not begun to work after a few days, the question of a different approach is raised.

For the older equipment, probably the easiest way to alter the pull on the joints is to raise or lower the attachments at one or both ends of the couch. Where the apparatus does not permit such flexibility, the same effect can be achieved by altering the strapping or the patient's posture.

Numerous different positions are possible. The patient may lie face down or face up, hips flexed, hips straight, and whether prone or supine the straps can be applied in four different ways, fastened to either the top or underside of the thoracic and lumbar harnesses.

Thus both straps may be pulling from beneath, both from above, the lumbar strap may be up and the thoracic down and vice versa. The variation in pull may be minimal but in difficult cases it can mean all the difference between success and failure.

Caudal epidural local anaesthesia

This is the treatment of choice for an irreducible lumbar displacement. Thus its application is restricted to large displacements that cannot be shifted by manipulation or traction. Most patients supposed to require operation merely need this injection to get well and stay well.

A solution of 1 : 200 procaine 50ml in normal saline is injected via the sacral hiatus into the sacral canal (*Figure 13.82*). This bathes the external aspect of the dura mater, nerve roots and adjacent structures in anaesthetic, so although the displacement remains the patient can no longer feel the pain. In suitable cases – with a couple of back-up injections if necessary – full and lasting relief is to be expected.

It is a simple outpatient procedure and does not require general anaesthetic. Lateral epidurals are of no effect except with the extremely rare L3 lesions.

Results

Immediately following a successful injection the patient regains painless (though not necessarily full) lumbar mobility and improved straight-leg raise.

After the first hour or so the symptoms may or may not return. A week should elapse before assessing the injection's long-term results unless severe pain makes it imperative to see the patient sooner.

The effect of the injection is very variable during the days immediately following infiltration. Some patients lose their symptoms for a couple of days and then relapse, whereas others get well and stay well. A few undergo increased pain for a day or two and then recover rapidly.

The injection should be repeated at the end of a week or 10 days if either:

(1) Pain is diminished.
(2) Lumbar mobility or straight-leg raise has improved (even though the pain remains unaltered).

A total of three further injections may be required at, for example, weekly or fortnightly intervals.

If there is no improvement at the end of the first week, treatment by injection is abandoned. Alternatively, if at that date the patient has full painless range, then no further treatment is called for except in the event of subsequent deterioration.

In 1963 Coomes (see page 155) estimated the relative value of recumbency and epidural local anaesthesia in a series of 50 patients. All had sciatica with severe pain and

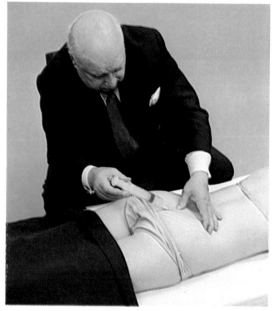

13.82 *Injection of procaine via the sacral hiatus anaesthetizes the lower extent of the dura mater. Often the relief from pain is permanent.*

signs of impaired conduction along the nerve root. Half were hospitalized and the others received one or two injections and rested at home. The injected patients largely recovered within 10 days, whereas the recumbent took 30 days to reach the same degree of comfort. In Canada, Fraser (1976) contrasted the duration and cost of acute lumbago treated by epidural anaesthesia and by traditional measures (e.g. recumbency, traction in bed, heat, analgesics) and came up with figures of 3.8 days for the injection and 15.6 for the other methods.

Anaesthetic

The solution is 1 : 200 procaine 50ml in normal saline without adrenaline – pure water must not be used otherwise really severe pain results for about 24 hours. Other solutions of marcaine or xylocaine/lignocaine may be used with appropriate alteration in dosage to avoid motor paralysis. Only surface anaesthesia is needed.

Procaine achieves better results than the more modern anaesthetics.

Indications

The injection is the main weapon for disposing of root pain with absent or sluggish reflex, one or more weak muscles or analgesic skin (not mere pins and needles).

Indications are:

(1) *Hyperacute lumbago.* Both manipulation and traction are strongly contraindicated. The patient experiences severe twinges on the slightest movement and is generally immobilized in bed. The injection affords immediate complete relief for about 90 minutes during which free mobility of the joint is restored and spontaneous reduction begins. The patient must get home and into bed before the end of this interlude and should lie prone. Not much pain returns and by the following morning the patient is normally well enough for reduction by manipulation.

(2) *Root pain with neurological signs.* Neither manipulation nor traction will work.

The injection does not work so well on:

(a) Patients over 60, but good results can be obtained.

(b) Third lumbar disc lesions (relatively rare) with root pain.

(3) *Root pain without neurological signs.* The injection is useful for six categories:

(a) Root pain that has continued for too long. It should clear up spontaneously in a year at most. Epidural local anaesthesia is indicated if the pain – usually accompanied by limited straight-leg raise – obstinately refuses to go.

(b) Primary posterolateral disc protrusions. The displacement is nuclear so manipulation will fail, and although traction succeeds there is a high rate of recurrence. The injection is only successful when the protrusion has stabilized in the position of maximum displacement, designated by stabilization of the limitation of straight-leg raise, usually with a range of about 30–60°.

(c) Recurrent sciatica after a root palsy. Relapse at the same level from sciatica with neurological signs is uncommon following recovery, whether achieved spontaneously or by epidural injection. However, if the pain returns within the year, then epidural local anaesthesia is given. It is more often successful than treating the attack as a new displacement by starting off again with manipulation or traction.

(d) Root pain without physical signs. A patient may complain of root pain and yet have full painless range of both straight-leg raise and lumbar movements. If the history suggests a disc lesion, epidural local anaesthesia is induced diagnostically and in many cases secures lasting relief. The cause of pain may be bruising of the dural sleeve persisting from a past disc lesion.

(e) Recovering sciatica. If sciatic pain without backache and reasonably intense root symptoms are subsiding, it is best to steer clear of manipulation and traction. The patient is over the worst and suffers little more than an ache in the limb and limited straight-leg raise.

(f) Nocturnal cramp. Severe cramp in the calf of the affected leg coming on each night may wake a patient long after sciatica has ceased. Epidural local anaesthesia serves to desensitize the nerve root and the injection may need repeating some six months later.

(4) *Pregnancy.* In the last month of pregnancy, the injection is to be preferred to manipulation or traction.

(5) *Intractable backache.* A low lumbar disc lesion which, in the absence of contraindications, proves refractory to both manipulation and traction should be treated by injection. The pain may be lastingly abolished or diminished.

(6) *Chronic backache.* This condition may present with no articular signs. Manipulation of such a disc lesion will fail, whereas injection may relieve dural bruising.

(7) *Matutinal or nocturnal backache.* The patient can do everything, even heavy work by day, but is regularly woken in the small hours or early morning by backache severe enough to force him out of bed. The symptoms last for about an hour and examination during the day reveals nothing. The only diagnostic indication may be that during his attack a cough causes pain.

(8) *Diagnostic.* It is chiefly in early cases with slight symptoms and physical signs difficult to interpret that the injection helps diagnostically. It is also helpful with patients with uncharacteristic backache in medico-legal disputes. If, following the injection, the symptoms abate and full straight-leg raise is practicable, the lesion must be connected with the exterior surface of the dura mater or the lower lumbar nerve roots. They are the only material tissues rendered anaesthetic.

Translumbar epidural

It is possible that this is more effective for L3 discs (rare), but the technique is potentially more dangerous as the needle is aimed at, and indeed may touch, the dura. There is no evidence that it is more effective for disc lesions at lower levels.

Disc surgery and epidural local anaesthesia

Operation can leave the patient with a permanently weakened back. As the worst that can result from unsuccessful injection is for the patient to be no better, it makes sense to try it before resorting to surgery, the more so since conservative treatments are less likely to work after the operation. This argument is further bolstered on grounds of time and expense – minimal in the case of the injection – and because the results compare well.

Findings

Ombregt's findings, although without controls, amply substantiate the indications for injection arrived at on clinical grounds (International Symposium on Low Back Pain, Antwerp, 1982). Although they do not of course establish the injection's comparative efficacy, they nevertheless provide an excellent prognostic rule-of-thumb. Over a period of two years he injected 94 patients. Of these, 69 were restored to full painless range. A total of 208 injections were given without side-effects. His findings were:

(1) Hyperacute lumbago. Five cases. All pain-free within five days. The injection was supplemented by one to four sessions of manipulation.
(2) Backache. Twenty-one cases, producing 12 recoveries and nine failures. Chronic low back pain thus remains a difficult problem. The category was subdivided as follows:
   (a) Intractable backache (i.e. manipulation and traction failed to secure any or adequate relief). Nine cases – three failures, three pain-free after injection and subsequent manipulation, and three pain-free after injection alone.
   (b) Chronic backache with no clear articular signs. Nine cases – three well (previous mean duration of pain two and a half years) and six no better (previous mean duration of pain four years).
   (c) Matutinal backache. Three patients – all rendered pain-free.
(3) Root pain without neurological deficit. Twenty-three cases. Nineteen recoveries and four failures, subdivided as follows:
   (a) Root pain for six months or longer (previous mean duration of pain 20 months). Thirteen cases – 10 pain-free within an average of 5.1 weeks after an average of 2.7 injections each, and three no better.
   (b) Primary posterolateral onset. Four cases – all recovered after one or two injections.
   (c) No results from traction or manipulation. Six cases – five recoveries and one failure.
(4) Root pain with neurological deficit. Thirty-nine cases – 31 recoveries and eight no better. Of the failures, four required operation. Of the 33 patients with L5, S1 or S2 palsies, a total of 29 were rendered pain-free, but one of the two L3 palsies was unimproved as were three out of the four L4 palsies.
(5) Root pain, post-laminectomy. Six cases – two well (12 months elapsed since operation) and four no better (4–12 years since operation).

Contraindications

These are remarkably few:

(1) *Sensitivity to local anaesthetic.* Inquiry should be made of any history of adverse reaction to procaine. If a patient does state she is sensitive to procaine, it is more probable that adrenaline is the trouble and a test injection should be made into, for example, the buttock.
(2) *Strict asepsis must be observed.* Introduction of bacteria into the neural canal would be disastrous and the injection must be postponed if the neighbouring skin is not clear from sepsis. Should a needle have to be inserted twice, a fresh one must be used.
(3) *The proper procedure should be followed*:
   (a) The injection is never given under general anaesthesia. The patient cannot then report on any untoward symptoms.
   (b) Only 50 ml is run in slowly over the course of some minutes.
   (c) A check is made to ensure the needle has not penetrated the theca. An injection into the cerebrospinal fluid would prove fatal.

It is probably best to wait a few days after a myelogram before giving the injection. A pre-1950 laminectomy militates against success as diffuse fibrosis – which the anaesthetic cannot penetrate – resulted from the talcum powder in which the surgeons' gloves were then packed. A post-1950 laminectomy or arthrodesis of any period have no such deleterious consequences.

Dangers of epidural injection have been greatly exaggerated. In the many thousands of injections given by Dr Cyriax, a total of four patients were encountered with a semi-permeable dura mater and developed a paraplegia lasting two hours. Two of these cases were recorded 35 years ago before central sterilization and may have been attributable to some pollution in the water in which the instruments lay. No case of sepsis has yet occurred.

Technique

The object of the injection is to insert the needle through the sacral hiatus and inject some 50 ml of 1 : 200 procaine into the sacrum. As the injection proceeds the fluid ascends to the third lumbar level, thus anaesthetizing the dura mater and nerve roots (*Figure 13.83*).

The patient lies prone with buttocks exposed. The skin at the lower sacrum and intergluteal cleft is sterilized and the buttocks are held stretched well apart (*Figure 13.84*).

The operator is seated on the patient's left and the left hand is used to palpate for the two cornua, bony prominences just to either side of the mid-line at the fourth sacral level (*Figure 13.85*). The gap between the cornua indicates the position of the sacral hiatus through which the needle will be inserted.

A small amount of the procaine solution is injected into the overlying skin.

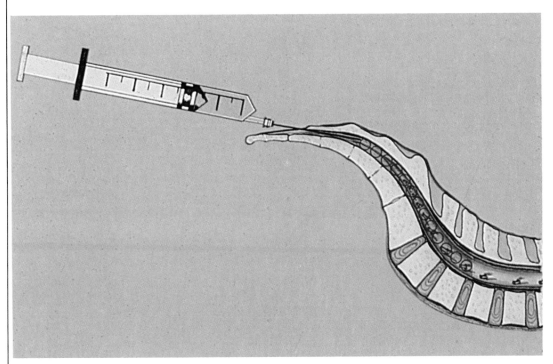

13.83 *Injection into the neural canal. The needle stops well short of the theca; the anaesthetic rises to L3.*

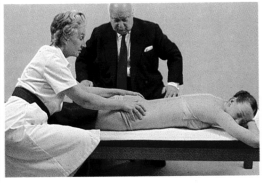

13.84 *The assistant's arms are horizontal, out of the physician's way, as the gluteal masses are held apart.*

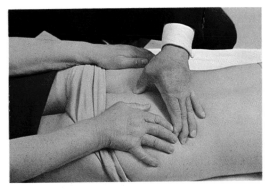

13.85 *Palpating for the cornua.*

An ordinary lumbar puncture needle with stylet is passed through the anaesthetic area of skin and on into the intercornual space (*Figure 13.86*).

The difficult part of the insertion is to assess correctly the angle at which to thrust the needle further. If it is blocked by bone, a different angle must be tried. While palpating for the cornua the physician gauges the slope on the flat surface presented by the fifth sacral segment. This affords some guidance on the relevant angulation, which varies widely from patient to patient.

In the ordinary case the needle passes in without hindrance to some 4–5 cm. In most patients the theca ends at the lower level of the first sacral vertebra and the needle must stop short of this line.

The sole check on whether the integrity of the dura has been breached occurs on withdrawal of the stylet (*Figure 13.87*). But it provides a clear and unambiguous indicator. If cerebrospinal fluid escapes, the needle is lying intrathecally, almost certainly because the dura mater extends to an abnormally low level. In this case, the level at which the flow ceases is noted as the needle is withdrawn, and the injection is deferred until the following day by which time the puncture will have sealed.

If nothing flows back, the injection commences. If blood issues, the needle lies in a vein or haematoma and must be edged into a harmless position.

The injection proceeds very slowly: infiltration of the entire amount takes 5–10 minutes. At first the patient feels an ache at each side of the mid-sacrum; later the symptoms may be reproduced in the leg. Finally the pain ceases.

The injection raises the pressure in the cerebrospinal fluid, which is transmitted upwards to the brain. The first indication of labile cerebral circulation is often faltering speech, so throughout the infiltration the patient is tenaciously engaged in conversation. If her speech falters unduly – or if she complains of giddiness or intolerable pain – the injection is stopped for a few minutes before resuming slowly.

Aspiration is repeated every 10 ml to make sure the tip of the needle has not moved.

If on entry the needle missed the space between the cornua it must lie extrasacrally, and as the injection continues a swelling is felt rising at one side of the sacral spinous processes. Thus throughout the first half of the injection the operator's left hand rests on the sacrum in order to detect the appearance of any such mound (*Figure 13.88*), and any doubt can be resolved by a rapid injection of 2 ml air which can be palpated in the soft tissue.

After the injection, the patient lies prone for some 20 minutes, continuously accompanied, an essential precaution as it is only by the end of this period that adverse effects would have appeared. Thereafter, the patient can go home, returning next week for re-examination. For results and the appropriate follow-up procedure see page 226.

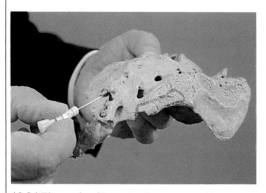

13.86 *The angle of insertion is a matter of fine judgement and experience.*

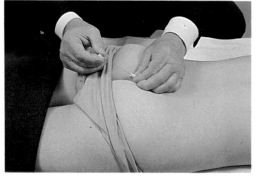

13.87 *Withdrawing the stylet. Were the theca penetrated, cerebrospinal fluid would escape. Accordingly, this is a vital check.*

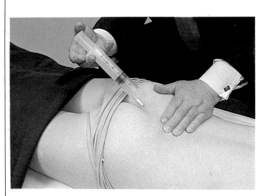

13.88 *A faulty insertion can lead to the needle lying superficial to the sacrum; the operator feels for any extrasacral swelling.*

Pain modulation

Although epidural local anaesthesia is probably the definitive treatment for irreducible disc lesions, secondary alternatives exist in the form of pain modulation techniques, for example transcutaneous electrical neural stimulation, interferential and, in particular, electro-acupuncture at the posterior ramus.

The latter technique is applicable between L3 and S1. It is easier than and may be preferable to the sinuvertebral block and involves delivering low-frequency electrical stimulation via acupuncture needles to the emergent posterior rami of the affected segment. Precise technique varies from level to level as the L3 to L5 posterior rami are intercepted at the edge of the relevant lamina, and S1 in the first sacral foramen.

Initially the treatment is given for some 10 minutes and if necessary repeated as soon as the patient has stabilized from the previous treatment. Treatment duration may be progressed in 10-minute increments. If improvement ceases, there is occasionally increased stiffness the next day, normally followed by improvement. Treatment is discontinued as soon as significant improvement has been achieved, normally after 1–6 sessions. It would seem that the effect of this technique is to reduce or abolish C fibre input, which can continue long after the causative trauma and is associated with spasm – for example diminished straight-leg raising and motor inhibition. Hence the treatment frequently restores full range of straight-leg raising and motor function to muscles involved in a root palsy. It may be useful as a speedy alternative to traction or (as with the epidural) where signs and symptoms suggest that neither traction nor manipulation will work.

Prophylaxis

At the lumbar spine there are three main methods of prophylaxis:

(1) Ligamentous sclerosants.
(2) Corset.
(3) Posture.

All three approaches depend on enhanced lumbar stability in the correct position.

Sclerosants

For general information on intention, method and sclerosant solution the reader is referred to the corresponding section on the thoracic spine on page 195. It will be remembered that any displacement must first be reduced.

The ligaments are infiltrated at both ends at their point of insertion to periosteum; no fluid is introduced unless the tip of the needle is felt to impinge against bone. At each point, 1 ml is injected.

Injections are given at weekly intervals and the following ligaments are infiltrated:

(1) First week: supraspinous and interspinous ligaments at the fourth level and the interspinous at the fifth lumbar levels.

(2) Second week: the posterior ligaments of the facet joints.
(3) Third week: deep lumbar fascia.

The injections smart as the solution goes in. Then the local anaesthetic takes effect, and the ache ceases for at least an hour. After that the pain returns, but by the next day the symptoms have ceased.

The patient comes back a week later for re-examination and the succeeding injection. If any displacement is found, manipulative reduction is carried out immediately. Only when this is achieved is the patient ready for the next infiltration.

Until tissue contracture is established, the patient must avoid flexing her back. This takes about six weeks but continues to an optimum at about 9 months to a year. Thereafter the tendency to relapse is greatly diminished, although after some years the injections may have to be repeated.

Alternatively, all three groups may be injected concurrently on three separate weekly occasions with a total of 5 ml P2G and 5 ml local anaesthetic on each visit. In this case the procedure may be intolerably painful, and pre-injection analgesics or even a sedative anaesthetic or gas and oxygen may be required.

The first injection: supraspinous and interspinous ligaments

There is no need for a skin drawing. The operator palpates directly for the declivity between the spinous processes and the needle is inserted half-way between the fifth spinous process and the first sacral spinous process. First the tip points superiorly until it meets bone and a series of droplets are deposited along the inferior surface of the fifth lumbar spinous process (*Figures 13.89* and *13.90*). Then the needle is half-withdrawn and the procedure repeated along the upper surface of the first sacral spinous process (*Figure 13.91*).

The entire procedure is repeated at the fourth lumbar level.

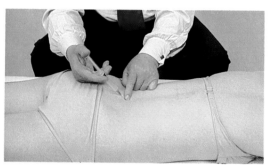

13.90

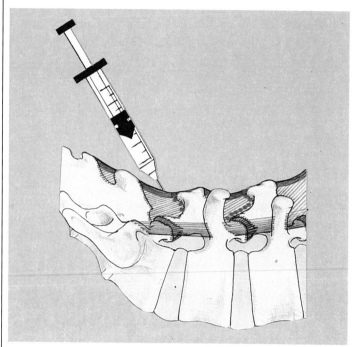

13.89

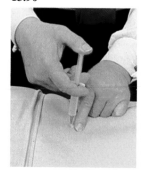

13.89, 13.90, 13.91 *One ml P2G is injected at varying angles of insertion along the ligamento-periosteal junctions at L4 and L5. Injections are never made unless the operator is clinically certain the displacement is reduced.*

13.91

The second injection: facet ligaments

This time a skin drawing is made (*Figures 13.92* and *13.93*) with the long side-to-side line as a marker running between the iliac crests. The L4/5 joint lies directly underneath. The mid-line is intersected by three cross-bars, each half-way between the spinous processes. The lateral boundaries of the grid are some 2.5 cm to either side of the mid-line and overlie the facet joints.

The needle is inserted directly downwards at the corner of the grid (*Figures 13.94* and *13.95*) and should encounter tough ligamentous resistance before reaching bone. Then 1 ml is injected partly into the ligament and partly into the joint.

The process is repeated at the other side and then at the other level.

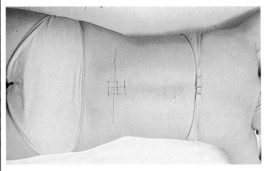

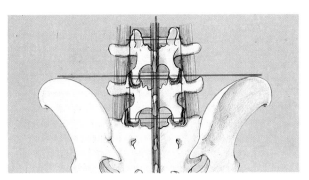

13.92, 13.93 *The grid is identical for injection of the facet ligaments and the deep lumbar fascia. The procedures are difficult but by no means impossible. Sites of infiltration for both are shown in Figure 13.93 marked in red.*

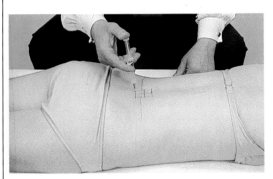

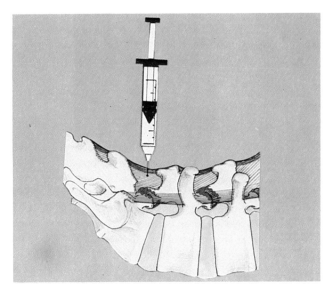

13.94, 13.95 *The needle enters vertically at the outer corners of the grid to inject 1 ml P2G into capsule and ligaments of the facet joints.*

The third injection: deep lumbar fascia

The final injection is given a week later into the medial edge of the deep lumbar fascia. A spot is chosen level with the relevant spinous process on the boundary of the grid (*Figure 13.96*) and the needle thrust in until it runs into the lamina (*Figure 13.97*). It is half-withdrawn and inserted obliquely until the bony lamina is no longer tangible; the medial edge of the deep lumbar fascia lies just laterally. Then 1 ml is injected in a single load.

The procedure is duplicated on the other side and at the adjacent level.

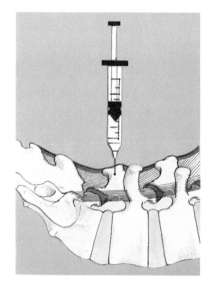

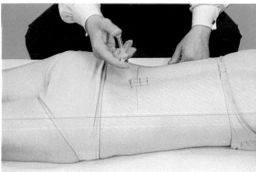

13.96, 13.97 *One ml P2G is injected into one spot at each of the four edges of the grid.*

A corset

Recurrent attacks from an unstable fragment of disc may be prevented by use of a properly made corset. This is much to be preferred to the plaster cast which, apart from many other drawbacks, cannot be sufficiently tight to take effect. It must be emphasized that a corset is not a means of reducing a displacement. It is for maintaining reduction once achieved.

The corset is of fabric with two posterior steels accurately moulded to the patient's lumbar curve. An exact fit of the steels is essential.

The corset extends as far above as below the level requiring support and must span at least 12 inches. It can be worn indefinitely, but to be really effective must be tight enough to prevent lumbar movement.

Posture

Nachemson's findings (see page 155) have demonstrated that intervertebral pressure is at its greatest when the patient flexes her spine. Moreover, when the spine is in flexion the disc is pushed posteriorly (i.e. towards the dura mater) by the tilt on the surfaces of the vertebrae. As these two effects frequently combine to produce a displacement, the moral is clear. The patient must:

(1) Flex her trunk as little as possible, particularly when lifting.
(2) Maintain her lumbar lordosis.

These precepts should govern deportment throughout life, whether at work, rest or play, in the office or the home, standing, sitting, lying or lifting. This regimen, together with its rationale and implications, must be driven home. Modern chair designs with the seat itself angled forwards may play a significant role in the comfort of sedentary workers with chronic back problems. Other than swimming, exercises play no useful role and are very likely to be harmful. Back conditions are not of muscular origin, nor can an intra-articular displacement be favourably affected by exercises directed at increased 'suppleness'. A quest for greater range, if achieved, simply exposes the spine to increased loads and increased liability to prolapse.

Differential diagnosis

A large number of non-disc lesions give rise to pain in the back, groin or lower limb, but even in the aggregate they are much less common than a disc lesion. Some are considered briefly below.

Afebrile osteomyelitis
In acute cases, the history resembles lumbago, but straight-leg raise is full. If the condition is chronic, the pain encroaches for some weeks with no diagnostic signs until the onset of bilateral limitation of side flexion. In both cases the capsular pattern is found.

Ankylosing spondylitis
The symptoms come and go irregularly, irrespective of activity, and may alternate from one side of the body to the other. An X-ray of the sacroiliac joints is diagnostic; the capsular pattern is present and an HLA-B27 test confirmatory. See also page 80.

Aortic occlusion
The pain occurs only on walking. Usually claudication in one or both limbs overshadows the minor backache.

Brucellosis
The symptoms are a chronic backache with minor fever. In the later stages an X-ray is diagnostic.

Fractured transverse process
The unilateral pain follows direct injury to the back and abates after two weeks. Resisted side flexion usually hurts and an X-ray is diagnostic.

Fractured vertebral body
The central pain is constant for the first few weeks but ceases after a month or so. At first the capsular pattern is marked and kyphosis is palpable at the level of the fracture. An X-ray is diagnostic.

Gastric ulcer adherent to the lumbar spine
The symptoms are connected both with posture and eating. An X-ray of the stomach is diagnostic.

Ligamentous overstretching
Ligaments, mainly the superspinous, iliolumbar and posterior sacroiliac, may on occasion be individually or generally involved in a chronic sprain, giving rise to widespread and ill-defined pain. Treatment is by local injection and attention to posture.

The symptoms seem only to occur in spondylolisthesis and the rare sacroiliac strain.

Neoplasm, lumbar
The history in the middle aged or elderly is of steady aggravation (unlike disc lesions) and of major root signs and minor root pain (disc lesions present the reverse) in a distribution not corresponding to any one root. The capsular pattern and an X-ray are both informative and further investigation with CT scan or NMR helpful.

Neoplasm, sacral
Full painless lumbar range is accompanied by gross weakness of the muscles of one or both feet, but in the average case there is no root pain. An X-ray is diagnostic, as are CT and NMR scans.

Neuroma, lumbar
The condition is rare and should be considered if, for example, the history is unusual or if L1 or L2 root signs are discovered. The capsular pattern is sometimes present and a myelogram reveals the growth, especially with CT and NMR scan.

Neurosis
The alleged history, signs and symptoms are inconsistent and contradictory.

Nutritional osteomalacia
The gait – a characteristic waddle – is suggestive.

Osteitis deformans
Movement of the lumbothoracic spine is restricted and the pain pervades the entire back. An X-ray is diagnostic.

Osteochondrosis, adolescent
The condition appears harmless of itself. In 1962 Ross (see page 155) X-rayed the spines of 5000 police candidates aged 20. He found evidence of osteochondrosis in two-thirds but only 4.2% of the group had experienced backache.

Osteophytosis, posterior
In contrast to anterior osteophytosis, pain may result from compression of the dura mater by a posterior osteophyte. An X-ray is diagnostic.

Osteoporosis, senile
Pain results only if the condition is accompanied by a disc lesion or if the wedging comes on suddenly, in which case the ache is severe for a week or two and goes after a couple of months. An X-ray is diagnostic. Sometimes repeated micro-fractures cause pain. Recent research suggests the condition is much more common in men than previously thought.

Spinal claudication
Walking (cf. standing) causes backache, typically with pins and needles in both feet.

Spondylolisthesis
This may be painless or may be responsible for a disc lesion at the unstable joint. In the latter case there is an enhanced tendency to relapse for slight reasons. Alternatively, pain can result from the sustained stretching of the intervertebral ligaments. The ache is then central and largely unconnected with lumbar movements, but if the nerve roots are caught against the bony edge of the vertebra below, then root pain is engendered, generally bilateral with pins and needles. See page 200.

Tuberculous caries
Kyphos is detectable where bone is eaten away; there is fixation and pain here and at adjacent levels. The X-ray is diagnostic and the capsular pattern is present.

Vertebral hyperostosis
This can be symptomless and is primarily a radiological finding, but elderly patients with ache in the entire trunk and marked limitation at every spinal joint may be the victims of this condition.

Zygapophyseal joints
Subject to arthritis (traumatic/degenerative/primary inflammatory disease), producing the capsular pattern. Pain from the facet joints is commonly an expression of spinal degenerative disease. The pain may be bilateral and more than one level may be involved. The pain may occur on extension and passive rotations. Tenderness on deep palpation is suggestive.

Referred pain
Pain referred to the back from, for example, an intra-abdominal or pelvic viscus, will allow full painless range of lumbar movement.

The lumbar nerve roots
Monoradicular and polyradicular symptoms

The table below sets out the roots which may be affected by a disc lesion at any given level:

L1 disc	L1 root only
L2 disc	L2 root only
L3 disc	L3 root only
L4 disc	L4 root by itself
	L4 and L5 roots together
	L5 root by itself
	S3 root by itself (extremely rare)
	S4 root by itself
L5 disc	L5 root by itself
	L5 and S1 roots together
	S1 root by itself
	S1 and S2 roots together
	S2 root by itself
	S3 root by itself (extremely rare)
	S4 root by itself

Lumbar root signs

The maximum root signs at each level are detailed below.
A disc lesion may affect two roots simultaneously (see over); involvement of three would arouse grave disquiet.

L1 root pressure

Disc lesions at both L1 and L2 are very rare and root pressure even rarer, as the nerve roots emerge high up and pass well lateral to the disc.

Pain in the dermatome (*Figure 13.98*) and numbness in the groin.

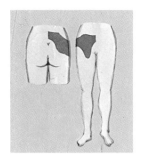

13.98 *The L1 dermatome.*

L2 root pressure

A displacement at L2 is commoner than L1, although still highly unusual.

Pain in the dermatome (*Figure 13.99*).
Weak psoas – resisted hip flexion.
Analgesia from groin to knee.
In addition to a disc lesion consider:

(1) Secondary malignant deposits (psoas grossly weak *and* spinal movements grossly limited).
(2) Meralgia paraesthetica (analgesia at outer aspect of thigh; the lumbar movements have no bearing on the pain).

Pain at the front of the thigh may also be caused by lesions of the hip joint, psoas, abductor and quadriceps muscles, psoas bursa, femur or a loose body in the hip joint.

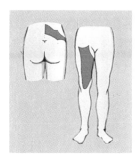

13.99 *The L2 dermatome.*

L3 root pressure

Disc lesions are fairly common at the L3 joint. As the nerve root is stretched by lumbar extension and relaxed on flexion, extension is the movement predisposed to hurt in the thigh. Pain in the dermatome (*Figure 13.100*).

Weak quadriceps — resisted knee extension.
Weak psoas — resisted hip flexion.
Painful prone-lying knee flexion.
Pain at front of knee on full straight-leg raise (occasionally).
Sluggish or absent knee jerk.
Analgesia from patella to ankle.
For alternative causes of pain at the front of the thigh see L2.

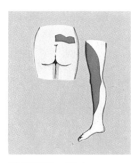

13.100 *The L3 dermatome.*

L4 root pressure

Disc lesions abound at both the L4 and L5 joints; in either case the pattern may be polyradicular. Thus a lateral displacement pinches the L4 root, one protruding just at the edge of the posterior longitudinal ligament (i.e. more medially) pinches L5 and a large displacement will compress both roots. Pain in the dermatome (*Figure 13.101*).

Weak tibialis anterior – resisted dorsiflexion.
Weak extensor hallucis – resisted extension of the hallux.
Analgesia at outer part of lower leg running to the big toe.
Limitation of straight-leg raise (occasionally bilateral).
Jerks unaffected.

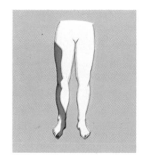

13.101 *The L4 dermatome. Both L4 and L5 include the big toe.*

L5 root pressure

The L5 root can be compressed by either the L4 or the L5 disc. The pattern may be polyradicular. Pain in the dermatome (*Figure 13.102*).

Weak extensor hallucis – resisted extension of the hallux.
Weak peronei – resisted eversion of the foot.
Weak gluteus medius – resisted abduction of the thigh.
Analgesia at outer leg running to the inner three toes.
Unilateral limitation of straight-leg raise.
Sluggish or absent ankle jerk.

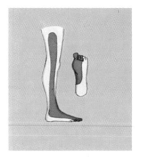

13.102 *The L5 dermatome.*

S1 root pressure

The S1 root can be affected by the L5 disc. The pattern may be polyradicular. Pain in the dermatome (*Figure 13.103*).

Weak peronei – resisted eversion of the foot.
Weak calf muscles – rising on tiptoe.
Weak hamstrings – resisted knee flexion.
Wasting of, and inability to contract, the gluteal mass.
Unilateral limitation of straight-leg raise.
Sluggish or absent ankle jerk.
Analgesia of the outer two toes, the outer foot and the
    outer leg as far as the lateral aspect of the knee.

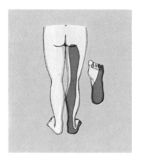

13.103 *The S1 dermatome.*

S2 root pressure

This is as for S1 except:

(1) The peronei are not involved.
(2) The analgesia ends under the heel, not extending to the foot.

    The dermatome is shown in *Figure 13.104*.

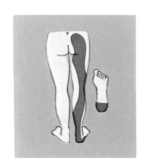

13.104 *The S2 dermatome.*

S3 root pressure

It is highly unusual for other roots to be affected at the same time as the S3 root, and pain in the dermatome (*Figure 13.105*) is the only symptom. There is no muscle weakness, no limitation of straight-leg raise, no analgesia, and the bladder and rectal functions are normal – as are the jerks.

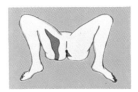

13.105 *The S3 dermatome.*

S4 root pressure

The S4 root may be compressed by either the L4 or the L5 disc protruding centrally, unlike other roots which are only threatened by lateral protrusions. S4 root pressure is an absolute bar to manipulation (see also page 207) and even traction is not wholly safe. Pain is felt in the saddle area, scrotum or vagina (*Figure 13.106*) with analgesia of the anus, loss of rectal expulsive power and difficulty in passing or retaining urine. By contrast the articular signs may be unobtrusive and it is thus the history rather than the examination which alerts. Permanent bladder paralysis may ensue if the condition is left untreated and immediate laminectomy is the rule. Bilateral sciatica threatens the posterior longitudinal ligament, rupture of which might endanger the S4 root.

    Rectal, penile, scrotal, testicular, vaginal and bladder disorders are by far the commonest causes of fourth sacral pain.

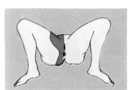

13.106 *The S4 dermatome.*

PART FOUR

APPENDICES

I THE DERMATOMES

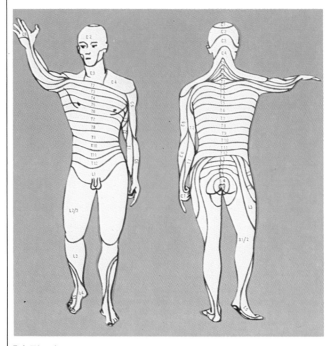

I.1 *The dermatomes.*

After the first month, the fetus starts to divide into 40 segments. With the passage of time each segment becomes differentiated into dermatome (skin), myotome (muscles and other soft tissues) and scleratome (bone and fibrous septa). The dermatomes govern the distance that pain arising from any point in the myotome may travel distally.

The shape of each dermatome varies considerably from one individual to another. Those illustrated on this and the ensuing pages are substantially based on the work of Foerster who, in 1933, mapped out the dermatomes anew. But minor refinements are incorporated where clinical experience has consistently shown discrepancies with the original.

The opening diagrams are included by way of a general overview, as they depict only the central part of many of the skin segments and cannot represent the considerable areas of overlap.

The dura mater refers pain not on a segmental but on an extrasegmental basis. The areas to which pain may be referred from cervical, thoracic and lumbar disc lesions are illustrated in Figure I.7.

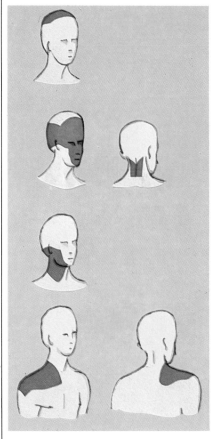

I.2 *The upper cervical dermatomes. C1 (top), C2 (upper centre), C3 (lower centre), C4 (bottom).*

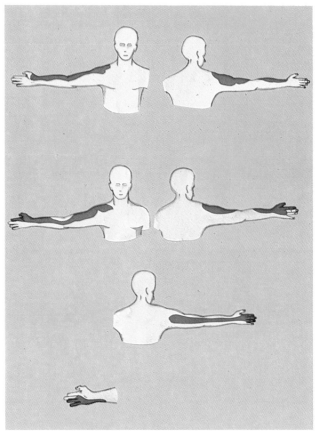

I.3 *The lower cervical dermatomes. C5 (top), C6 (upper centre), C7 (lower centre), C8 (bottom).*

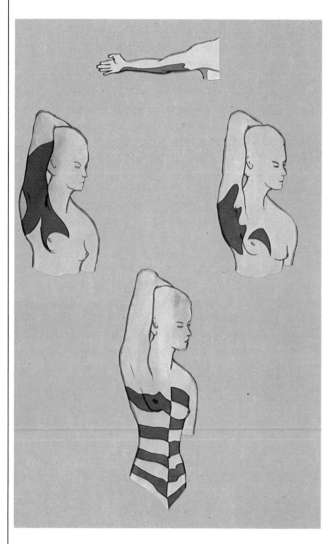

I.4 *The thoracic dermatomes. T1 (top), T2 (centre left), T3 (centre right), T4–12 (bottom).*

I.5 *The lumbar dermatomes. L1 (top left), L2 (top centre), L3 (top right), L4 (lower left), L5 (lower right).*

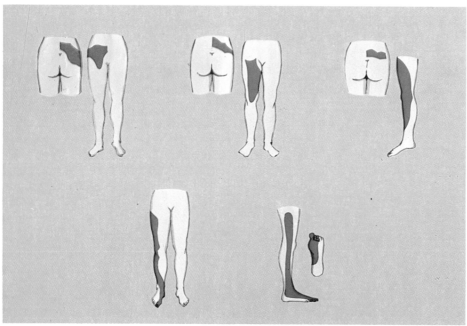

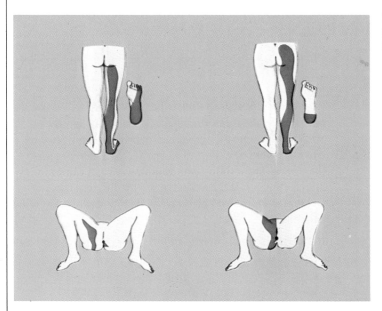

I.6 *The sacral dermatomes. S1 (top left), S2 (top right), S3 (lower left), S4 (lower right).*

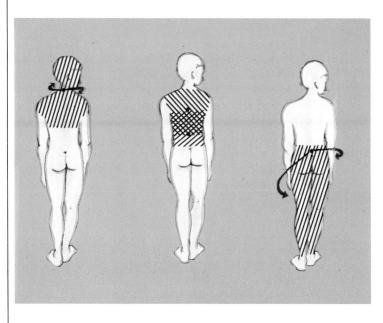

I.7 *Extrasegmental reference. The maximum areas in which pain may be felt as a result of interference with the dura mater at cervical (left), thoracic (centre) and lumbar levels (right).*

II PINS AND NEEDLES

Pins and needles in all four limbs characterize disorders such as peripheral neuritis, diabetes, pernicious anaemia and central cervical disc lesions.

Pressure on the spinal cord: no pain; pins and needles referred extrasegmentally.

Pressure on the dural sleeve to a nerve root: pain; numbness; pins and needles (neither edge nor aspect).

Pressure on a nerve trunk: no pain; pins and needles (a release phenomenon; aspect but no edge).

Pressure on a small nerve: no pain; numbness; slight pins and needles (aspect and edge).

Where symptoms are present, the whole nerve must be examined from the spine distally. The lists below set out the various areas (often with alternatives) that can be affected by pins and needles caused by different types of lesion; the indications given are probabilities not certainties.

The hand

When an area that does not correspond to any one nerve is described, the lesion must lie above the differentiation of the brachial plexus.

C5 disc lesion (C6 root): Thumb, index and long finger. Thumb and index finger (the more common).

C6 disc lesion (C7 root): Index, long, ring and little finger. Index, long and ring finger (the most common). Index and long finger. Long finger alone. Long and ring finger.

C7 disc lesion (C8 root): Long, ring and little finger. Ring and little finger.

Carpal tunnel syndrome: Thumb, index, long and radial side of the ring finger; palmar surface.

Cervical rib (compressing the lower trunk of the brachial plexus prior to division into median and ulnar nerve): All five digits of one hand. Thumb, index, long and radial side of the ring finger.

Median nerve, compression: Thumb, index, long and radial side of the ring finger; palmar surface.

Radial nerve, compression: As above, dorsal surface.

Cervical central disc lesion: All five digits of both hands.

Thoracic outlet syndrome: All five digits of one hand. All five digits of both hands.

Ulnar nerve, compression: Little finger and ulnar side of ring finger.

Numbness of the thumb alone is likely to be caused by occupational pressure on the digital nerve at the outer side of the thumb, whereas pins and needles normally stem from contusion of the thenar branch of the median nerve.

The thigh

L2 root pressure: front of thigh.
L3 root pressure: front of thigh.
L4 root pressure: outer side.
L5 root pressure: outer side.
S1 root pressure: back of thigh.
S2 root pressure: back of thigh.
Meralgia paraesthetica: outer side only.
Pregnancy or large uterine fibromyoma: outer side.

Lower leg

S1 root pressure: back of calf.
S2 root pressure: back of calf.
Entrapment of the saphenous nerve just below the knee: along front of leg to big toe.
Entrapment of the tibial nerve as it emerges half-way down the tibia: down front of leg and first and second toes.

The feet

The cause of pins and needles in the feet usually lies in the spine.

Cervical disc lesion: Cord signs (bilateral).

Thoracic disc lesion: Cord signs (bilateral).

Lumbar disc lesion: Root pressure (unilateral, see list opposite).

Spinal claudication: Lack of arterial blood supply on walking (bilateral).

Spondylolisthesis: Root pressure (bilateral).

Root pressure

L4 root: The hallux.

L5 root: First, second and third toes, inner half of the sole, dorsum of whole of foot.

S1 root: Outer two toes and outer half of the sole.

S2 root: Plantar aspect of the heel (and the whole of the back of the leg up to the buttock).

Pressure on the popliteal nerve at the neck of the fibula produces pins and needles in the foot.

III THE CAPSULAR PATTERNS

Shoulder

So much limitation of abduction, more than that of lateral rotation, less than that of medial rotation.

Elbow

Flexion usually more limited than extension, rotations full and painless except in advanced cases.

Wrist

Equal limitation of flexion and extension, little limitation of deviations.

Trapezio-first metacarpal joint

Only abduction limited.

Sign of the buttock

Passive hip flexion more limited and more painful than straight-leg raise.

Hip

Marked limitation of flexion and medial rotation, some limitation of abduction, little or no limitation of adduction and lateral rotation.

Knee

Gross limitation of flexion, slight limitation of extension.

Ankle

More limitation of plantiflexion than of dorsiflexion.

Talocalcanean joint

Increasing limitation of varus until fixation in valgus.

Mid-tarsal joint

Limitation of adduction and internal rotation, other movements full.

Big toe

Gross limitation of extension, slight limitation of flexion.

Cervical spine

Equal limitation in all directions except for flexion which is usually full.

Thoracic spine

Limitation of extension, side flexion and rotations, less limitation of flexion.

Lumbar spine

Marked and equal limitation of side flexions, limitation of flexion and of extension.

IV FACT SHEETS

The shoulder

Summary

A straightforward joint producing clear findings. History of little importance diagnostically. Exclude neck as source of pain before proceeding to examination of shoulder. Nearly all shoulder structures are of C5 derivation.

For convenience, the acromio- and sternoclavicular joints are included in the following table.

Capsular pattern

Some limitation of medial rotation (except in a very mild case), greater limitation of passive abduction, greatest limitation of passive lateral rotation.

End-feel

A hard end-feel on elevation suggests arthritis.

DIAGNOSIS, Shoulder	SIGNS AND SYMPTOMS	TREATMENT
A. Pain on passive movement		
1. Capsular conditions Traumatic arthritis	Trauma plus capsular pattern Patient aged 45 or over	Stage 1: stretch Stage 2: injection 2 ml steroid suspension *or* distract Stage 3: stretch
Steroid-sensitive arthritis	Capsular pattern, no trauma	Injection 2 ml steroid suspension
Osteoarthrosis	Normally symptomless of itself	No treatment warranted
2. Non-capsular conditions Acute subdeltoid bursitis	Incapacity to abduct arm, rapid onset	Stage 1: morphine plus injection 2×5 ml steroid suspension (N.B. possible subacromial extent) Stage 2: figure of eight bandage
Chronic subdeltoid bursitis	Painful arc only	Injection 0.5% procaine 5–10 ml, possibly subacromial
Subluxation	'Dead arm'	Muscle rehabilitation
B. Pain on resisted movement		
Supraspinatus – 4 sites	Painful resisted abduction with/without painful elevation and/or painful arc (localizing signs)	Injection 1 ml steroid suspension *or* massage (except at musculotendinous junction, where only massage is effective)
Infraspinatus – 3 sites	Painful resisted lateral rotation (N.B. localizing signs)	Injection 1 ml steroid suspension *or* massage
Subscapularis – 2 sites	Painful resisted medial rotation (N.B. localizing signs)	Injection 1 ml steroid suspension *or* massage
Biceps – 5 sites (2 at elbow)	Painful resisted elbow flexion and usually painful resisted supination	Glenoid origin: injection 2 ml steroid suspension Bicipital groove: massage Belly: massage
Acromioclavicular joint	Passive movements, especially adduction, painful at extreme of range	Injection 1 ml steroid suspension *or* massage
Sternoclavicular joint	Painful neck and scapular movements	Injection 1 ml steroid suspension

Examination

Active elevation I: willingness.
Passive elevation: joint capsule, psychogenic limitation.
Active elevation II: painful arc (lesion lies in a pinchable position).
Passive abduction: glenohumeral range (cf. active elevation I).
Passive lateral rotation: joint capsule.
Passive medial rotation: joint capsule.
Resisted abduction: supraspinatus.
Resisted adduction: pectoralis major, latissimus dorsi (both rare).
Resisted lateral rotation: infraspinatus.
Resisted medial rotation: subscapularis.
Resisted elbow flexion: biceps.
Resisted elbow extension: triceps (rare).

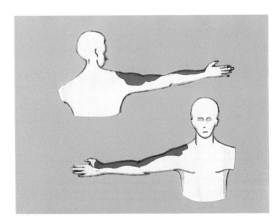

IV.1 *The C5 dermatome.*

The elbow

Summary
The patient can normally distinguish between referred pain and pain of local origin. Commence with examination of neck and shoulder if necessary.

Capsular pattern
Flexion is more limited than extension; rotations are free except in advanced arthritis.

End-feel
A softer end-feel on extension suggests a displacement, as does a hard end-feel on flexion. A hard end-feel on pronation or supination suggests severe arthritis. A hard end-feel on extension is found both in the normal joint (full range) and in arthritis (limited range).

Examination

Passive flexion: joint capsule.
Passive extension: joint capsule.
Passive pronation: upper radio-ulnar joint or accessory sign for the biceps.
Passive supination: upper radio-ulnar joint or accessory sign for the biceps.
Resisted flexion: biceps.
Resisted extension: triceps (rare).
Resisted pronation: accessory sign for common flexor tendon (golfer's elbow) or pronator teres (rare).
Resisted supination: biceps if resisted flexion also painful or supinator brevis (rare).
Resisted wrist flexion: golfer's elbow.
Resisted wrist extension: extensores carpi radialis (tennis elbow).

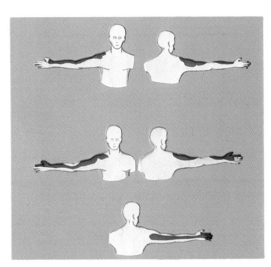

IV.2 *The C5, C6 and C7 dermatomes (top, centre and bottom). Nerve root pain or symptoms originating from the shoulder may be felt in the arm.*

DIAGNOSIS, Elbow	SIGNS AND SYMPTOMS	TREATMENT
A. Pain on passive movement		
1. Capsular conditions Traumatic arthritis	Trauma plus capsular pattern	Injection 2 ml steroid suspension *or* rest in flexion. No forced movement
Rheumatoid arthritis	Capsular pattern, no trauma	Injection 2 ml steroid suspension. No forced movement
Osteoarthrosis	Normally symptomless of itself	No treatment warranted
2. Non-capsular conditions Displacement in adolescence	Intermittent attacks, limitation of extension or flexion	Operate
Displacement in adults	Intermittent attacks, limitation of extension or flexion	Manipulative reduction if extension limited
Radial nerve entrapment	Nocturnal pain	Surgery?
Olecranon fossa impingement	Painful passive and active extension	Injection
B. Pain on resisted movement		
Biceps – 5 sites (3 at shoulder)	Painful resisted flexion and painful resisted supination; if passive pronation also painful the site is at the tenoperiosteal junction	Lower musculotendinous junction: massage Lower tenoperiosteal junction: injection 2 ml steroid suspension *or* massage
Tennis elbow – 4 sites	Painful resisted wrist extension	Tenoperiosteal junction (common): injection 1 ml steroid suspension *or* massage and Mills's manipulation *or* tenotomy Belly (rare): injection 0.5% procaine 10 ml Tendinous (very rare): massage Supracondylar (very rare): massage
Golfer's elbow – 2 sites	Painful resisted wrist flexion and sometimes painful resisted pronation	Tenoperiosteal site: injection 1 ml steroid *or* massage Musculotendinous junction: massage
Triceps	Painful resisted elbow extension	Injection *or* massage
Pronator teres	Painful resisted pronation	Injection

The wrist and hand

Summary
With the exception of pins and needles, symptoms are not referred appreciably. For RSI, treat the individual condition diagnosed

Capsular patterns
Lower radio-ulnar joint: pain but no limitation on both passive rotations.

Wrist: equal limitation of flexion and extension.

Thumb: limitation of passive abduction, pain on passive backward movement during extension.

Interphalangeal joints: about equal limitation of flexion and extension with rotations painful at extreme of range.

Examination

Wrist
Passive pronation: capsule, radio-ulnar joint.
Passive supination: capsule, radio-ulnar joint.
Passive wrist flexion: capsule, wrist joint; dorsal ligaments.
Passive wrist extension: capsule, wrist joint; carpal subluxation.
Passive radial deviation: ulnar collateral ligament.
Passive ulnar deviation: radial collateral ligament.
Resisted wrist flexion: flexor tendons.
Resisted wrist extension: extensor tendons.
Resisted ulnar deviation: ulnar deviators.
Resisted radial deviation: radial deviators.

Thumb
Passive backward movement during extension: capsule, trapezio-first metacarpal joint.

Resisted thumb extension: abductor longus and extensor brevis pollicis.
Resisted thumb flexion: flexor pollicis longus (rare).
Resisted thumb abduction: abductor longus and brevis (rare).
Resisted thumb adduction: thumb adductor (rare).

Fingers
Resisted finger abduction: interosseous muscles.
Resisted finger adduction: interosseous muscles.
Resisted finger extension: extensors.
Resisted finger flexion: flexors.
Passive finger extension: interphalangeal joints.
Passive finger flexion: interphalangeal joints.

The last four movements are normally performed for all fingers simultaneously.

DIAGNOSIS, Wrist and hand	SIGNS AND SYMPTOMS	TREATMENT
WRIST **A. Pain on passive movement**		
1. Capsular conditions Rheumatoid or traumatic arthritis, radio-ulnar joint	Capsular pattern	Injection 1 ml steroid suspension
Arthritis, wrist: 1. Traumatic	Capsular pattern plus fracture	Immobilization
2. Rheumatoid	Capsular pattern	Immobilization *or* injection 2 ml steroid suspension
3. Osteoarthrosis		No treatment warranted
2. Non-capsular conditions Carpal capitate subluxation	Passive extension slightly limited, flexion full and painful	Manipulative reduction
Lunate capitate ligament	Passive wrist flexion painful at extreme of range	Massage
Radial collateral ligament	Painful passive ulnar deviation at extreme of range	Injection 1 ml steroid suspension *or* massage
Ulnar collateral ligament	Painful passive radial deviation	Injection 1 ml steroid suspension
Carpal tunnel syndrome	Pins and needles, 3½ digits	Injection 2 ml steroid suspension (diagnostic and sometimes curative)

B. Pain on resisted movement		
Extensores carpi radialis	Painful resisted wrist extension and radial deviation	Injection 1 ml steroid suspension *or* massage
Extensores carpi ulnaris	Painful resisted wrist extension and ulnar deviation	Injection 1 ml steroid suspension *or* massage
Flexor carpi ulnaris	Painful resisted wrist flexion and ulnar deviation	Injection 1 ml steroid suspension *or* massage
Flexor carpi radialis	Painful resisted wrist flexion and radial deviation	Injection 1 ml steroid suspension *or* massage
Flexor digitorum – upper site	Painful resisted finger flexion	Injection 2 ml steroid suspension *or* massage (except if rheumatoid)

THUMB
A. Pain on passive movement

Arthritis, trapezio-first metacarpal joint	Capsular pattern	Injection 1 ml steroid suspension *or* massage

B. Pain on resisted movement

Abductor longus and extensores pollicis, tenosynovitis – 2 sites	Painful resisted extension and painful resisted abduction	Upper site: massage Lower site: injection 1 ml steroid suspension
Flexor pollicis longus: 1. Tenosynovitis – 2 sites	Painful resisted flexion	Upper site: injection 1 ml steroid suspension *or* massage Lower site: injection 1 ml steroid suspension
2. Trigger thumb	Thumb locks	Injection 1 ml steroid suspension *or* operation

HAND
A. Pain on passive movement

Arthritis, finger joints	Capsular pattern	If rheumatoid, injection 0.5–1 ml steroid suspension

B. Pain on resisted movement

Dorsal interossei	Painful resisted abduction	Massage
Palmar interossei	Painful resisted adduction	Massage
Flexor digitorum – lower site 1. Trigger finger	Finger locks	Injection 1 ml steroid suspension *or* operation
2. Rheumatoid inflammation	Painful resisted finger flexion	Injection 1 ml steroid suspension

The sacroiliac, buttock and hip

Summary
As symptoms in the buttock, thigh or hip are frequently referred from the spine, preliminary examination and history must exclude this possibility. The sacroiliac joint itself is rarely at fault.

The sign of the buttock
This indicates a major lesion. It is some limitation and pain on straight-leg raise and more limitation and pain on passive hip flexion.

Examination
SIJ strain (supine): anterior sacroiliac ligaments.
SIJ strain (side lying): posterior sacroiliac ligaments.
SIJ strain (prone): anterior sacroiliac ligaments.
Passive hip flexion: joint capsule; the sign of the buttock; loose body; bursitis.
Passive medial rotation: joint capsule.
Passive lateral rotation: joint capsule; loose body; bursitis.
Passive hip extension: joint capsule.
Straight-leg raise: the sign of the buttock if passive hip flexion more limited and more painful.
Resisted hip flexion: psoas and quadriceps, malignant disease.
Resisted lateral rotation: gluteal bursitis (accessory sign); quadratus femoris.
Resisted medial rotation: gluteal bursitis (accessory sign).
Resisted abduction: gluteal bursitis (accessory sign).
Resisted extension: gluteal bursitis (accessory sign).
Resisted adduction: adductors ('rider's sprain').
Resisted knee extension: quadriceps.
Resisted knee flexion: hamstrings.

Capsular pattern
Hip: marked limitation of medial rotation, some limitation of flexion and abduction.

End-feel
If the hip joint is normal, the end-feel on all four passive movements is elastic; in arthritis, the end-feel is hard. A prematurely empty end-feel on passive hip flexion accompanies the sign of the buttock.

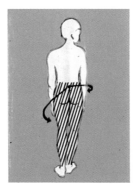

IV.3 *The maximum area to which pain may be referred by a lumbar disc lesion compressing the dura mater.*

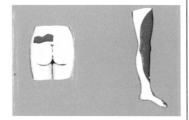

IV.4 *The L3 dermatome. The hip is of L3 derivation.*

DIAGNOSIS, Sacroiliac, buttock and hip	SIGNS AND SYMPTOMS	TREATMENT
SACROILIAC		
Ankylosing spondylitis	Painful SIJ strain(s)	Phenylbutazone or indomethacin during attack
BUTTOCK		
Serious disorders, e.g. osteomyelitis, ischiorectal abscess, etc.	The sign of the buttock	As appropriate
Psoas bursitis	Painful passive adduction in flexion, sometimes painful passive lateral rotation	Injection 0.5% procaine 50 ml *or* possibly 5 ml steroid suspension
Gluteal bursitis	Painful passive movements in a non-capsular way	Injection 0.5% procaine 50 ml *or* possibly 5 ml steroid suspension
Claudication	Pain on sustained active hip extension	Operation
HIP **A. Pain on passive movement**		
1. Capsular conditions Rheumatoid, traumatic or spondylitic arthritis	Capsular pattern	Injection 5 ml steroid suspension
Osteoarthrosis	Capsular pattern	Early stage: stretch
Serious disorders in children, e.g. congenital dislocation, pseudocoxalgia, etc.	Mostly visible radiographically	As appropriate
2. Non-capsular conditions Loose body with or without osteoarthrosis	Severe momentary twinges	Manipulative reduction – 2 methods
B. Pain on resisted movement		
Psoas	Painful resisted hip flexion when hip at right angles	Massage
Adductor longus	Painful resisted hip adduction	Tenoperiosteal junction: injection 2 ml steroid suspension *or* massage Musculotendinous junction: massage
Rectus femoris	Painful resisted knee extension	Massage
Hamstrings	Painful resisted knee flexion	Ischial origin: injection 5 ml steroid suspension Belly: injection 50 ml local anaesthetic during first few days, thereafter massage plus Faradism

The knee

Summary
History is particularly important and in cases of traumatic origin must establish the precise strain imposed on the joint. Capsular limitation is often a secondary response to ligamentous sprain. The capacity for localization is good.

Examination

Passive flexion: joint capsule.
Passive extension: joint capsule.
Valgus strain: medial collateral ligament.
Varus strain: lateral collateral ligament.
Passive lateral rotation: medial coronary ligament.
Passive medial rotation: lateral coronary ligament.
Forwards shearing: anterior cruciate ligament.
Backwards shearing: posterior cruciate ligament.
Lateral shearing: posterior cruciate ligament (secondary sign), meniscus.
Resisted flexion: hamstrings.
Resisted medial rotation and flexion: semitendinosus or popliteal muscles (rare).
Resisted lateral rotation and flexion: biceps.
Resisted extension: quadriceps.

Test for fluid, heat, synovial thickening and ligamentous laxity; consider cause of painless weakness, particularly on resisted extension.

Capsular pattern
More limitations of flexion than of extension with rotations free.

End-feel
In arthritis the end-feel on passive flexion is usually hard.

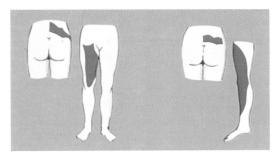

IV.5 *The L2 (left) and L3 dermatomes (right).*

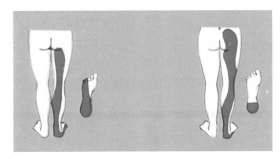

IV.6 *The S1 (left) and S2 dermatomes (right).*

DIAGNOSIS, Knee	SIGNS AND SYMPTOMS	TREATMENT
A. Pain on passive movement		
1. Capsular conditions Secondary traumatic arthritis	Trauma plus capsular pattern	Diagnose and treat causative lesion
Rheumatoid arthritis	Capsular pattern, no trauma	Injection 5 ml steroid suspension
Osteoarthrosis	Visible radiographically	No treatment warranted
Baker's cyst	Cyst in upper calf following rheumatoid arthritis	Aspirate
Haemarthrosis	Capsular pattern, joint distended	Aspirate
2. Non-capsular conditions Medial collateral ligament	Painful passive valgus strain plus marked capsular pattern	Acute and subacute stage: massage in maximum flexion and maximum extension followed by gentle mobilization Chronic stage: manipulative rupture
Stieda–Pellegrini's disease	Visible radiographically following valgus strain	No treatment
Medial coronary ligament	Painful passive lateral rotation plus capsular pattern	Massage
Cruciate ligaments – 4 sites (anterior cruciate, anterior or posterior end; posterior cruciate, anterior or posterior end)	Some/all passive movements painful at extreme of range	Injection 2 ml steroid suspension
Meniscus	Immediate disabling pain, knee locks	Manipulative reduction probably followed by operation
Loose body with or without osteoarthrosis	Intermittent attacks, often full passive extension hurts and flexion is limited	Manipulative reduction – 4 methods
Anterior knee pain syndrome		Exercises, orthotics
	Painful resisted extension	
B. Pain on resisted movement		
Suprapatellar tendon	Painful resisted extension	Injection 2 ml steroid suspension *or* massage
Infrapatellar tendon	Painful resisted extension	Injection 2 ml steroid suspension *or* massage
Quadriceps expansion	Painful resisted flexion Lesion at bicipital tendon if resisted lateral rotation also painful	Massage
Hamstrings	Painful resisted flexion and painful resisted medial rotation	Bellies: massage followed by Faradism Bicipital tendon: massage
Popliteal tendon		Belly: massage Tendinous origin: injection steroid suspension *or* massage
Ileotibial tract	Painful resisted hip abduction	Massage

The leg

Summary
Soft-tissue lesions of the leg present few problems either of
diagnosis or treatment.

Examination
Standing on tiptoe: gastrocnemius and soleus.
Resisted dorsiflexion: tibialis anterior.
Resisted plantiflexion: gastrocnemius and soleus.
Resisted inversion: tibialis posterior.
Resisted eversion: peronei.
    Short plantiflexor muscles may produce any one of a
number of conditions in the ankle or foot.

DIAGNOSIS, Leg	SIGNS AND SYMPTOMS	TREATMENT
Pain on resisted movement Gastrocnemius – 'tennis leg'	Painful resisted plantiflexion, except when knee flexed	Injection 0.5% procaine 50 ml *and* active exercises *and* raised heel and massage
Tendo Achillis	Painful resisted plantiflexion	Massage *or* injection 2 ml steroid suspension
Intermittent claudication	Pain in calf on walking, relieved by rest	Operation
Peroneal tendon – 4 sites	Painful resisted eversion	Massage
Tibialis posterior – 3 sites	Painful resisted inversion	Support and massage *or* massage
Tibialis anterior	Painful resisted dorsiflexion and painful resisted inversion	Massage
Tibiofibular joint	Local symptoms	Desensitization
Stress fracture	Incongruous pattern	Avoidance/management of activity

The ankle and foot

Summary
Despite the intricacy of the foot joints, the lesions are easy
to identify and respond well to treatment.

Capsular patterns
Ankle: more limitation of plantiflexion than dorsiflexion.
Talocalcanean joint: increasing limitation of varus until it
fixes in valgus.
Mid-tarsal joint: limitations of adduction and internal
rotation, other movements full.
Big toe: gross limitation of extension, slight limitation of
flexion.

Examination
Passive dorsiflexion: ankle joint.
Passive plantiflexion: ankle joint, anterior tibiotalar ligament.
Passive inversion during plantiflexion: talofibular,
calcaneofibular and mid-tarsal ligaments.
Passive eversion during plantiflexion: deltoid ligament.
Varus strain: tibiofibular ligament, talocalcanean joint,
calcaneofibular ligament.
Valgus strain: talocalcanean joint.
Mid-tarsal passive dorsiflexion: mid-tarsal joint.

Mid-tarsal passive plantiflexion: mid-tarsal joint.
Mid-tarsal passive adduction: mid-tarsal joint (capsular
pattern).
Mid-tarsal passive abduction: mid-tarsal joint.
Mid-tarsal passive medial rotation: mid-tarsal joint
(capsular pattern), calcaneocuboid ligament.
Mid-tarsal passive lateral rotation: mid-tarsal joint.
    The examination proceeds to the toes if necessary. The
resisted movements of the leg must also be tested.

DIAGNOSIS, Ankle and foot	SIGNS AND SYMPTOMS	TREATMENT
ANKLE **Pain on passive movement**		
1. Capsular conditions Osteoarthrosis	Capsular pattern	Arthrodesis if warranted
2. Non-capsular conditions Anterior talofibular ligament — 2 sites	Painful passive inversion during plantiflexion	First day or so: injection 1 ml steroid suspension. Thereafter massage only
Calcaneofibular ligament	Painful varus strain	First day or so: injection 1 ml steroid suspension. Thereafter massage only
Calcaneocuboid ligament	Painful passive inversion and mid-tarsal medial rotation	First day or so: injection 2 ml steroid suspension. Thereafter massage only
Adhesions, talofibular or calcaneocuboid ligaments	Pain following exertion	Manipulative rupture
Anterior tibiofibular ligament: 1. Sprain	Painful varus strain	Massage
2. Unstable mortice joint	History, foot turns over easily. Click and excessive range on varus strain	Sclerosis *or* operation
Deltoid ligament	Painful passive eversion during plantiflexion	Support and injection 2 ml steroid suspension
Anterior tibiotalar ligament Loose body	Painful passive plantiflexion Erratic twinges on plantiflexion	Massage Manipulative reduction
TALOCALCANEAN JOINT		
Pain on passive movement *1. Capsular conditions* Osteoarthrosis	Capsular pattern	Operation if warranted
Rheumatoid or sub-acute traumatic arthritis	Capsular pattern	Injection 2 ml steroid suspension
Sudeck's atrophy	Visible radiographically	No treatment avails
2. Non-capsular conditions Dancer's heel	Painful passive plantiflexion at full range	Injection 2 ml steroid suspension
Immobilization limitation	Fixation in mid-position following immobilization	Mobilization
Subcutaneous nodules	Nodules palpable in subcutaneous fascia	Tenotomy *or* adapted footwear
Plantar fasciitis	Examination negative apart from tender spot. History of pain on first few steps of walking	Support *or* injection 2 ml steroid suspension

MID-TARSAL JOINT
Pain on passive movement

1. Capsular conditions Osteoarthrosis	Normally symptomless of itself	No treatment warranted
Monarticular rheumatoid arthritis	Capsular pattern	Immobilization
Sub-acute arthritis in middle age	Any movement towards inversion restricted by muscle spasm	Injection 2 ml steroid suspension *or* support
Sub-acute arthritis in adolescence	Valgus of the heel and abduction of the forefoot maintained by muscle spasm	Support and strapping
2. Non-capsular conditions Mid-tarsal ligaments: 1. Strain	Pain at extremes of passive range	Support, exercises *and* mobilization. Injection steroid suspension if necessary
2. Contracture	History and limitation at mid-tarsal joint; no muscle spasm	Injection 2–5 ml steroid suspension

CUNEO-FIRST METATARSAL JOINT

Osteoarthrosis	History of adolescent osteochondrosis	Adapted footwear *or* operation

METATARSAL SHAFTS

Marching fracture	Pain on walking, localized warmth, oedema and tenderness	Spontaneous recovery six weeks from onset

FIRST METATARSOPHALANGEAL JOINT

Capsular conditions Arthritis in adolescence	Capsular pattern	Adapted footwear
Rheumatoid arthritis	Capsular pattern	Injection 1 ml steroid suspension
Osteoarthrosis	Capsular pattern	Injection 1 ml steroid suspension
Gout	Capsular pattern	Phenylbutazone, indomethacin

SESAMO-FIRST METATARSAL JOINT

Traumatic arthritis	Pain on resisted flexion of the hallux	Injection 1 ml steroid suspension

OTHER METATARSOPHALANGEAL JOINTS

1. Capsular conditions Rheumatoid or traumatic arthritis	Capsular pattern	Injection 1 ml steroid suspension
2. Non-capsular conditions Acute metatarsalgia	Pain on walking, at outer border of forefoot. Characteristic history (attacks); examination negative	Support *or* operation
Chronic metatarsalgia	Pain on walking at plantar aspect of forefoot (middle three toes)	Support *and* exercises

The cervical spine

Summary
Nearly all pain of cervical origin is caused by a disc lesion compressing the dura mater or nerve roots. The symptoms and signs are usually unilateral scapular pain and limitation in the non-capsular pattern. Because compression of the parenchyma will produce weakness in the upper limb, after the cervical movements the arm is examined against resistance. A root palsy of the seventh cervical root is much the commonest.

Nearly all cervical disc lesions respond to manipulation, but the most careful differential diagnosis is required to sift out those rare cases where manipulation could prove dangerous.

Capsular pattern
Approximately equal limitation of all six movements except flexion.

Non-capsular pattern characteristic of internal derangement
Pain/limitation on two, three or four movements.

End-feel
A hard end-feel accompanies the capsular pattern except in rheumatoid arthritis.

Differential diagnosis

Pancoast's tumour	Neuralgic amyotrophy
Neurofibroma	Acroparaesthesia
Basilar ischaemia	Thoracic outlet syndrome
Drop attacks	Carpal tunnel syndrome
Osteophytic root palsy	Soft-tissue lesion at shoulder

Examination

Six active cervical movements (extension, both side-flexions, both rotations, flexion): pain of cervical origin.
Five passive cervical movements (as above excluding flexion): painful/limited in non-capsular pattern characteristic of internal derangement.
Six resisted cervical movements (as above): painless if displacement present.
Active shoulder girdle elevation: scapular mobility.
Resisted shoulder girdle elevation: C2, C3 or C4 root palsy if weak.
Scapular approximation: dural mobility.
Shoulder girdle forwards: dural mobility.
Active arm elevation: lesion at shoulder.
Resisted abduction: C5 root palsy if weak (or supraspinatus if painful).
Resisted adduction: C7 root palsy.
Resisted medial rotation: rupture of subscapular tendon (rare).
Resisted lateral rotation: C5 root palsy, neuritis (or infraspinatus if painful).
Resisted elbow flexion: C5 or C6 root palsy (or biceps if painful).
Resisted elbow extension: C7 root palsy.
Resisted wrist extension: C6 root palsy (or extensores carpi radialis if painful).

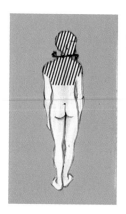

IV.7 *The maximum area within which pain may be referred by a cervical disc lesion compressing the dura mater*

Resisted wrist flexion: C7 root palsy (or common flexor tendon if painful).
Resisted ulnar deviation: C8 root palsy.
Resisted thumb adduction: C8 root palsy.
Resisted thumb extension: C8 root palsy.
Resisted thumb abduction: Cervical rib.
Resisted finger adduction: T1 root palsy.
Brachioradialis jerk: C5 root palsy.
Biceps jerk: C5 or C6 root palsy.
Triceps jerk: C7 root palsy.
Plantar response: Cord sign.

TREATMENT OF A CERVICAL DISPLACEMENT

Manipulation
This is the treatment of choice for a cartilaginous displacement. Nearly all cervical displacements are cartilaginous. After each manoeuvre the patient is re-examined to assess progress.

Technique
The object is to reduce the displacement. One assistant is required to supply traction; a high couch is used.

Straight pull
Rotation during traction 1
Rotation during traction 2
Side-flexion during traction
Anteroposterior gliding – if extension remains painful
Lateral gliding – if residual ache
Traction with leverage – posterocentral displacement
Bateman's – acute torticollis, nuclear displacement

Contraindications to manipulation – danger
Cord signs
Basilar ischaemia
Drop attacks
Rheumatoid arthritis
Gross cervical deformity
Posterocentral protrusion } special technique practicable
Patient on anticoagulants

Contraindications – ineffective
1. Root palsy
2. Brachial pain after first two months
3. Cervical movements cause pain down arm
4. Primary posterolateral displacement

The thoracic spine

Summary
Some thoracic pain is caused by disc lesions compressing the dura mater or nerve roots. The ache may be anterior only. There are no root signs and consequently examination is confined to the trunk with resisted movements playing their part to detect muscular lesions.

It is not always easy to differentiate visceral disorder from a disc lesion and history must be given its full weight. With a displacement the passive rotations are the movements most likely to hurt; disc lesions are particularly responsive to manipulative reduction, repeated as necessary on relapse.

Capsular pattern
Equal and severe limitations of movement in every direction.

Non-capsular pattern characteristic of internal derangement
Pain and/or limitation on some but not all movements.

Differential diagnosis
Visceral disorder
Neuroma
Adolescent osteochondrosis
Adult osteochondrosis
Senile osteoporosis
Ankylosing spondylitis
Osteitis deformans
Fractured rib
Neuritis
Neuralgic amyotrophy
Diaphragmatic or cardiac pain
Thrombosis of the lower aorta
Cervical disc lesion

Examination

Neck flexion: dural mobility.
Scapular approximation: dural mobility.
T1 stretch: T1 nerve root.
Six active thoracic movements (extension, both side-flexions, both rotations, flexion): painful/limited in non-capsular pattern characteristic of internal derangement.
Passive rotations: extreme of range often painful if displacement present.
Six resisted thoracic movements (as above): contractile structures.
Plantar response: cord signs.

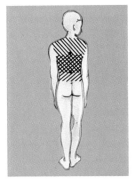

IV.8 *The maximum area within which pain may be referred by a thoracic disc lesion compressing the dura mater.*

TREATMENT OF A THORACIC DISPLACEMENT

Manipulation
The treatment of choice for a cartilaginous displacement is manipulation. Nearly all thoracic displacements are cartilaginous. After each manoeuvre the patient is re-examined to assess progress. Relapse frequently occurs and may be countered either by manipulative reduction or sclerosants

Contraindications – danger
Cord signs
Patient on anticoagulants

Contraindications – ineffective
None

Technique
The object is to reduce the displacement. Two assistants are required to supply traction; a low couch is used,

Extension during traction 1
Extension during traction 2
Rotation during traction 1 ⎫
Rotation during traction 2 ⎬ Rotary manipulations of
Rotation during traction 3 ⎪ increasing strength
Rotation during traction 4 ⎭
Upper thoracic rotation – for upper thoracic disc lesions (rare)

Prophylaxis
Sclerosants: The object is to shorten the posterior ligaments, thus forestalling relapse. The displacement must first be reduced.
Technique: Injection 1 ml P2G solution into each ligamentoperiosteal junction at both ends of the supraspinous ligaments and into the outlying facet joints. The injections at each site are given a total of three times at weekly intervals.

The lumbar spine

Summary
Much pain of lumbar origin is caused by minor and remediable displacements of disc material compressing the dura mater or nerve roots. Disc lesions are particularly common at the L4 and L5 levels. Compression of the parenchyma produces weakness in the lower limb; this is examined by resisted movements after the lumbar movements have been tested. Root signs may be polyradicular.

Most displacements are cartilaginous and respond to manipulation. Some displacements are of nuclear material and require sustained traction. The pain from an otherwise irreducible (i.e. large) displacement can be abolished or permanently diminished by an injection of epidural local anaesthetic. Operation is hardly ever called for. History is particularly important.

Capsular pattern
Approximately equal limitation of both side-flexions; extension and flexion also limited.

Non-capsular pattern characteristic of internal derangement
Pain and/or limitation on some but not all movements or asymmetric limitation in all directions (e.g. lumbago).

Examination

Inspection, palpation: bony signs.
Four active lumbar movements (extension, both side-flexions, flexion): capsular pattern, or non-capsular pattern characteristic of internal derangement.
Standing on tiptoe: S1 or S2 root palsy.
Straight-leg raise: dural mobility (bilateral limitation); nerve root mobility at L4, L5, S1 and S2 (unilateral limitation).
SIJ strain (supine): anterior sacroiliac ligaments.
Resisted hip flexion: L2 or L3 root palsy.
Resisted ankle dorsiflexion: L4 root palsy.
Resisted toe extension: L4 or L5 root palsy.
Resisted eversion: L5 or S1 root palsy.
Knee jerk: L3 root palsy.
Ankle jerk: S1, S2 or L5 (rare) root palsy.
Passive knee flexion: nerve root mobility at L3.
Resisted knee extension: L3 root palsy.

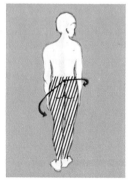

IV.9 *The maximum area within which pain may be referred by a lumbar disc lesion compressing the dura mater.*

Resisted knee flexion: S1 or S2 root palsy.
Wasting of glutei: S2 root palsy.
Plantar response: cord signs.
Cutaneous analgesia: sensory defect.

TREATMENT OF A LUMBAR DISPLACEMENT

Manipulation	Traction	Epidural local anaesthesia
The treatment of choice for a small cartilaginous displacement is manipulation. Most lumbar displacements are cartilaginous. After each manoeuvre the patient is re-examined to assess progress.	The treatment of choice for a small nuclear displacement is traction. This reduces intervertebral pressure, creating negative pressure within the joint and sucking the semi-liquid protrusion back	The treatment of choice for a large lumbar displacement is epidural local anaesthesia. This desensitizes the dura mater and nerve roots.

Manipulation

The treatment of choice for a small cartilaginous displacement is manipulation. Most lumbar displacements are cartilaginous. After each manoeuvre the patient is re-examined to assess progress.

Technique
The object is to reduce the displacement. No assistants are required; a low couch is used.

Rotation strain ⎫
Reverse rotation strain ⎪ rotary
Rotation strain 2 ⎬ manipulations
Rotation strain 3 ⎪ of increasing
Rotation strain 4 ⎭ strength

Forced extension 1 ⎫ extension
Forced extension 2 ⎪ manipulations
Forced extension 3 ⎬ normally
Forced extension 4 ⎪ reserved for
Forced extension 5 ⎭ the elderly

Correction of lateral deviation 1
Correction of lateral deviation 2

Contraindications – danger
Cord signs
S4 signs
Bilateral sciatica
Spinal claudication
Hyperacute lumbago

Contraindications – ineffective
1. Root signs (i.e. weakness)
2. Root pain for 6 months plus (if patient under 60)
3. Sciatica with patient fixed in lateral deviation or flexion
4. Trunk movements suggest a nuclear protrusion
5. Post-laminectomy

Traction

The treatment of choice for a small nuclear displacement is traction. This reduces intervertebral pressure, creating negative pressure within the joint and sucking the semi-liquid protrusion back

Technique
The distracting force is the maximum the patient can stand without discomfort (min. 30 kg, max. 80 kg for manual couches). Treatment is sustained for half an hour daily for a minimum of two weeks. The patient is re-examined before each treatment.

Contraindications – danger
Acute lumbago
Sciatica with gross lumbar deformity
Respiratory embarrassment
S4 signs

Contraindications – ineffective
1. Root signs (i.e. weakness)
2. Root pain for 6 months plus

Epidural local anaesthesia

The treatment of choice for a large lumbar displacement is epidural local anaesthesia. This desensitizes the dura mater and nerve roots.

Technique
Injection via the sacral hiatus, using 50 ml 1:200 procaine. General anaesthesia is not required and the injection proceeds over several minutes. Strict asepsis must be observed. The patient is re-examined after a week and the injection is repeated as necessary up to, say, three times

Contraindications – danger
Sensitivity to local anaesthetic. Follow procedure and observe strict asepsis

Contraindications – ineffective
1. Indications that manipulation or traction will succeed
2. Pre-1950 laminectomy

Consider also pain modulation

Prophylaxis
1. Posture – maintain lumbar lordosis
2. Corset to maintain (not achieve) reduction, cf. a plaster cast
3. *Sclerosants*
   The object is to shorten the posterior ligaments thus forestalling relapse. The displacement must first be reduced.

Technique
Injection 1 ml P2G solution into each end of:
    Week 1 – supraspinous and interspinous ligaments
    Week 2 – facet ligaments
    Week 3 – deep lumbar fascia

INDEX